OXFORD MEDICAL PUBLICATIONS

ORAL PATHOLOGY

Oral Pathology

Third Edition

•

J. V. SOAMES

Professor of Oral Pathology
University of Newcastle upon Tyne

AND

J. C. SOUTHAM

Emeritus Professor of Oral Medicine and Oral Pathology
University of Edinburgh

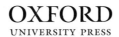

OXFORD
UNIVERSITY PRESS

OXFORD
UNIVERSITY PRESS

Great Clarendon Street, Oxford OX2 6DP

Oxford University Press is a department of the University of Oxford.
It furthers the University's objective of excellence in research, scholarship,
and education by publishing worldwide in

Oxford New York

Athens Auckland Bangkok Bogotá Buenos Aires Calcutta
Cape Town Chennai Dar es Salaam Delhi Florence Hong Kong Istanbul
Karachi Kuala Lumpur Madrid Melbourne Mexico City Mumbai
Nairobi Paris São Paulo Singapore Taipei Tokyo Toronto Warsaw

with associated companies in Berlin Ibadan

Oxford is a registered trade mark of Oxford University Press
in the UK and in certain other countries

Published in the United States
by Oxford University Press Inc., New York

First published 1985
Reprinted 1988, 1989, 1990 (with corrections), 1991
Second edition 1993
Reprinted 1995, 1996
Third edition 1998
Reprinted 1999

A catalogue record for this book is available from the British Library

Library of Congress Cataloging in Publication Data
Soames, J. V.
Oral Pathology / J.V. Soames and J.C. Southam. — 3rd ed.
Includes bibliographical references and index.
1. Mouth—Diseases. 2. Teeth—Diseases I. Southam, J. C.
II. Title.
[DNLM: 1. Stomatognathic System—pathology. WU 140 S6760 1998]
RC815.S59 1998
617.5'22—dc21
DNLM/DLC
for Library of Congress   97–34803   CIP

ISBN 0 19 262 895 X (hbk)
      0 19 262 894 1 (pbk)

Printed in Hong Kong

PREFACE TO THE FIRST EDITION

Oral pathology is that part of pathology concerned with the scientific study of the causes and effects of oral disease, an understanding of which is essential for diagnosis and for the development of rational treatment and preventive programmes. The main purpose of this book is to provide the undergraduate dental student with sufficient information, as a foundation on which to build such as understanding, but it is also hoped that it will be of value to postgraduate students preparing for higher clinical qualifications.

Since this is essentially an undergraduate text we have consciously omitted or treated only briefly some of the rarer oral diseases. With regard to the commoner conditions we have endeavoured to interpret and incorporate recent advances in knowledge and in some cases even speculation. Where controversy exists we have attempted to provide an outline of the main arguments or at least a consensus view, but it is inevitable that in some cases we have had to be dogmatic.

Limitation of space and constraints imposed by costs have restricted the number of illustrations, but photographs are no substitute for practical experience and it is hoped that students will have the opportunity and be encouraged to study many of the diseases covered in this book in clinical and laboratory classes. Similarly, the reference at the end of each chapter are in no sense comprehensive but either provide the reader with more detailed accounts of specific topics or are major review articles or specialized texts which themselves contain a more extensive bibliography.

We have much pleasure in acknowledging the help we have received from our many colleagues either directly or through their writings. The thoughts and ideas contained within the book partly reflect the authors' initial training in oral pathology in Manchester and Sheffield. The writing started when both authors worked together in Edinburgh and progress slowed when one of the authors moved to Newcastle. We would particularly wish to thank Yvonne Stables for her skill in deciphering and typing the drafts of the manuscripts, Gordon Bolas for much help with the indexing, Brian Conroy for his expertise in photomicrography, and David Sales for the line drawings.

Newcastle upon Tyne   J. V. S.
Edinburgh   J. C. S.
July 1985

PREFACE TO THE SECOND EDITION

In the eight years that have passed since the publication of the First Edition of *Oral pathology* there have been many advances in our understanding of basic disease processes that particularly reflect the enormous progress in molecular biology. These have had their impact on research in oral pathology and on the day-to-day practice of diagnostic oral histopathology where, for example, immunohistochemical techniques are now routinely used. There have also been important changes in the patterns of oral and dental diseases associated, for example, with AIDS, the oral manifestations of which are important early diagnostic features, and the increasing numbers of elderly patients retaining their natural dentition. Several new clinicopathological entities have been described and others such as the odontogenic and salivary gland tumours have undergone changes in nomenclature and classification.

This Second Edition has been thoroughly revised and updated with several chapters being extensively rewritten. Diseases which are becoming increasingly important such as those associated with HIV infection are now fully described and illustrated. Our aim, as with the First Edition, has been to produce a compact and readable text aimed primarily at undergraduate students, but we hope that it will also be of value to postgraduates studying for higher clinical qualifications, more so now that we have included information on some of the less common oral diseases. In addition, we have been mindful of the needs of general dental practitioners and of colleagues in other fields of medicine who wish to update their knowledge and understanding of oral diseases.

In response to criticism of the First Edition, this edition is extensively illustrated with over 400 photographs, some 190 of which are in colour, and we hope the book satisfies its purpose the better for this change. The illustrations have been drawn from our departmental collections but it is inevitable that over the years these have been enhanced by material 'collected' from elsewhere. Where this could be identified we have sought approval for its inclusion; we apologize for any that have escaped our notice but hope that colleagues will be pleased with the results.

Once again, we wish to acknowledge the advice and help we have had from our many colleagues. We particularly wish to express our gratitude for the assistance and skills of Mrs Diane Burgess for the typing and wordprocessing needed in the preparation and reorganization of the revised text; to David Sales for the line drawings and photomicrography; and to Brain Hill and Jan Howarth of the Department of Medical Illustration, Newcastle upon Tyne Dental Hospital, for most of the clinical photographs.

Newcastle upon Tyne   J. V. S.
Edinburgh   J. C. S.
November 1992

PREFACE TO THE THIRD EDITION

In undertaking the third edition our aim, as before, has been to provide a text primarily for undergraduate students, but with sufficient breadth and depth to be of value both to postgraduates studying for higher clinical qualifications, and to the continuing professional development of general dental practitioners. We have been aware of the impact of advances in molecular biology and genetics relevant to the understanding of basic disease processes, such as neoplasia, and of their application in oral pathology. We have also taken the opportunity to amend the classification and nomenclature of diseases, particularly the salivary gland tumours and odontogenic tumours, in line with current opinion.

To encompass these developments we have revised and updated the text, expanding some sections, editing others, and deleting concepts no longer generally accepted, so that the overall length of the book has not been significantly increased. One or two relatively new and rare entities, such as the glandular odontogenic cyst, have been included for completeness and the references recommended for further reading have been extensively updated. We have retained the general format and chapter headings adopted for the second edition but the revised text is now considerably enhanced by being illustrated throughout in colour and by the inclusion of key points which, we hope, will help the reader identify important aspects of particular diseases.

As with the first two editions we are much indebted to the help and comments we have had from colleagues and students, and hope their criticisms have been addressed. We also wish to acknowledge the word processing and typing skills of Mrs Sylvia Bohan in preparing the revised text and owe special thanks to Joan for her patience, and for the many hours spent cutting, pasting, and proof reading.

Newcastle upon Tyne   J. V. S.
Edinburgh   J. C. S.
November 1997

CONTENTS

oral Paths

1 - 2 - 3 - 4 for Test tomorrow.

1 Disorders of development of teeth

1 Disorders of development of teeth

Disorders of development of teeth may be prenatal or postnatal in origin and may be inherited or acquired. Their recognition and evaluation require a thorough knowledge of the normal chronology of the human dentition and of the normal development and structure of the teeth.

Disorders of development of teeth may be due to abnormalities in the differentiation of the dental lamina and the tooth germs, causing anomalies in the number, size, and form of teeth (abnormalities of morphodifferentiation) or to abnormalities in the formation of the dental hard tissues resulting in disturbances in tooth structure (abnormalities of histodifferentiation). Abnormalities of histo-differentiation occur at a later stage in development than abnormalities of morphodifferentiation; in some disorders both stages of differentiation are abnormal.

DISTURBANCES IN NUMBER OF TEETH

Hypodontia, anodontia, and associated syndromes

The congenital absence of teeth may be referred to as hypodontia, when one or several teeth are missing, or anodontia when there is a complete absence of one or both dentitions.

Hypodontia is more common in the permanent than in the primary dentition occurring in about 3–7 per cent of the population (excluding absent third molars), and may be symmetrical when particular teeth or groups of teeth are involved, or haphazard when no pattern is discernible. It is very unusual for deciduous teeth to be congenitally absent, but it is likely in such cases that the permanent successional tooth will also fail to form. Third molars, permanent maxillary lateral incisors, and mandibular second premolars are the teeth most frequently involved in symmetrical forms, and a hereditary trait can sometimes be shown with missing maxillary lateral incisors. Hypodontia is more common in females. There are also racial differences in the prevalence of missing teeth, permanent mandibular central incisors, for example, apparently being absent in Japanese and Swedish populations much more frequently than in other groups studied. Hypodontia may also be associated with other craniofacial anomalies and developmental syndromes (Table 1.1).

Hypohidrotic ectodermal dysplasia

Anodontia is rare and in most cases is associated with other defects, the most frequent being hereditary hypohidrotic ectodermal dysplasia which is characterized by the congenital absence of ectodermal structures. The disorder is rare and is

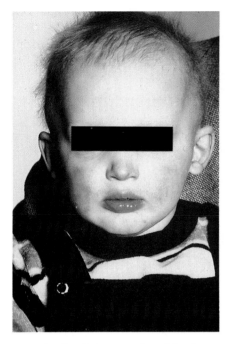

Fig. 1.1 Hypohidrotic ectodermal dysplasia.

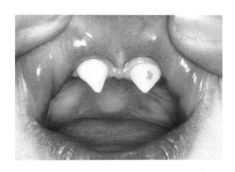

Fig. 1.2 Hypodontia associated with hypohidrotic ectodermal dysplasia.

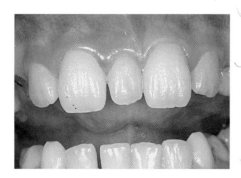

Fig. 1.3 Mesiodens.

usually inherited as an X-linked recessive trait, although a very rare autosomal recessive form has been described and sporadic cases have been reported. Affected patients have smooth, dry skin with fine, scanty hairs (Fig. 1.1) and partial or total absence of sweat glands which leads to hyperthermia. Some have a few teeth present, but these are often retarded in eruption, deformed, and frequently have conical crowns (Fig. 1.2). Female carriers usually show only mild manifestations that may be restricted to minimal hypodontia, such as absent maxillary lateral incisors, but carriers may be detected by a reduced sweat pore count.

Supernumerary teeth (hyperdontia)

These are teeth additional to those of the normal series. They may develop in any tooth-bearing area but occur most frequently in the anterior and molar regions of the maxilla followed by the premolar region of the mandible. Occasionally, they are associated with other defects, such as cleft palate or cleidocranial dysplasia (see Table 1.1). They may prevent the eruption, or cause malposition or resorption of adjacent teeth, and may develop dentigerous cysts if unerupted. Supernumerary teeth are more common in females, are usually single and occur in about 1–3 per cent of the population in the permanent dentition. They are unusual in the deciduous dentition.

Supernumerary teeth occurring at certain sites may be referred to by special terms. A mesiodens (Fig. 1.3) is a supernumerary tooth developing between the maxillary central incisors and is the most common of all supernumerary teeth.

Table 1.1 Examples of craniofacial anomalies and developmental syndromes associated with abnormalities in the number of teeth

Syndrome/anomaly	Associated features
A. Hypodontia	
Cleft lip/palate	Possible deafness and other cranial and skeletal abnormalities
Crouzon syndrome	Craniosynostosis, maxillary hypoplasia, hypertelorism
Down syndrome (trisomy 21)	Multiple, e.g. mental retardation, maxillary hypoplasia macroglossia
Hypohidrotic ectodermal dysplasia	Hypotrichosis, hypohidrosis, saddle-nose
Ellis-van Creveld syndrome (chondroectodermal dysplasia)	Dwarfism, polydactyly, cardiac malformations
Oral-facial-digital syndrome	Cleft palate, hypoplasia of the nose, digital malformations
B. Hyperdontia	
Cleft lip/palate	Possible deafness and other cranial and skeletal abnormalities
Cleidocranial dysplasia	Aplasia of clavicles, delayed ossification of fontanelles, cranium
Gardner syndrome	Multiple osteomas of jaws, skin cysts and fibromas, intestinal polyposis
Oral-facial-digital syndrome	Cleft palate, hypoplasia of the nose, digital malformations

The majority have conical crowns and short roots. A paramolar (Fig. 1.4) arises alongside the maxillary molars and is usually buccally placed, and a distomolar develops distal to a third molar. Supernumerary teeth which morphologically resemble those of the normal series are called supplemental teeth but most are reduced in size.

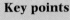

Key points

Hypodontia
- more common in permanent than primary dentition
- absence of primary teeth associated with absence of permanent successors
- may be associated with other developmental abnormalities

Anodontia
- rare
- associated most frequently with hypohidrotic ectodermal dysplasia (HED)
- HED usually X-linked recessive

Hyperdontia (supernumerary teeth)
- more common in maxilla than mandible
- more common in females than males
- relatively uncommon in primary dentition

DISTURBANCES IN SIZE OF TEETH

Macrodontia and microdontia

The size of both the teeth and the jaws is determined predominantly by genetic factors, and great variations occur in the ratio of tooth size to jaw size. The terms macrodontia and microdontia are used to describe teeth which are larger or smaller than normal, respectively, but what might be accepted within the limits of normal variation has never been adequately defined. Both macrodontia and microdontia may involve the entire dentition, or only one or two teeth symmetrically distributed in the jaws. Microdontia of the whole dentition may be associated with other defects, for example Down syndrome and congenital heart disease.

Whilst it is convenient to consider abnormalities in the number and the size of teeth separately the anomalies often occur together. For example, hypodontia and microdontia may occur together in several of the conditions listed in Table 1.1. More common examples are seen in patients with one missing permanent maxillary lateral incisor, in which case the contralateral tooth is frequently peg-shaped.

DISTURBANCES IN FORM OF TEETH

Disturbances in tooth form may involve the crown, the root, or both. The most frequent variations of the crowns of teeth affect maxillary permanent lateral incisors, which may be peg-shaped or show an accentuated cingulum — either variation sometimes being associated with an invagination. Premolars or molars with an increased or decreased number of cusps are also frequently seen. Variations in the number, course, form, and size of roots are particularly common.

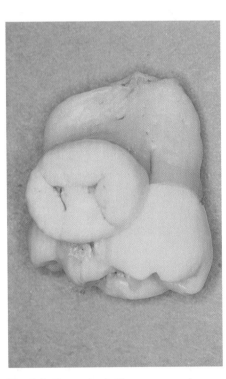

Fig. 1.4 Paramolar (with concrescence).

Dilaceration

The term dilaceration is used to describe a deformity in which the crown of the tooth is displaced from its normal alignment with the root, so that the tooth is severely bent along its long axis (Figs 1.5, 1.6). Dilaceration is usually the result of acute mechanical trauma and most frequently involves the maxillary incisors.

Taurodontism

A taurodont tooth (bull-like tooth) is one in which the pulp chamber has a greater apico-occlusal height than in normal teeth, with no constriction at the level of the amelocemental junction with the result that the chamber extends apically well beyond the cervix (Fig. 1.7). The anomaly affects multirooted teeth and is thought to be caused by the failure of Hertwig's sheath to invaginate at the proper horizontal level. It is rare in the primary dentition. Taurodont teeth may occur as incidental findings or be associated with other rare craniofacial or dental anomalies. There is also an association with abnormalities in the number of the sex chromosomes such as in Klinefelter and poly-X syndromes.

Double teeth (connated teeth)

Double teeth and connated teeth are descriptive terms used to describe a developmental anomaly where two teeth appear joined together. The degree of union is variable and may involve the crown, the roots, or both. It is very unusual for teeth to be united by enamel only, joining of the dentine and also the pulp chamber being much more frequent.

A variety of other terms have been applied to this anomaly based on its supposed aetiology, such as fusion and gemination. These have been defined as:

Fusion — the union between dentine and/or enamel of two or more separate developing teeth.

Gemination — the partial development of two teeth from a single tooth bud following incomplete division.

However, the aetiology remains unclear although a genetic basis has been suggested. For this reason, general terms such as double teeth or connated teeth

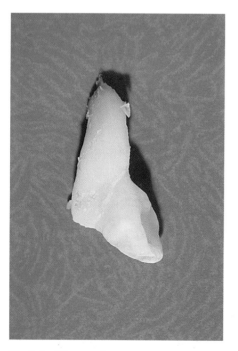

Fig. 1.5 Dilacerated permanent maxillary lateral incisor.

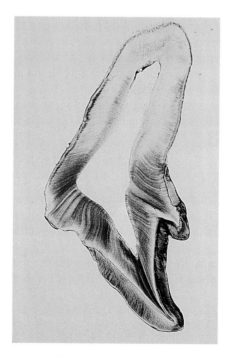

Fig. 1.6 Ground section of dilacerated tooth shown in Fig. 1.5.

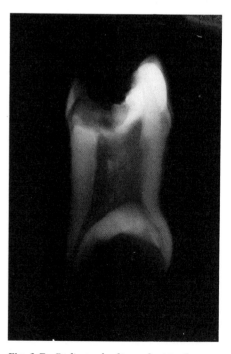

Fig. 1.7 Radiograph of taurodont tooth.

(meaning developed or born together), which describe the appearance with no implication regarding aetiology, are preferred. The developmental anomaly of double teeth must be distinguished from concrescence which is an acquired condition where teeth are joined by cementum only (see below).

Double or connated teeth are more common in the primary than in the permanent dentition, the prevalence in different series ranging from 0.5–1.5 per cent for the primary and 0.1–0.2 per cent for the permanent dentitions. The incisors (and also the canines in the primary dentition) are most frequently involved and the condition may be bilaterally symmetrical (Fig. 1.8).

Concrescence

Concrescence is an acquired disorder in which the roots of one or more teeth are united by cementum alone after formation of the crowns (Figs 1.4, 1.9). This is most frequently seen in the permanent dentition where the roots of teeth develop close together (for example, between maxillary second and third molars) or following hypercementosis associated with chronic inflammation.

Double or connated teeth   **Key points**

- developmental anomaly
- union of enamel and/or dentine (with or without pulp)
- more common in primary than permanent dentition
- anterior teeth mainly involved

Concrescence

- acquired anomaly
- union by cementum alone
- more common in permanent than primary dentition

DISTURBANCES IN STRUCTURE OF TEETH

Disturbances in structure of enamel

Enamel normally develops in two stages. In the first, or secretory, stage, the ameloblasts perform the dual function of matrix production and initial mineralization. Matrix production involves the synthesis and secretion of matrix proteins, the amelogenins and enamelins. Initial mineralization appears immediately

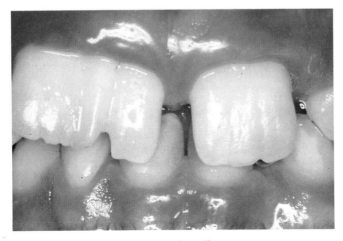

Fig. 1.8 Connation (gemination) of maxillary incisors.

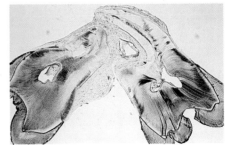

Fig. 1.9 Concrescence of maxillary molars.

after secretion and crystals abut the plasma membrane of the ameloblast. In the second stage, the maturation stage, there is withdrawal of water and protein from the enamel with a concomitant increase in mineral content before the tooth erupts. Most classifications of disturbances in enamel formation distinguish between those that affect matrix formation and those that affect initial mineralization and maturation, producing hypoplastic and hypomineralized enamel, respectively. This distinction may at times be hard to sustain as some disturbances affect both matrix formation and mineralization, but it remains a useful clinical division.

Key points	**Defective amelogenesis**
	• matrix formation — enamel hypoplasia
	• mineralization — hypomineralized enamel
	• maturation — hypomineralized enamel

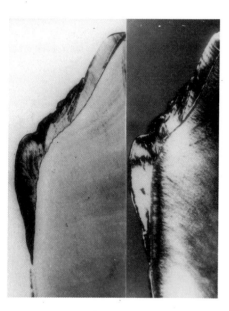

Fig. 1.10 Ground section of a tooth viewed with normal (left) and polarized (right) light showing chronological enamel hypoplasia and corresponding prominent incremental lines in dentine.

The primary changes in enamel hypoplasia occur in the ameloblasts which subsequently fail to produce a normal volume of matrix. However, any matrix which is produced generally becomes as fully mineralized as normal enamel. Enamel hypoplasia presents clinically as pits or grooves in the enamel surface (Fig. 1.10), or as a general reduction in the thickness of the whole of the enamel. The apparently haphazard distribution and variation in depth of pitting in some forms of hypoplasia reflect the varying sensitivity of ameloblasts to injury. Examination of ground sections shows that the defective enamel has fewer prisms than normal and that these may run in abnormal directions. In some cases no prism structure can be seen.

Hypomineralized enamel results from a failure of the ameloblasts to fully calcify the previously formed matrix, and generally such enamel appears clinically as white and opaque. After eruption it may become pigmented buff, orange, or brown and be quickly chipped and worn away. Much of the organic matrix of hypomineralized enamel remains acid-insoluble and is often preserved in sections of decalcified specimens.

Hypoplastic and hypomineralized enamel may result from disturbances affecting a single tooth, a group of teeth, or all of the teeth, and the structure of the enamel formed depends on the severity and duration of the disturbance as well as its nature. Most disturbances of ameloblast function can produce both hypoplasia and hypomineralization, but clinically one type usually predominates in a particular patient.

The classification given in Table 1.2 is based on the aetiology of hypoplastic and hypomineralized enamel. It is not exhaustive but includes the common causes.

Localized causes

Local infection or trauma

Enamel hypoplasia or hypomineralization involving a single tooth is most commonly seen in permanent maxillary incisors, or maxillary or mandibular premolars. The usual cause of these abnormalities is infection or trauma related to the deciduous predecessor resulting in damage to the ameloblasts of the permanent successor. Such teeth are often called Turner teeth. Clinically, the defects range from yellowish or brownish pigmentation of the enamel to extensive pitting and irregularity of the surface, the crowns often being smaller than normal. The yellowish colour is sometimes due to the deposition of cementum on the enamel surface.

Table 1.2 Aetiology of developmental abnormalities of enamel

Local causes
Infection
Trauma
Radiotherapy
Idiopathic (enamel opacities)

General causes
(a) *Environmental/systemic*
        (chronological hypoplasias)
    (i)   Prenatal   — infections, e.g. rubella, syphilis
                      — maternal disease
                      — excess fluoride ions
    (ii) Neonatal   — haemolytic disease of the newborn
                      — hypocalcaemia
                      — premature birth/prolonged labour
    (iii) Postnatal — severe childhood infections especially the viral exanthemata
                      — chronic diseases in childhood, e.g. congenital heart disease,
                          gastrointestinal and endocrine diseases
                      — nutritional deficiencies, e.g. vitamin D
                      — cancer chemotherapy
                      — excess fluoride ions
(b) *Genetic*
    (i)   Teeth only affected
          — amelogenesis imperfecta
    (ii) Teeth affected in association with generalized defects
          — ectodermal dysplasia syndromes
          — Down syndrome (trisomy 21)

Enamel opacities

These are white, opaque spots seen in smooth-surface enamel, some of which become brown-stained after eruption (Fig. 1.11). The opacities are common and are seen in as many as one in three children aged 12–14 years. They have a random distribution, and teeth in both the deciduous and the permanent dentition are affected. The maxillary permanent central incisor is most frequently involved. The cause is not known but the opacities are thought to be due to local rather than systemic factors. The prevalence is less in areas with one part per

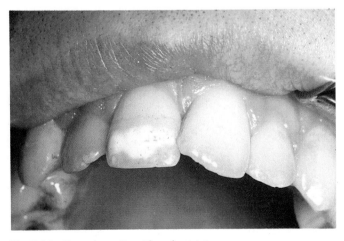

Fig. 1.11 Enamel opacity with early staining.

million of fluoride in the drinking water. Histological examination of the enamel shows the opaque spots to be hypomineralized.

Key points	Developmental abnormalities of enamel — aetiology
	• local causes
	• generalized causes
	— environmental/systemic disturbances (chronological hypoplasia)
	— genetically determined

Generalized causes

Chronological hypoplasias

Any serious nutritional deficiency or systemic disease occurring during the time of formation of the teeth is capable of leading to enamel hypoplasia or hypomineralization, because ameloblasts are amongst the most sensitive cells in the body in terms of metabolic requirements. Such time-related disturbances are called chronological hypoplasia and most enamel hypoplasias due to environmental causes are of this type. A pitting type of hypoplasia usually results from such disturbances and produces a horizontal band of hypoplasia, the distribution of which is related to that enamel which was forming at the time of the disturbance (Figs 1.10, 1.12). Thus a disturbance occurring at or soon after birth may affect the incisal edges of the permanent central incisors and the occlusal surfaces of the first permanent molars in addition to the deciduous teeth (Fig. 1.13).

Congenital syphilis

This disease produces characteristic hypoplastic changes in the enamel of permanent incisors and first molars due to infection of the tooth germ by spirochaetes. The mesial and distal surfaces of the incisors taper towards the incisal edges rather than toward the cervical margin, giving a 'screw-driver' appearance, and the incisal edges usually have a central notch (Hutchinson's incisors) (see Chapter 11). These changes are most obvious in the maxillary central incisors. The occlusal surfaces and occlusal thirds of the crowns of the first molars are covered by small globular masses of enamel (Moon's molars or mulberry molars).

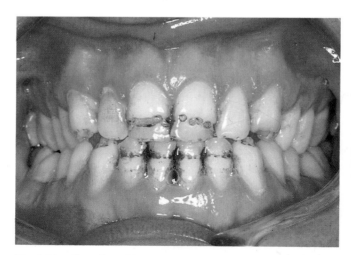

Fig. 1.12 Chronological hypoplasia of enamel associated with measles in early childhood.

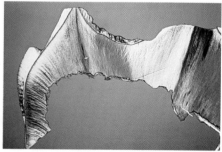

Fig. 1.13 Enamel hypoplasia associated with neonatal hypocalcaemia. A prominent step-like defect separates the thin prenatal enamel from the normal postnatal enamel following restoration of normal calcium levels. Ground section of a deciduous molar viewed with polarized light.

Fluoride ions

Ingestion of fluoride during the period of tooth formation may result in hypomineralized or hypoplastic enamel. This is not usually clinically evident with one part per million or less of fluoride in the drinking water, but it becomes progressively apparent above this level. Fluoride opacities occur symmetrically around the arch but vary in severity from tooth to tooth. They are found mainly in the permanent dentition, but the deciduous teeth may be involved in severe cases and in areas of endemic fluorosis. The premolars, upper incisors, and second molars are most severely affected. Dental fluorosis (Fig. 1.14) is characterized by faint white flecking of the enamel, white patches or striations, or in more severe cases by yellow, black, or brown staining (particularly in teeth most exposed to light) and by hypoplasia of varying degree. In severe cases the hypoplasia may lead to confluent pitting with associated loss of the normal tooth form. Histological examination of fluorosed enamel shows subsurface areas of diffuse hypomineralization deep to a well-calcified surface layer. The term 'mottling' has been used to describe the appearances of the enamel resulting from a high fluoride intake during the period of tooth formation. It must be realized that fluorosed enamel is clinically and histologically indistinguishable from other types of hypomineralized and hypoplastic enamel.

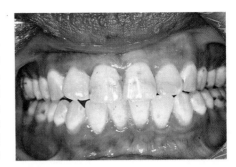

Fig. 1.14 Dental fluorosis.

Amelogenesis imperfecta

This inherited developmental abnormality of enamel is usually classified into two distinct types based on whether the abnormality is related to defective mineralization (hypomineralized type) or defective matrix formation (hypoplastic type). In the hypomineralized form, which is further subdivided into hypocalcified and hypomaturation types, matrix formation is normal, but calcification is abnormal, whereas in hypoplastic types matrix formation is defective but any formed is normally mineralized. However, electron microscopic and microradiographic studies suggest that in all types of amelogenesis imperfecta there are disturbances in both calcification and matrix formation, indicating a generalized disturbance of amelogenesis. Autosomal dominant, autosomal recessive, and X-linked patterns of inheritance are identified, but these are not related to the clinical manifestations (phenotype) which show either predominantly hypomineralization, hypoplasia, or a combination of both. Based on differences in patterns of inheritance and clinical manifestations 14 subtypes have been described. The main types and patterns of inheritance are shown in Table 1.3.

The majority of forms of amelogenesis imperfecta are inherited as autosomal dominant or X-linked traits, although varying expressivity of the involved gene may make genetic interpretation difficult. An amelogenin gene is located on the short arm of the X chromosome and it is probable that mutations in X-linked

Table 1.3   Amelogenesis imperfecta: main types and patterns of inheritance

Hypocalcified types
  Autosomal dominant form

Hypomaturation types
  Autosomal dominant forms, (including snow-capped teeth)

Hypoplastic types
  Autosomal dominant, smooth, rough, or pitted forms
  X-linked form

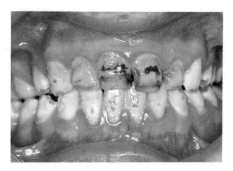

Fig. 1.15 Amelogenesis imperfecta, hypocalcified type.

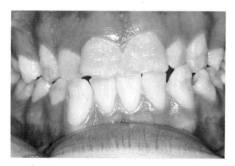

Fig. 1.16 Amelogenesis imperfecta, hypoplastic type with generalized roughening of the enamel.

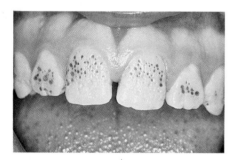

Fig. 1.17 Amelogenesis imperfecta, hypoplastic type with generalized pitting of the enamel.

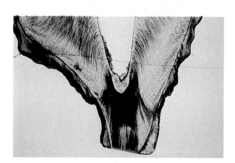

Fig. 1.18 Amelogenesis imperfecta, hypoplastic type. Ground section showing generalized pitting/roughness of the enamel.

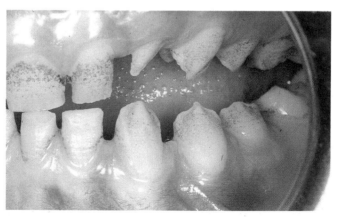

Fig. 1.19 Amelogenesis imperfecta, hypoplastic type, smooth form.

forms of amelogenesis imperfecta result in defective amelogenin synthesis, producing hypoplasia or hypomineralization depending upon the expression in different individuals. Recently, an autosomal dominant form of amelogenesis imperfecta has been mapped to chromosome 4q, but the related biochemical defect is presently unknown. All types of amelogenesis imperfecta affect the deciduous and permanent dentitions and most of the enamel on all of the teeth is usually involved. The teeth are no more prone to dental caries than normal teeth.

The hypocalcified type is the most common form. Newly erupted teeth appear normal in size and shape and have enamel of normal thickness, although there may be mild hypoplasia. However, the enamel is of a soft, chalky consistency (Fig. 1.15) and is rapidly lost by abrasion and attrition exposing the dentine. Gross attrition is a feature of the hypocalcified type and the teeth may be worn down to gum level. Because of the deficient mineralization, the enamel has a similar density to dentine on radiographs. In the hypomaturation types of amelogenesis imperfecta the enamel is generally of normal thickness on eruption but exhibits variable opaque, mottled, brownish-yellow to white appearances. The enamel is soft and attrition occurs, but not as severely as in the hypocalcified type. In one form, the incisal edges and occlusal surfaces, especially of the maxillary teeth are particularly affected by flecks or larger areas of opaque white enamel giving a 'snow-capped' appearance.

In the hypoplastic types of amelogenesis imperfecta the enamel does not reach normal thickness and there is considerable variation in clinical appearances. In some cases, localized areas of hypoplasia are randomly distributed over the surface of the enamel producing generalized roughness and pitting or irregular vertical grooving and wrinkling (Figs 1.16–1.18). In the smooth form, the enamel over the whole of the crown is affected and the teeth have sharp, needle-like cusps (Fig. 1.19). The enamel is very thin but hard and glassy. It lacks a normal prismatic structure and may be laid down in incremental bands parallel to the surface.

In the X-linked form, heterozygous females are less severely affected than males or homozygous females and tend to show alternating irregular vertical bands of normal and defective enamel, reflecting the random inactivation of one or other of the X chromosomes in different groups of ameloblasts (Lyonization effect).

Amelogenesis imperfecta

Main types

- hypomineralized
  — hypocalcified types
  — hypomaturation types
- hypoplastic

Main patterns of inheritance

- autosomal dominant
- X-linked
- mode of inheritance not related to a particular clinical type

Disturbances in structure of dentine

Dentine is the first-formed dental hard tissue, the cells of the internal enamel epithelium inducing the adjacent mesenchymal cells of the dental papilla to differentiate into odontoblasts. Both the odontoblasts and subodontoblastic cells influence the development of the first-formed or mantle dentine, the subodontoblastic cells forming part of the collagenous matrix which is embedded in a ground substance rich in glycosaminoglycans. As more matrix is formed the odontoblasts migrate centripetally and their processes remain in the matrix which begins to mineralize when it is about 5 μm thick. Calcification is initiated by small crystallites (which at first are probably budded from the odontoblasts) and completed by subsequent growth and fusion of discrete globules called calcospherites. Where fusion of calcospherites does not occur, hypomineralized areas of interglobular dentine remain. The matrix of circumpulpal and root dentine is synthesized by odontoblasts, a layer of uncalcified matrix (predentine) normally being present at the pulpal surface. Peritubular dentine consisting of calcium phosphate and a non-collagenous matrix is formed along the internal surfaces of the dentinal tubules throughout life, the tubule diameter being progressively reduced or even obliterated.

Most of the clinically significant disturbances of dentinogenesis have a genetic aetiology, but some environmental or systemic disturbances affecting calcium metabolism or calcification may also produce abnormal dentine. The developmental abnormalities of dentine are listed in Table 1.4. Many are rare.

Dentinogenesis imperfecta Type II (hereditary opalescent dentine)

This is an autosomal dominant disorder with variable expressivity, appearing in equal frequency in males and females involving approximately 1 in 8000 individuals. It has been mapped to chromosome 4q (see also autosomal dominant amelogenesis imperfecta). Both the deciduous and permanent dentitions are affected. On eruption the teeth have a normal contour but an opalescent amber-like appearance (Fig. 1.20). Subsequently, they may have an almost normal colour, following which they become translucent, and finally grey or brownish with bluish reflections from the enamel. Although in most cases the enamel is structurally normal it is rapidly lost and the teeth then show marked attrition (Fig. 1.21). In some cases the enamel includes hypomineralized areas.

Radiological examination shows short, blunt roots with partial or even total obliteration of the pulp chambers and root canals by dentine (Fig. 1.22) Histological examination shows that apart from a thin layer of normal tubular

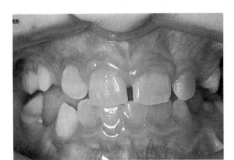

Fig. 1.20 Dentinogenesis imperfecta showing opalescent amber-like appearance of the teeth.

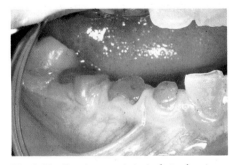

Fig. 1.21 Dentinogenesis imperfecta showing marked attrition of deciduous dentition.

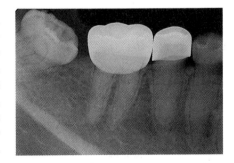

Fig. 1.22 Radiograph of teeth in dentinogenesis imperfecta showing obliteration of the pulp chambers and root canals and stunting of the roots.

Table 1.4 Developmental abnormalities of dentine

Local causes
Trauma — e.g. Turner teeth; radiotherapy

General causes
Dentinogenesis imperfecta
Type I   — associated with osteogenesis imperfecta
Type II   — teeth only affected (including 'shell-teeth')
Type III — Brandywine isolate

Dentine dysplasia
Type I   — radicular dentine dysplasia (rootless teeth)
Type II   — coronal dentine dysplasia

Environmental/systemic
Vitamin D-dependent rickets
Vitamin D-resistant rickets (hypophosphataemia)
Hypophosphatasia
Juvenile hypoparathyroidism
Other mineral deficiencies
Drugs, e.g. chemotherapeutic agents

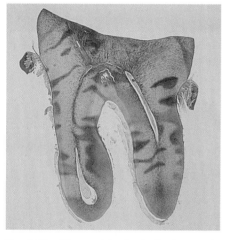

Fig. 1.23 Abnormal dentine in dentinogenesis imperfecta with partial obliteration of the pulp chamber.

mantle dentine (i.e. the dentine immediately adjacent to the enamel or cementum), the dentine contains a reduced number of tubules, many of which are wide and irregular, and areas of atubular dentine may be present. This abnormal dentine partly or totally obliterates the pulp chamber and root canal (Fig. 1.23). Vascular inclusions are often found in the dentine, representing remnants of odontoblasts and pulp tissue. The amelodentinal junction (ADJ) is straight rather than scalloped.

Biochemical analysis of the dentine shows an increased water content and a decreased mineral content when compared with normal dentine. The microhardness of the dentine is low, explaining the rapid attrition of the teeth which occurs following loss of enamel. The latter may be due to the abnormal configuration of the amelodentinal junction and to the abnormal physical properties of the dentine which render it less able to withstand distortional forces. Caries is unusual in affected teeth, presumably due to the reduced number of invasion pathways in the dentine, with the caries being confined to the superficial layers which are quickly worn away. The pulp cavities in deciduous teeth may not be obliterated, the dentine may remain thin and the pulps may become exposed by attrition (see 'shell-teeth' below).

A similar anomaly to dentinogenesis imperfecta type II occurs in some patients with osteogenesis imperfecta (see Chapter 16 and Fig. 16.2), and although the two defects are closely related it would appear that they are separate conditions. The appearances of the deciduous dentition in types I and II are indistinguishable, but the involvement of the permanent dentition in type I (associated with osteogenesis imperfecta) is very variable.

'Shell teeth' is a rare variant of dentinogenesis imperfecta type II in which the pulp chamber is not obliterated, the dentine being quite thin and forming a shell around the pulp which contains coarse collagen fibres and no odontoblasts. The roots of the teeth are usually short. It has been suggested that the condition represents a homozygote form of dentinogenesis imperfecta. Several similar cases have occurred in a particular racial isolate group in southern Maryland, USA (the Brandywine isolate; dentinogenesis type III).

Dentinal dysplasia

Two forms of this rare autosomal dominant disease are identified. In type I (root-less teeth) the permanent teeth have normal crowns associated with roots composed of dysplastic dentine containing numerous calcified, spherical bodies with consequent displacement and disarrangement of the dentinal tubules resembling water streaming round boulders. The pulp chamber and root canals are largely obliterated and the roots are usually very stunted. The abnormality is due to a defect in Hertwig's root sheath which fragments and is incorporated into the dental papilla where it induces formation of fused globular masses of abnormal dentine.

In type II dentinal dysplasia (coronal dentine dysplasia) the primary teeth have an amber colour similar to that seen in dentinogenesis imperfecta and their pulp chambers are obliterated. Permanent teeth are of normal colour, have thistle or flame-shaped pulp chambers and multiple pulp stones, but normal root length.

Metabolic disturbances affecting dentinogenesis

In the active phase of rickets the width of the predentine is increased and the recently formed dentine is incompletely calcified. Subsequently, bands and areas of interglobular dentine corresponding to the period of illness are seen in the dentine. Pronounced interglobular dentine is also a feature of vitamin D-resistant rickets (hypophosphataemia) (Fig. 1.24), but large pulp chambers and long pulp horns which may extend as clefts to the amelodentinal junction are also seen. The overlying enamel may also be cracked or defective allowing direct access of bacteria to the pulp, resulting in pulpitis and periapical sequelae without carious attack. Increased amounts of interglobular dentine and widening of the predentine may be seen in other environmental disorders affecting mineralization such as hypophosphatasia (see also hypocementosis) and nutritional deficiencies. The effects of drugs varies with the nature of the drug and period of administration. Cytotoxic agents often produce increased prominence of incremental lines coinciding with drug administration.

The teeth in juvenile hypoparathyroidism may be small with hypoplastic enamel covering dentine which shows prominent incremental lines. The roots may be stunted and there may be structural abnormalities in the radicular dentine with vascular inclusions.

Regional odontodysplasia (ghost teeth)

This is an uncommon developmental disorder of unknown aetiology associated with abnormalities of enamel, dentine, pulp, and the dental follicle. Both deciduous and permanent dentitions are affected and the number of teeth and number of quadrants involved varies. The defect occurs most frequently in the anterior part of the maxilla and is usually unilateral.

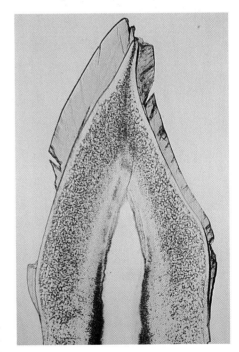

Fig. 1.24 Ground section of a tooth from a patient with hypophosphataemia showing prominent interglobular dentine.

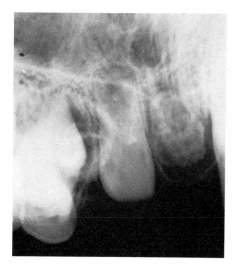

Fig. 1.25 Radiograph of anterior maxillary teeth in regional odontodysplasia showing their ghostly appearance.

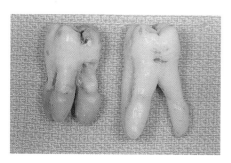

Fig. 1.26 Hypercementosis of maxillary molars.

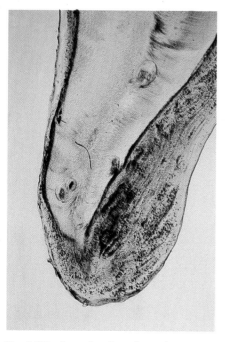

Fig. 1.27 Ground section of a tooth root showing hypercementosis.

The teeth are delayed in eruption and generally have a very irregular shape with hypoplastic and irregularly mineralized enamel. The dentine is thinner than normal and contains large areas of interglobular dentine. Wide, open apices, pulp stones, and abnormal foci of calcification scattered throughout the follicle are also features. Radiological examination shows reduced radiopacity of the teeth with loss of distinction between the enamel and dentine, described as a 'ghostly' appearance (Fig. 1.25).

Disturbances in structure of cementum

The coronal third of the root is normally covered only by a narrow layer of acellular (primary) cementum, whereas the apical two-thirds and furcation areas are covered by an additional thicker layer of cellular (secondary) cementum. Cellular cementum continues to be formed throughout the life of the tooth and typically shows incremental lines of growth. The thickness of the cementum varies considerably between individuals, but generally increases with age and to compensate for occlusal wear.

Hypercementosis

In certain circumstances cementogenesis may be abnormally increased to produce hypercementosis (Figs 1.26, 1.27) which may be the result of local or general disorders and which may affect one or many teeth. Hypercementosis may be associated with root ankylosis, when the cementum is directly continuous with the alveolar bone, or with concrescence (see Fig. 1.9). Some cases of hypercementosis are idiopathic but others may be associated with certain conditions:

Periapical inflammation

Although resorption of cementum may occur close to the centre of the inflammatory focus, apposition of cementum may be stimulated a little further away. This produces a generalized thickening of the cementum or a localized knob-like enlargement.

Mechanical stimulation

Excessive forces applied to a tooth may produce resorption, but mechanical stimulation below a certain threshold may stimulate apposition of cementum (Fig. 1.28).

Functionless and unerupted teeth

Such teeth may show areas of cementum resorption, but excessive apposition of cementum may also occur. In unerupted teeth the cementum may even extend over the surface of the enamel if the reduced enamel epithelium is lost.

Paget's disease of bone

Hypercementosis is often seen in teeth of patients with Paget's disease, the thickened cementum showing a mosaic appearance analogous to that seen in the bone. The cementum forms irregular masses and ankylosis is common (see Fig. 17.7).

Hypocementosis

Hypoplasia and aplasia of cementum are uncommon. In cleidocranial dysplasia there is a lack of cellular cementum following the deposition of acellular cementum. Aplasia of cementum is seen in hypophosphatasia (Fig. 1.29): a recessive autosomal disease, characterized by a reduced serum alkaline phosphatase level with deformities of the extremities similar to those of rickets and failure of calcification of the calvarium. Premature loss of some or all deciduous and permanent teeth is seen, aplasia of cementum preventing normal periodontal attachment. Dentine formation may also be abnormal.

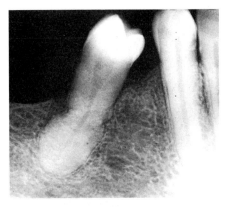

Fig. 1.28 Hypercementosis associated with mechanical stimulation.

FURTHER READING

Aldred, M. J. and Crawford, P. J. (1995). Amelogenesis imperfecta — towards a new classification. *Oral Diseases*, **1**, 2–5.

Aldred, M. J., Crawford, P. J., Roberts, E., Gillespie, C. M., Thomas, N. S., Fenton, I., Sandkuigl, L. A., and Harper, P. S. (1992). Genetic heterogeneity in X-linked amelogenesis imperfecta. *Genomics*, **14**, 567–73.

Brook, A. H. (1974). Dental anomalies of number, form and size: their prevalence in British schoolchildren. *Journal of the International Association of Dentistry for Children*, **5**, 37–53.

Brook, A. H. (1984). A unifying aetiological explanation for anomalies of human tooth number and size. *Archives of Oral Biology*, **29**, 373–8.

Crawford, P. J. M. and Aldred, M. J. (1989). Regional odontodysplasia: a bibliography. *Journal of Oral Pathology and Medicine*, **18**, 251–63.

Deutsch, D., Catalano-Sherman, J., Dafni, L., David, S., and Palmon, A. (1995). Enamel matrix proteins and ameloblast biology. *Connective Tissue Research*, **32**, 97–107.

Fearne, J. M., Bryan, E. M., and Brook, A. H. (1990). Enamel defects in the primary dentition of children born weighing less than 2000 g. *British Dental Journal*, **168**, 433–7.

Forsman, K., Lind, L. Backman, B., Westermark, E., and Holmgren, G. (1994). Localization of a gene for autosomal dominant amelogenesis imperfecta (ADAI) to chromosome 4q. *Human Molecular Genetics*, **3**, 1621–5.

Godfrey, J. L. (1973). A histological study of dentine formation in osteogenesis imperfecta congenita. *Journal of Oral Pathology*, **2**, 95–111.

Kupietzsky, A. and Houpt, M. (1995). Hypohidrotic ectodermal dysplasia: characteristics and treatment (1995). *Quintessence International*, **26**, 285–91.

Raghoebar, G. M., Boering, G., Vissinka, A., and Stegenga (1991). Eruption disturbances of permanent molars: a review. *Journal of Oral Pathology and Medicine*, **20**, 159–66.

Shields, E. D., Bixler, D., and El-Kafrawy, A. M. (1973). A proposed classification of heritable human dentine defects with a description of a new entity. *Archives of Oral Biology*, **18**, 543–53.

Thakkar, N. S. and Sloan, P. (1990). Dental manifestations of systemic disease. In *Oral manifestations of systemic diseases* (2nd edn) (ed. J. H. Jones and D. K. Mason), pp. 480–511. W. B. Saunders, London.

Winter, G. B. (1997). Anomalies of tooth formation and eruption. In *Paediatric dentistry* (ed. R. R. Welbury), pp. 255–80. Oxford University Press, Oxford.

Witkop, C. J., Jr. (1975). Hereditary defects of dentine. *Dental Clinics of North America*, **19**, 25–45.

Witkop, C. J., Jr. (1989). Amelogenesis imperfecta, dentinogenesis imperfecta and dentine dysplasia revisited: problems in classification. *Journal of Oral Pathology*, **17**, 547–53.

Zhu, J. F., Marcushamer, M., King, D. L., and Henry, R. J. (1996). Supernumerary and congenitally absent teeth: a literature review. *Journal of Clinical Pediatric Dentistry*, **20**, 87–95.

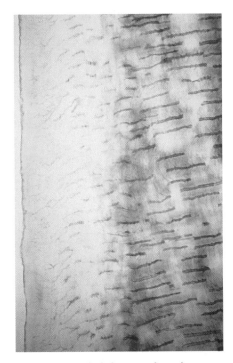

Fig. 1.29 Decalcified section through a root showing aplasia of cementum associated with hypophosphatasia.

2 Dental caries

2 Dental caries

Loss of tooth substance may result from the action of oral microorganisms as in dental caries, or be due to non-bacterial causes. The latter include mechanical factors associated with attrition and abrasion, chemical erosion, and pathological resorption.

Dental caries may be defined as a bacterial disease of the calcified tissues of the teeth characterized by demineralization of the inorganic and destruction of the organic substance of the tooth. It is a complex and dynamic process involving, for example, physicochemical processes associated with the movements of ions across the interface between the tooth and the external environment, as well as biological processes associated with the interaction of bacteria in dental plaque with host defence mechanisms.

Dental caries has been recognized throughout history and exists around the world, although the prevalence and severity varies in different populations. In industrialized countries there was a sharp increase in disease activity in the first half of this century, but since the early 1970s there has been a steady and continued decrease in the prevalence of dental caries among children. Epidemiological studies have also shown that this is continued into adult life. As a result, more people are retaining more teeth for much longer than before and this is reflected in the increase in the prevalence of root surface caries as people grow older.

Despite the encouraging and sustained reduction in dental caries in industrialized countries, the prevalence is increasing in certain developing countries and is associated with urbanization and the increased availability of refined carbohydrates.

AETIOLOGY OF DENTAL CARIES

Various theories for the aetiology of dental caries have been proposed, but there is now overwhelming support for the acidogenic theory. This theory, which has remained virtually unchanged since first postulated by W. D. Miller in 1889, proposes that acid formed from the fermentation of dietary carbohydrates by oral bacteria leads to a progressive decalcification of the tooth substance with a subsequent disintegration of the organic matrix (Fig. 2.1). Alternative theories have largely been discarded because of the lack of experimental evidence. Some of the evidence supporting the acidogenic theory is discussed below.

Role of bacteria and dental plaque

Experiments with germ-free animals have shown that bacteria are essential for the development of dental caries. Bacteria are present in dental plaque which is

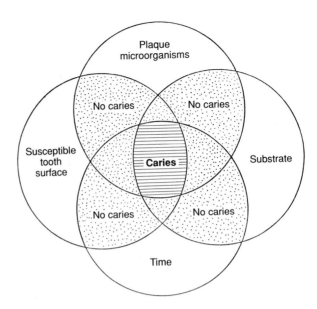

Fig. 2.1 Diagrammatic representation of the parameters involved in the aetiology of dental caries.

found on most tooth surfaces. Plaque consists predominantly of bacteria suspended in an amorphous matrix derived from salivary mucoids and extracellular bacterial polysaccharides (glucans). Leucocytes and desquamated epithelial cells may become entrapped.

A clean enamel surface is covered within a few seconds by an adsorbed layer of glycoprotein from the saliva (the pellicle), on to which coccal bacteria adhere over the following 2 hours. After 24 hours streptococci comprise up to 95 per cent of the total cultivable flora of plaque. During this time the pioneer bacteria have multiplied, formed microcolonies, and become enmeshed in plaque matrix which contains many substances of host, bacterial, and dietary origin. When there is an excess of sugar in the environment the principal components of the matrix are extracellular glucans synthesized by plaque bacteria. Otherwise the matrix consists mainly of salivary glycoprotein partially degraded by bacteria. Streptococci remain the dominant group of organisms in plaque for about 7 days, after which time anaerobic filamentous bacteria become evident, and by 14 days microscopy shows them to be the dominant organisms. The organisms are often arranged in parallel units or palisades commencing at the deep surface of the plaque, the palisades consisting of coccal, bacillary, filamentous, or spirochaetal forms. Organisms are most closely packed adjacent to the enamel surface, becoming more widely spaced towards the salivary surface. Many of the organisms close to the enamel surface may be dead.

Plaque is important in the aetiology of caries because acid is generated within its substance to such an extent that enamel may be dissolved. Dietary sugars diffuse rapidly through plaque where they are converted to acids (mainly lactic acid but also acetic and propionic acids) by bacterial metabolism. The pH of the plaque may fall by as much as 2 units within 10 minutes after the ingestion of sugar, the high density of bacteria in the plaque contributing to this rapid fall in pH. Some 30 to 60 minutes later the pH of the plaque slowly rises to its original figure, due to the diffusion of the sugar and some of the acid out of the plaque, and the diffusion into the plaque of buffered saliva which helps to dilute and neutralize the acid. At a critical pH, which varies in different plaques but is usually about 5.5, mineral ions are liberated from the hydroxyapatite crystals of the surface enamel, and diffuse into the plaque. The pH curves of plaque in response to sugar (Stephan's curves) are similar in shape in caries-free and caries-active individuals. However, since the starting pH may be lower in caries-active mouths, the reduction in pH will be greater and the pH will be depressed below the critical level for a greater period of time. Around a neutral pH the plaque is supersaturated with mineral ions because of the extra ions from the enamel, and some of the excess ions in the plaque may be redeposited on the enamel crystal surfaces. The reprecipitation of mineral is aided by fluoride ions which can substitute for hydroxyl ions, resulting in deposition of fluorapatite. There is, therefore, a see-sawing of ions across the plaque-enamel interface as the chemical environment within the plaque changes (Fig. 2.2). However, mineral ions may be lost from the system by diffusion out of the plaque and into the saliva during the acid phase, and repeated episodes lead to an overall de-mineralization and the initiation of enamel caries. Obviously the frequency and duration of the acid phase of plaque will affect the rate of development of caries, and this is why the reduction of carbohydrate intake between meals has such a beneficial effect in caries prevention. Once enamel caries has progressed to cavity formation, the plaque becomes progressively more removed from saliva and probably remains acidic for longer periods. Many plaque bacteria store carbohydrate as an intracellular glycogen-like polysaccharide which may be formed from a variety of sugars, and this may be broken down to acid when other sources of carbohydrate are absent, such as between meals. In addition, as mentioned above, plaque organisms can synthesize extracellular glucans from dietary sugars which may also be metabolized to acid when other sources of carbohydrate are absent. However, abundant extracellular polysaccharides have other important consequences in that they markedly increase the bulk of the plaque, thereby interfering with the outward diffusion of acids and the inward diffusion of saliva and its buffering systems. Such plaques are likely to be more cariogenic because they favour retention of acid at the plaque–enamel interface.

Fluoride ions are present in relatively high concentration in plaque compared with saliva. Fluoride favours the precipitation of calcium and phosphate ions from solution, and so when present at the plaque–enamel interface the deposition of free mineral ions in the plaque as hydroxy- and fluorapatite on the remaining enamel crystals is encouraged. Fluorapatite crystals may also be formed during enamel development if fluorides have been administered systemically (for example by water fluoridation). Fluorapatite is less soluble in acid than hydroxyapatite. Systemic fluoride also promotes the formation of hydroxyapatite crystals with a more stable crystal lattice. Fluoride ions in plaque inhibit bacterial metabolism and this provides an additional mechanism for the preventive action of fluoride in enamel caries.

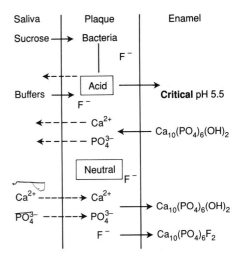

Fig. 2.2 Ionic exchanges at the saliva–plaque–enamel interface. Mineral ions are able to ebb and flow both from the enamel surface into the plaque and vice versa.

In dental plaque   **Key points**

- cariogenic bacteria ferment carbohydrate to acid
- cariogenic bacteria can store carbohydrate intra and extracellularly
- extracellular polysaccharides increase plaque bulk
- bulky plaques interfere with outward diffusion of acid and inward diffusion of salivary buffers
- ions see-saw across the plaque–enamel interface depending on pH
- fluoride ions encourage reprecipitation of minerals into enamel and inhibit bacterial metabolism

Acid is a general product of bacterial metabolism and no single bacterial species is uniquely associated with the development of enamel caries. Members of the 'mutans streptococci' group are the most efficient cariogenic organisms in animal experiments, and epidemiological data in humans indicates an association between the presence of *S. mutans* and *S. sobrinus* in plaque and the prevalence of caries. Some of the factors supporting an aetiological role for *S. mutans* in dental caries are summarized in Table 2.1. However, caries of enamel may develop in the absence of *S. mutans* and in some individuals high levels of *S. mutans* may be present on a tooth surface without the subsequent development of caries. The significance of *S. mutans* in the evolution of a carious lesion is not fully resolved, but it appears that the organism is important, but not essential, for the initiation of enamel caries. Other bacteria, for example lactobacilli, may be important in the further progression of the lesion. Lactobacilli are also the pioneer organisms in dentine caries (see later).

Other plaque bacteria associated with caries are species of streptococci such as *S. sanguis*, *S. mitis*, and *S. oralis* and members of the genera *Actinomyces* and *Lactobacillus*, all of which can induce experimental caries in animals. Actinomyces have been associated particularly with root surface caries, but the results from several studies show that other organisms including mutans streptococci and lactobacilli are involved. Because of the strong evidence that *S. mutans* and lactobacilli are major organisms associated with dental caries, simple screening tests to estimate the salivary levels of these bacteria have been developed as predictors of caries activity. Their reliability and validity require further testing and threshold values for distinguishing between high- and low-risk patients need to be better defined. Infants become colonized by mutans streptococci from their mothers, and there is evidence that children of high-risk mothers become colonized at an earlier age and develop more carious lesions than children of low-risk mothers.

Table 2.1 Factors supporting a role for *S. mutans* in the aetiology of dental caries

Rapid generation of acid from sucrose

Synthesis of extracellular polysaccharides
—adhesion to tooth
—increase in plaque bulk

Synthesis of intracellular polysaccharides
—acid production when sucrose absent from diet

Present in high numbers in plaque associated with developing lesions

High numbers at a particular tooth site predispose to subsequent caries

Highly cariogenic in animal models of experimental caries

Immunization against *S. mutans* reduces caries incidence in animal models

---

Key points

Microbiology of dental caries
- species strongly implicated:
  —mutans streptococci, e.g. *S. mutans*; *S. sobrinus*
  —lactobacilli, e.g. *L. casei*; *L. acidophilus*
- species possibly associated:
  —other streptococci, e.g. *S. mitis*
  —actinomyces, e.g. *A. viscosus*

Although experiments in germ-free animals have shown the importance of certain specific organisms in caries, the microbial flora of human dental plaque is extremely complex. In such a mixture of bacteria, interactions between different organisms will occur which may reduce or enhance the pathogenicity of individual species. However, at present, there is a lack of data as to how such interactions may affect the initiation and progression of dental caries.

Role of carbohydrates

Numerous epidemiological studies have demonstrated a direct relationship between fermentable carbohydrate in the diet and dental caries. The evidence includes:

1. The increasing prevalence of dental caries in developing countries and previously isolated ethnic groups associated with westernization, urbanization, and the increasing availability of sucrose in their diet. Examples include Inuit, native North and South Americans, African tribes, and the rural population in countries in the Far East.
2. The decrease in the prevalence of caries during World War II because of sugar restriction, followed by a rise to previous levels when sucrose became available in the post-war period.
3. The Hopewood House study—a children's home in Australia where sucrose and white bread were virtually excluded from the diet. The children had low caries rates which increased dramatically when they moved out of the home.

Different carbohydrates have different cariogenic properties. Sucrose is significantly more cariogenic than other sugars, partly because it is readily fermented by plaque bacteria and partly because of its conversion by bacterial glucosyl transferase into extracellular glucans. Sucrose is also readily converted into intracellular polymers. Glucose, fructose, maltose, galactose, and lactose are also highly cariogenic carbohydrates in experimental caries in animals, but the principal carbohydrates available in human diets are sucrose and starches. Dietary sugars can be divided into intrinsic (mainly fruit and vegetables) and extrinsic sources (added sugars, milk, fruit juices). Dietary advice recommends that consumption of extrinsic sugars (except milk) should be reduced. Much of the epidemiological data incriminates sucrose. Its relative importance is also well illustrated in patients with hereditary fructose intolerance who cannot tolerate fructose or sucrose (ingestion may lead to coma and death) but who are able to consume starches. Such individuals have little or no caries. Starch solutions applied to bacterial plaque produce no significant depression in pH, due to the very slow diffusion of the polysaccharide into the plaque which must be hydrolysed by extracellular amylase before it can be assimilated and metabolized by plaque bacteria. Other carbohydrates, such as sorbitol and xylitol, are very low cariogenic agents, partly because of their slow rate of fermentation.

Diet and dental caries   **Key points**

- caries prevalence increases when populations become exposed to sucrose-rich diets
- extrinsic sugars are more damaging than intrinsic sugars
- sucrose is the most cariogenic sugar
- frequency of sugar intake is of more importance than total amount consumed

Whilst there is no doubt that there is a direct relationship between dietary carbohydrates and caries, experimental evidence in humans has shown that the manner and form in which the carbohydrate is taken and the frequency of consumption are more important than the absolute amount of sugar consumed. The risk of caries is greatest if sugar is consumed between meals thus supplying plaque bacteria with (in the case of habitual 'snackers') an almost constant supply of carbohydrate. It is also increased if the sugar is consumed in a sticky form likely to be retained on the surfaces of the teeth.

Aetiological variables

Not all teeth or tooth surfaces are equally susceptible to caries, nor is the rate of progression of carious lesions constant. Factors influencing site attack and rates of progression in dental caries are largely unknown but may include:

Factors intrinsic to the tooth

Enamel composition—There is an inverse relationship between enamel solubility and enamel fluoride concentration. A graded increase in enamel resistance with age might account for selectivity of site attack.

Enamel structure—Developmental enamel hypoplasia and hypomineralization may affect the rate of progression but not the initiation of caries.

Tooth morphology—Deep, narrow pits and fissures favour the retention of plaque and food.

Tooth position—Malaligned teeth may predispose to the retention of plaque and food.

Factors extrinsic to the tooth

Saliva—Flow rate, viscosity, buffering capacity, availability of calcium and phosphate ions for mineralization, and the presence of antimicrobial agents such as immunoglobulins, thiocyanate ion, lactoferrin, and lysozyme may affect caries pattern.

Diet—There is evidence that the presence in the diet of phosphates, either organically bound or inorganic, may reduce the incidence of caries. Increasing the proportion of fat in the diet reduces the cariogenic effect of sugar, possibly by a physical effect. Evidence suggests that traces of molybdenum and vanadium in the diet may reduce caries.

Immunity—See later.

PATHOLOGY OF DENTAL CARIES

Clinically, dental caries may be classified according both to the location of the lesion on the tooth and to the rate of attack.

Classification by site of attack

Pit or fissure caries

This occurs on the occlusal surfaces of molars and premolars, on the buccal and lingual surfaces of molars, and the lingual surfaces of maxillary incisors. Early caries may be detected clinically by brown or black discoloration of a fissure in which a probe 'sticks'. The enamel directly bordering the pit or fissure may appear opaque, bluish-white as it becomes undermined by caries. Recently, it has been suggested that early fissure caries is becoming more difficult to diagnose by probing. Enamel which appears clinically sound can overlay extensive caries of the dentine although a lesion extending to the amelodentinal junction must be present. This is thought to be due to the effect of topical fluorides, particularly in toothpastes, which help maintain the integrity of enamel undermined by dentinal caries.

Smooth surface caries

This occurs on the approximal surfaces, and on the gingival third of the buccal and lingual surfaces. Approximal caries begins just below the contact point as a well-demarcated chalky-white opacity of the enamel (Fig. 2.3). At this stage there is no loss of continuity of the enamel surface and the lesion cannot be detected by a probe or on routine radiographs. The white spot lesion may become pigmented yellow or brown and may extend buccally and lingually into the embrasures. As the caries progresses, the surrounding enamel becomes bluish-white. The surface of the lesion becomes roughened before frank cavitation occurs. There are no consistent radiographic features which enable unequivocal identification of enamel lesions that have cavitated from lesions where the surface is still intact. However, in general, an enamel radiolucency that reaches the amelodentinal junction is associated with a cavity and with involvement of underlying dentine whereas, in most cases, a radiolucency that does not extend to the amelodentinal junction does not represent a frank cavity and such a lesion is best treated by preventive measures. Cervical caries extends occlusally from opposite the gingival margin on buccal and lingual tooth surfaces. It has a similar appearance to approximal caries, but almost always produces a wide open cavity.

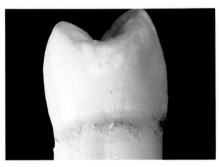

Fig. 2.3   White spot lesion of enamel caries involving an approximal surface of a premolar.

Diagnosis of caries   **Key points**
- early occlusal caries may be difficult to detect
- radiolucencies in approximal enamel that do not reach the amelodentinal junction do not usually indicate enamel cavitation

Cemental or root caries

This occurs when the root face is exposed to the oral environment as a result of periodontal disease. The root face is softened and the cavities, which may be extensive, are usually shallow, saucer-shaped, with ill-defined boundaries.

Recurrent caries

This occurs around the margin or at the base of a previously existing restoration.

Classification by rate of attack

Rampant or acute caries

This is rapidly progressing caries involving many or all of the erupted teeth, often on surfaces normally immune to caries. The rapid coronal destruction leads to early involvement of the pulp.

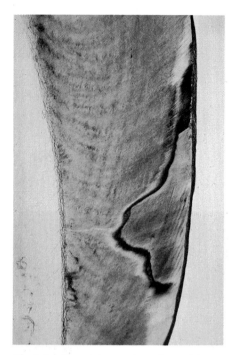

Fig. 2.4 Ground section through an early carious lesion in enamel showing zonation of the lesion.

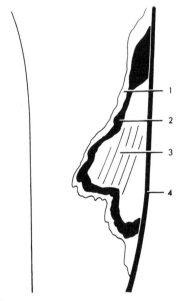

Fig. 2.5 Diagrammatic representation of the lesion in Fig. 2.4 showing: 1, translucent zone; 2, dark zone; 3, body of the lesion; 4, surface zone.

Slowly progressive or chronic caries

This is caries that progresses slowly and involves the pulp much later than in acute caries. It is most common in adults and the slow progress allows time for defence reactions of the pulpodentinal complex (sclerosis and reactionary dentine formation) to develop.

Arrested caries

This is caries of enamel or dentine, including root caries, that becomes static and shows no tendency for further progression.

Enamel caries

Ground sections of teeth have been used extensively in histopathological studies of enamel caries and have been examined by transmitted and polarized light, and by microradiography. Electron microscopy and biochemical analysis of microdissected pieces of carious enamel have also been carried out. Most research has concentrated on smooth surface caries to avoid the problems of interpretation of histological features imposed by the anatomy of pits and fissures. However, the pathological features are essentially similar in both sites. The established early lesion (white-spot lesion) in smooth surface enamel caries is cone-shaped, with the base of the cone on the enamel surface and the apex pointing towards the amelodentinal junction. The shape is modified in pit and fissure caries (see later). In ground sections it consists of a series of zones, the optical properties of which reflect differing degrees of demineralization (Figs 2.4, 2.5). These zones are described below.

Translucent zone

This is the first recognizable histological change at the advancing edge of the lesion. It is more porous than normal enamel and contains 1 per cent by volume of spaces, the pore volume, compared with the 0.1 per cent pore volume in normal enamel. The pores are larger than the small pores in normal enamel which approximate to the size of a water molecule. Chemical analysis shows that there is a fall in magnesium and carbonate when compared with normal enamel, which suggests that a magnesium–carbonate-rich mineral is preferentially dissolved in this zone. Dissolution of mineral occurs mainly from the junctional areas between the prismatic and interprismatic enamel. The prism boundaries, which are relatively rich in protein, allow ready ingress of hydrogen ions and the magnesium- and carbonate-rich mineral that is preferentially removed may represent the surface layers of crystallites at the prism boundaries. The translucent zone is sometimes missing, or present along only part of the lesion.

Dark zone

This zone contains 2–4 per cent by volume of pores. Some of the pores are large, but others are smaller than those in the translucent zone, suggesting that some remineralization has occurred due to reprecipitation of mineral lost from the translucent zone. It is thought that the dark zone is narrow in rapidly advancing lesions and wider in more slowly advancing lesions when more remineralization may occur.

Body of the lesion

This zone (Fig. 2.6) has a pore volume of between 5 and 25 per cent, and also contains apatite crystals larger than those found in normal enamel. It is suggested that these large crystals result from the reprecipitation of mineral dissolved from deeper zones. However, with continuing acid attack there is further dissolution of mineral both from the periphery of the apatite crystals and from their cores. The lost mineral is replaced by unbound water and to a lesser extent by organic matter, presumably derived from saliva and microorganisms. There is increased prominence of the striae of Retzius in the body of the lesion, the explanation for which is unknown.

Surface zone

This is about 40 μm thick and shows surprisingly little change in early lesions (see Fig. 2.6). The surface of normal enamel differs in composition from the deeper layers, being more highly mineralized and having, for example, a higher fluoride level and a lower magnesium level, and so interpretation of possible chemical changes in this zone is difficult. The surface zone remains relatively normal despite subsurface loss of mineral, because it is an area of active reprecipitation of mineral derived both from the plaque and from that dissolved from deeper areas of the lesion as ions diffuse outwards (see Fig. 2.2).

Histopathogenesis of the early lesion

The development of enamel caries can be traced through the following stages when ground sections are examined by transmitted light (Fig. 2.7).

1. Development of a subsurface translucent zone, which is unrecognizable clinically and radiologically.
2. The subsurface translucent zone enlarges and a dark zone develops in its centre.
3. As the lesion enlarges more mineral is lost and the centre of the dark zone becomes the body of the lesion. This is relatively translucent compared with sound enamel and shows enhancement of the striae of Retzius, interprismatic markings, and cross-striations of the prisms. The lesion is now clinically recognizable as a white spot.
4. The body of the lesion may become stained by exogenous pigments from food, tobacco, and bacteria. The lesion is now clinically recognizable as a brown spot.
5. When the caries reaches the amelodentinal junction it spreads laterally, and in this way the enamel may become widely undermined, giving the bluish-white appearance of the enamel seen clinically. Extension along the amelodentinal

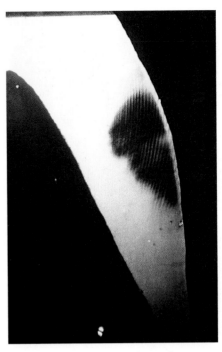

Fig. 2.6 Microradiograph of an early carious lesion in enamel showing loss of mineral from the body of the lesion, prominence of the striae of Retzius and intact surface zone.

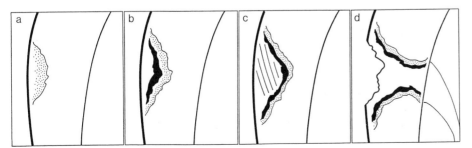

Fig. 2.7 Histopathogenesis of enamel caries: a, subsurface translucent zone; b, development of the dark zone; c, typical zoned structure of the early (white spot) lesion; d, cavitation of the surface, spread along the amelodentinal junction, reactive changes in dentine.

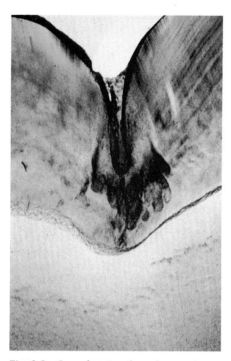

Fig. 2.8 Ground section through an early lesion of fissure caries in enamel.

junction may result in secondary undermining enamel caries. The time for caries to progress through enamel on the approximal surfaces of permanent teeth has been reported to be about 4 years but may be up to 8 years.

6. Breakdown of the surface zone with formation of a cavity. This stage may precede stage 5.

In some lesions dentine may be involved late in stage 3, while in other lesions it is not involved until stage 5 or 6. Bitewing radiographs do not show lesions until stage 4 or possibly late stage 3.

No unequivocal evidence for specific points of entry of the carious attack into the enamel has been found with light microscopy. Acid appears to diffuse in over a broad front. Ultrastructural studies suggest preferential dissolution initially along prism boundaries, but there is also a diffuse demineralization with an increase in intercrystallite distance affecting areas both within and between the prisms. These intercrystallite spaces presumably reflect the variation in pore volume in different areas of the lesion. Changes in crystal structure are thought to be due to both demineralization and reprecipitation of mineral.

Caries in a fissure does not start at the base, but develops as a ring around the wall of the fissure, the histological features of the lesion being similar to those seen on smooth surfaces. As the caries progresses it extends towards the dentine parallel to the enamel prisms and eventually coalesces at the base of the fissure (Figs 2.8, 2.9). This produces a cone-shaped lesion, but the base of the cone is directed towards the amelodentinal junction and is not on the enamel surface as in smooth surface caries. The area of dentine ultimately involved is therefore larger than with smooth surface lesions.

Key points	**Enamel caries**
	• a dynamic physicochemical process involving dissolution and reprecipitation of mineral
	• zonation of the early (white spot) lesion reflects different degrees of demineralization
	• surface zone is an area of active remineralization
	• the morphology of the lesion differs in pits and fissures compared with approximal surfaces

Dentine caries

Dentine differs from enamel in that it is a living tissue and as such can respond to caries attack. It also has a relatively high organic content, approximately 20 per cent by weight, which consists predominantly of collagen. In dentine caries it is, therefore, necessary to consider both the defence reaction of the pulpodentinal complex and the carious destruction of the tissue which involves acid demineralization followed by proteolytic breakdown of the matrix. The defence reaction

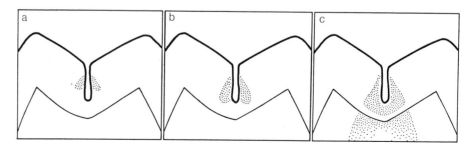

Fig. 2.9 Diagrammatic representation of the development of fissure caries.

may begin before the carious process reaches the dentine, presumably because of irritation to the odontoblasts transmitted through the weakened enamel, and is represented by the formation of reactionary (or tertiary) dentine and dentinal sclerosis (see later). However, in progressive lesions the defence reaction is progressively overtaken by the carious process as it advances towards the pulp.

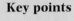

Processes in dentine caries

- defence reaction of pulpodential complex
  —sclerosis
  —reactionary dentine formation
  —sealing of dead tracts
- carious destruction
  —demineralization
  —proteolysis

Key points

Caries of the dentine develops from enamel caries: when the lesion reaches the amelodentinal junction, lateral extension results in the involvement of great numbers of tubules (Fig. 2.10). The early lesion is cone-shaped, or convex, with the base at the amelodentinal junction. Larger lesions may show a broadening of the apex of the cone as it approaches the circumpulpal dentine. This apparent slowing of the advancing front of the lesion suggests that circumpulpal dentine is more resistant to carious attack, possibly due to an increased fluoride content derived by diffusion of ions from tissue fluids in the pulp. In caries of dentine, demineralization by acid is always in advance of the bacterial front, the subsequent bacterial invasion being followed by breakdown of the collagenous matrix.

Because of the sequential nature of the changes, studies of ground and decalcified sections show a zoned lesion in which four zones are characteristically present (Fig. 2.11).

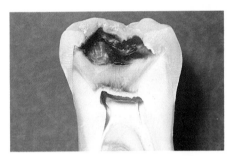

Fig. 2.10 Bisected grossly carious molar. Spread of caries along the amelodentinal junction has resulted in undermining of the enamel.

Zone of sclerosis

The sclerotic or translucent zone is located beneath and at the sides of the carious lesion. It is almost invariably present, being broader beneath the lesion than at the sides and is regarded as a vital reaction of odontoblasts to irritation. Two patterns of mineralization have been described. The first is the result of acceleration of the normal physiological process of centripetal deposition of peritubular dentine which eventually occludes the tubules. In the second, mineral first appears within the cytoplasmic process of the odontoblasts and the tubule is obliterated by calcification of the odontoblast process itself. Sclerosed dentine therefore has a higher mineral content. It has been suggested that the sclerotic zone at the side of the lesion may be due to passive deposition of mineral previously removed by the carious process from the body of the lesion rather than to the reaction of odontoblasts. Dead tracts, which, in contrast to sclerotic (translucent) zones, are opaque when ground sections are examined with transmitted light, may be seen within the zone of sclerosis. They are the result of death of odontoblasts, the empty dentinal tubules containing air and degenerate odontoblast processes. As such they provide ready access of bacteria and their products to the pulp. To prevent this the pulpal end of a dead tract is occluded by a thin layer of hyaline calcified material, sometimes called eburnoid, which is derived from pulpal cells. Beyond this, further, often very irregular, reactionary dentine may form following differention of odontoblasts or odontoblast-like cells from the pulp.

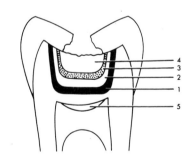

Fig. 2.11 Diagrammatic representation of the zones in established dentine caries: 1, sclerosis; 2, demineralization; 3, bacterial invasion; 4, destruction; 5, reactionary, tertiary dentine beneath the lesion.

Zone of demineralization

In the demineralized zone the intertubular matrix is mainly affected by a wave of acid diffusing ahead of the bacterial front. As this zone is in advance of the zone of bacterial invasion the soft dentine in the base of a deep cavity would not need to be removed if soft but sterile dentine could be distinguished from soft infected dentine. Although various caries-detector dyes have been developed their validity and reliability require further study and, at present, they are not recommended for routine use.

Zone of bacterial invasion

In this zone the bacteria extend down and multiply within the dentinal tubules (Fig. 2.12), some of which may become occluded by bacteria (Fig. 2.13). There are always, however, many empty tubules lying among tubules containing bacteria. The bacterial invasion probably occurs in two waves, the first wave consisting of acidogenic organisms, mainly lactobacilli, produce acid which diffuses ahead into the demineralized zone. A second wave of mixed acidogenic and proteolytic organisms then attack the demineralized matrix. The walls of the tubules are softened by the proteolytic activity and some may then be distended by the increasing mass of multiplying bacteria. The peritubular dentine is first compressed, followed by the intertubular dentine, resulting in elliptical areas of proteolysis–liquefaction foci. Liquefaction foci run parallel to the direction of the tubules and may be multiple, giving the tubule a beaded appearance (Fig. 2.14). These changes are enhanced in the zone of destruction. The bacteria may show varying degrees of degeneration.

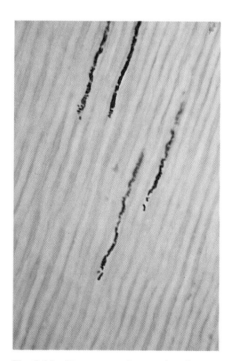

Fig. 2.12 Pioneer organisms at the advancing front of the zone of bacterial invasion in dentine caries.

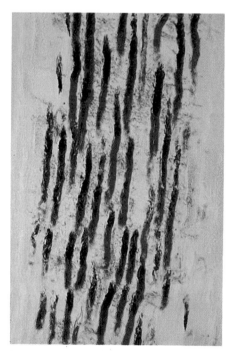

Fig. 2.13 Packing of the dentinal tubules by bacteria in the zone of bacterial invasion (Gram stain).

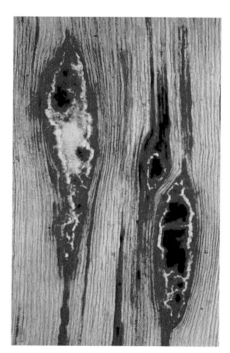

Fig. 2.14 Liquefaction foci in dentine caries.

Zone of destruction

In the zone of destruction the liquefaction foci enlarge and increase in number. Cracks or clefts containing bacteria and necrotic tissue also appear at right angles to the course of the dentinal tubules–transverse clefts (Fig. 2.15). The mechanism of formation of transverse clefts is uncertain. They may follow the course of incremental lines, or result from the coalescence of liquefaction foci on adjacent tubules, or arise by extension of proteolytic activity along interconnecting lateral branches of odontoblast tubules. Bacteria are no longer confined to the tubules and invade both the peritubular and intertubular dentine. Little of the normal dentine architecture now remains and cavitation commences from the amelodentinal junction. In acute, rapidly progressing caries the necrotic dentine is very soft and yellowish-white; in chronic caries it has a brownish-black colour and is of leathery consistency.

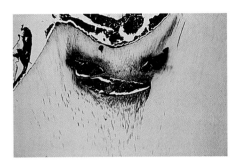

Fig. 2.15 Transverse clefts in dentine caries.

Carious destruction of dentine

- bacterial invasion of tubules
- acidogenic organisms—demineralization followed by:
- proteolytic organisms—destruction of demineralized matrix
- liquefaction foci
- transverse clefts

Key points

Reactionary (or tertiary) dentine

A layer of reactionary (or tertiary) dentine is often formed at the surface of the pulp chamber deep to the dentine caries, this dentine being localized to the irritated odontoblasts. It varies in structure but the tubules are generally irregular, tortuous, and fewer in number than in primary dentine, or may even be absent. The regularity of the tubules is thought to be inversely related to the degree of irritation of the odontoblasts. Decalcified sections may show basophilic incremental lines. Microradiography shows variations in mineralization, but areas of hypermineralization when compared with primary dentine may be present. Its formation effectively increases the depth of tissue between the carious dentine and the pulp, and in this way delays involvement of the pulp.

Reactionary dentine is a non-specific response to odontoblast irritation, also being formed in reaction to tooth wear and cavity and crown preparations.

Root caries

The primary tissue affected in root caries is usually the cementum. The development of cemental caries is preceded by exposure of the root to the oral environment as a result of periodontal disease followed by bacterial colonization. Although *Actinomyces* species are present in large numbers and have been implicated in the disease, other organisms including mutans streptococci and lactobacilli are also associated with root caries.

Microradiographs of developing lesions show subsurface demineralization of the root which may extend into dentine. The surface layer is hypermineralized and is analogous to that seen in the early enamel lesion. It represents a zone of reprecipitation of mineral removed from the subsurface and of remineralization from minerals present in plaque/saliva. Fluoride is readily taken up by carious root surfaces and this enhances remineralization.

Despite the initial hypermineralization of the surface, progressive softening occurs with time in active lesions. Root caries is clinically diagnosed by a softening and brownish discoloration of the tissues. Demineralization is rapidly followed by bacterial invasion along the exposed collagen fibres and fracture and loss of successive layers of cementum. These fractures frequently occur parallel to the root surface and are associated with invasion of bacteria along the incremental bands in cementum which run as concentric layers around the root. This extension results in lesions that spread laterally around the root and often coalesce with other lesions so that eventually the carious process may encircle the root.

As the cementum is lost the peripheral dentine is exposed. The basic reactions and carious destruction of this tissue are the same as those described previously. Sclerosis may lead to arrested lesions and the surface of the exposed dentine may be covered by a hypermineralized layer.

Arrested caries

Enamel

Arrest of an approximal smooth-surface lesion prior to cavity formation can occur when the adjacent tooth is lost so that the lesion becomes accessible to plaque control. Remineralization may then occur from saliva or from the topical application of calcifying solutions, but a normal crystalline structure is not necessarily re-formed.

Dentine

Arrest of coronal dentinal caries may occur in lesions where there is loss of the unsupported overlying enamel following extensive lateral spread of caries along the amelodentinal junction. The loss of enamel exposes the superficially softened carious dentine to the oral environment and it is then removed by attrition and abrasion, leaving a hard, polished surface. Such dentine is deeply pigmented, brown-black in colour. Its surface is hypermineralized due to remineralization from oral fluids and has a high fluoride content. The extensive lateral spread of caries along the amelodentinal junction is a major factor in the arrest of dentinal lesions and is, in part, due to marked sclerosis which is a feature of such lesions. The sclerosis limits the rate of inward spread of the caries. (In contrast, teeth involved by rampant caries show a minimal protective response.)

Arrested lesions of root caries have a similar clinical appearance and develop in a similar manner following loss of the superficially softened cementum.

IMMUNOLOGICAL ASPECTS OF DENTAL CARIES

Caries in man is associated with the development of serum and salivary antibodies against *S. mutans*, but in almost all individuals this natural active immunity appears to have little effect as caries is virtually universal in Western populations. This may be because *S. mutans* is only weakly antigenic.

However, artificial active immunity following experimental immunization of rats and monkeys with *S. mutans* using both live and dead organisms as well as cell-wall preparations has been shown to produce a significant reduction in caries. Immunization evokes a humoral response characterized by IgG, IgM, and IgA classes of antibodies and also induces cell-mediated immune responses. These effector systems can gain access to the oral cavity via the gingival crevice and saliva, but the immunological mechanisms involved in prevention of dental caries are unclear. However, in these experimental systems the reduction in the number of carious lesions appears to be associated with a reduction in the number of *S. mutans* organisms in plaque. The salivary immune mechanism would presumably act through secretory IgA and might prevent *S. mutans* from adhering to the tooth surface. Crevicular immune mechanisms could involve any or all of the humoral and cellular components of systemic immunity; immunoglobulins, complement, neutrophil leucocytes, sensitized lymphocytes, and macrophages may pass through the base of the sulcus and so reach the tooth surface. Although the relative importance of salivary and crevicular mechanisms has not been fully elucidated, the powerful immune components of the latter suggest it is the more important. Evidence suggests that protection is associated with IgG-mediated reactions and that IgA and IgM antibodies confer little or no protection and may interfere with the protective effect of IgG. The IgG antibody may act as an opsonin, facilitating phagocytosis and ultimately death of *S. mutans* by neutrophil leucocytes and macrophages. The role of the cell-mediated immune response is uncertain but helper T-cell function is probably important.

Vaccines composed of whole cells of *S. mutans* may induce antibodies that cross-react with heart tissue, and so subcomponents of the organism have been investigated which retain the capacity to protect against caries but which do not contain cross-reacting heart antigens. These include proteins purified from the cell wall of *S. mutans* that are involved in the attachment of the organism to tooth surfaces.

Several other antigen preparations have been tested in animal studies including the glucosyltransferases. These bacterial enzymes convert sucrose into glucans which are important for the accumulation of *S. mutans* on tooth surfaces. Although antibodies to glucosyltransferases can reduce the accumulation of plaque and the incidence of caries in rodents, they appear to have little protective value in primates. This may be because such antibodies are probably most effective against the development of smooth surface rather than pit and fissure caries.

FURTHER READING

Banting, D. W. (1986). Epidemiology of root caries. *Gerodontolgy*, **5**, 5–11.

Bowen, W. H. (1994). Food components and caries. *Advances in Dental Research*, **8**, 215–20.

Edgar, W. M. (1993). Extrinsic and intrinsic sugars: a review of recent UK recommendations on diet and caries. *Caries Research*, **27**, Suppl. 1, 64–7.

Hardie, J. M. (1992). Oral microbiology: current concepts in the microbiology of dental caries and periodontal disease. *British Dental Journal*, **172**, 271–8.

Johnson, A. R. (1985). The early carious lesion of enamel. *Journal of Oral Pathology*, **4**, 128–57.

Kidd, E. A. M. (1984). The diagnosis and management of the 'early' carious lesion in permanent teeth. *Dental Update*, **11**, 69–81.

Kidd, E. A. M. (1996). The carious lesion in enamel. In *The prevention of dental disease* (3rd edn) (ed. J. J. Murray), pp. 95–106. Oxford University Press, Oxford.

Kidd, E. A. M., Ricketts, D. N. J., and Pitts, N. B. (1993). Occlusal caries diagnosis: a changing challenge for clinicians and epidemiologists. *Journal of Dentistry*, **21**, 323–31.

Mellberg, J. R. (1986). Demineralization and remineralization of root surface caries. *Gerodontology*, **5**, 25–31.

Rugg-Gunn, A. J. (1996). Diet and dental caries. In *The prevention of dental disease* (3rd edn) (ed. J. J. Murray), pp. 3–31. Oxford University Press, Oxford.

Russell, M. W. (1992). Immunization against dental caries. *Current Opinion in Dentistry*, **2**, 72–80.

Schupbach, P., Guggenheim, B., and Latz, F. (1989). Human root caries: histopathology of initial lesions in cementum and dentin. *Journal of Oral Pathology and Medicine*, **18**, 146–56.

Schupbach, P., Osterwalder, V., and Guggenheim, B. (1995). Human root caries: micro-biota in plaque covering sound, carious and arrested carious root surfaces. *Caries Research*, **29**, 382–95.

Silverstone, L. M. (1973). Structure of carious enamel including the early carious lesions. *Oral Sciences Review*, **3**, 100–60.

Silverstone, L. M. (1983). Remineralization and enamel caries: new concepts. *Dental Update*, **10**, 261–73.

Stanley, H. R., Pereira, J. C., Spiegel, E., Broom, C., and Schultz, M. (1983). The detection and prevalence of reactive and physiologic sclerotic dentin, reparative dentin and dead tracts beneath various types of dental lesions according to tooth surface and age. *Journal of Oral Pathology*, **12**, 257–89.

Van Houte, J., Lopman, J., and Kent, R. (1994). The predominant cultivable flora of sound and carious human root surfaces. *Journal of Dental Research*, **73**, 1727–34.

3 Other disorders of teeth

3 Other disorders of teeth

DISORDERS OF ERUPTION AND SHEDDING OF TEETH

Premature eruption, natal, and neonatal teeth

Teeth erupted at birth (natal) are slightly more common than teeth which erupt within the first 30 days of life (neonatal) and are seen in approximately 1 in 3000 live births. Almost always one or two central incisors are involved, four times more frequently in the mandible than the maxilla. They are thought to arise from normal tooth germs developing in a superficial position in the jaw with subsequent premature eruption. Such teeth are usually either lost spontaneously or extracted to prevent them being inhaled and to prevent ulceration of the tongue or the mother's nipple. Coronal enamel and dentine structure is normal for the chronological age of the teeth, but the radicular dentine and cementum are generally irregular in structure due to the mobility of the tooth in the jaw (Fig. 3.1). However, if the teeth are left in the jaw the roots may sometimes continue to develop and the teeth become firm.

Premature eruption of other deciduous or permanent teeth is unusual and may be related to local factors such as a superficial location of a tooth germ or early shedding of deciduous teeth. Generalized early eruption of the permanent dentition may also be seen in children with endocrine abnormalities associated with an excess secretion of growth hormone or with hyperthyroidism.

Retarded eruption

Endocrinopathies (for example hypothyroidism), prematurity, nutritional deficiencies, and chromosome abnormalities, such as Down syndrome, may very occasionally be associated with retarded eruption of either the deciduous and/or permanent dentition. Idiopathic migration, traumatic displacement of tooth germs, or abnormally large crowns may also be associated with retarded eruption. Delayed eruption and multiple, impacted supernumerary teeth are also a feature of cleidocranial dysplasia (see Chapter 16).

Premature loss

This is usually the result of either dental caries and its sequelae, or chronic periodontal disease. Occasionally, premature loss of teeth is more specifically associated with diseases such as hypophosphatasia and hereditary palmar-plantar hyperkeratosis and other causes of prepubertal periodontitis (see Chapter 7).

Persistence of deciduous teeth

This occurs when deciduous teeth are not shed at the expected time, and is usually associated with the failure of eruption of the permanent successor

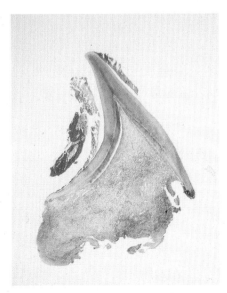

Fig. 3.1 Decalcified section through a neonatal incisor.

because it is missing or displaced. Persistence of the entire deciduous dentition is uncommon and usually has a systemic background, such as cleidocranial dysplasia when eruption of permanent teeth is impeded.

Impaction of teeth

An impacted tooth is one which remains unerupted, or only partly erupted, in the jaw beyond the time when it should normally be fully erupted. One or several teeth may be affected and the condition may be symmetrical. It is rarely seen in the primary dentition. In the permanent dentition the teeth most frequently involved are third molars, mandibular premolars, and maxillary canines. Local causes for impaction include abnormal position of the tooth germ, lack of space for the teeth in the jaws, supernumerary teeth, cysts, and tumours. As previously mentioned, cleidocranial dysplasia is almost always associated with multiple impacted teeth. Possible complications of impaction include resorption of the impacted tooth or adjacent erupted teeth, and the development of dentigerous cysts and odontogenic tumours.

Reimpaction of teeth

This term describes the situation in which a previously erupted tooth becomes submerged in the tissues. Alternative terms for the disorder are infraocclusion and submerged teeth. The deciduous second molar is most commonly affected and reimpaction occurs twice as frequently in the mandible than in the maxilla. The condition is associated with deficient development of the alveolar process around the reimpacted tooth which may, on rare occasions, become completely covered by oral mucosa. The roots of the tooth are usually partly resorbed and ankylosed to the bone. The cause is not known, but it is likely that the root first becomes ankylosed and that this is followed by lack of growth of the alveolar process. As the neighbouring teeth continue to move occlusally they tilt over the ankylosed tooth causing reimpaction.

NON-BACTERIAL LOSS OF TOOTH SUBSTANCE

Although it is convenient to discuss attrition, abrasion, and erosion separately, in many patients tooth wear involves elements of all three. For this reason terms such as 'tooth wear with a major component of attrition', are usually preferred as clinical diagnoses.

Key points	Non-bacterial loss of tooth substance
	● tooth wear
	—attrition
	—abrasion
	—erosion
	● resorption
	—internal
	—external

Attrition

This is loss of tooth substance as a result of tooth-to-tooth contact (Fig. 3.2). It may be physiological or pathological in origin, although clinically the distinction is often unclear. The pattern of tooth loss in physiological attrition is fairly constant; the incisal edges of the incisors are worn first, followed by the occlusal surfaces of the molars, the palatal cusps of the maxillary teeth, and the buccal cusps of the mandibular teeth. When the dentine becomes exposed it generally becomes discoloured brown. Because dentine is softer than enamel it is attrited at a greater rate and the lesions may become cup-shaped, surrounded by a rim of enamel. Approximal attrition leads to the transformation of contact points to contact areas and to the mesial migration of teeth which throughout life may amount to as much as 1 cm from third molar to third molar. Men generally show more severe attrition than women. The abrasive property of food is important in determining the rate of physiological attrition.

Pathological attrition may result from:

(1) abnormal occlusion—either developmental or following extractions;
(2) bruxism and habits such as tobacco and betel chewing;
(3) abnormal tooth structure, for example amelogenesis imperfecta, dentinogenesis imperfecta.

Exposure of dentinal tubules by attrition leads to the formation of reactionary dentine on the pulpal surface which protects the tooth against pulp exposure, and to the formation of translucent zones and dead tracts. The patient may complain of hypersensitive dentine.

Abrasion

This is the pathological wearing away of tooth substance by the friction of a foreign body independent of occlusion. Different foreign bodies produce different patterns of abrasion.

1. Toothbrush abrasion is common and is seen most frequently on exposed root surfaces of teeth. It is commonly associated with toothbrushing in a horizontal rather than a vertical direction and is made worse by an abrasive dentifrice. The maxillary teeth are more involved than the mandibular teeth, and the abrasion is most pronounced in the cervical regions of the labial surfaces of incisors, canines, and premolars (Fig. 3.3). The teeth on the left side are more involved in righthanded people and vice versa. The abrasion produces wedge-shaped grooves with sharp angles and highly polished dentine surfaces (Fig. 3.4).
2. Habitual abrasion may be seen in pipe-smokers.
3. Occupational abrasion develops when objects are held between or against the teeth during work, for example hair-grips.
4. Ritual abrasion of the teeth is uncommon today and is confined mainly to Africa.

Erosion

This is the loss of tooth substance by a chemical process that does not involve known bacterial action. It may render the teeth more susceptible to attrition and abrasion.

1. Dietary erosion may follow the excessive intake of acidic beverages or the habit of sucking citrus fruits. The erosions usually involve the gingival thirds of the teeth and are most commonly seen on the labial surfaces of the maxillary incisors. Shallow, broad concavities with polished surfaces are produced. Micro-radiography shows a gradual demineralization of the surface enamel to a depth of about 100 μm.

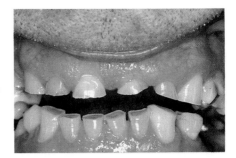

Fig. 3.2 Tooth wear with a large element of attrition.

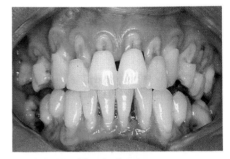

Fig. 3.3 Toothbrush abrasion.

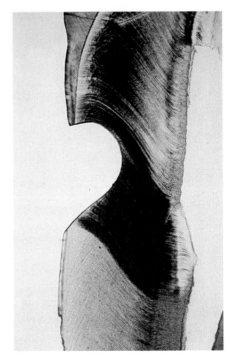

Fig. 3.4 Ground section through a toothbrush abrasion cavity showing underlying reactive changes in dentine and reactionary dentine formation.

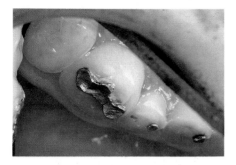

Fig. 3.5 Tooth wear with a large element of erosion.

2. Occupational erosion is seen in workers in contact with acids, for example those involved in making lead-acid batteries, and is usually due to atmospheric pollution. The incisal thirds of the incisors are usually involved because these are the surfaces most exposed to the atmosphere.

3. Regurgitation of stomach contents or persistent vomiting causes erosion in which the palatal surfaces of the maxillary teeth are primarily affected (Fig. 3.5). This may be associated with anorexia nervosa and bulimia nervosa. A similar pattern of erosion may also be seen in chronic alcoholics probably due to gastric reflux associated with chronic gastritis.

4. Idiopathic erosion. It has been reported that the saliva of patients with erosion, for which no cause can be found, has an increased citric acid content and an increased mucin content. This may interfere with the precipitation of minerals from saliva which would otherwise repair microscopic defects in the enamel.

As in attrition, reactionary dentine, translucent zones, and dead tracts develop in relation to the exposed dentinal tubules and the patients may complain of hypersensitive dentine.

Key points	**Tooth wear**
	• embraces attrition, abrasion, and erosion alone and in combinations
	• combined aetiologies modify clinical patterns of wear
	• stimulates protective responses of pulpodentinal complex

Resorption

The natural shedding of deciduous teeth follows the progressive resorption of the roots by cells resembling osteoclasts. This physiological resorption may be an inherent developmental process or it may be related to pressure from the permanent successor against the overlying bone or tooth.

Microscopic areas of superficial resorption of the roots of permanent teeth are extremely common, but resorption sufficient to be diagnosed radiologically is always pathological. Resorption is generally associated with some attempt at

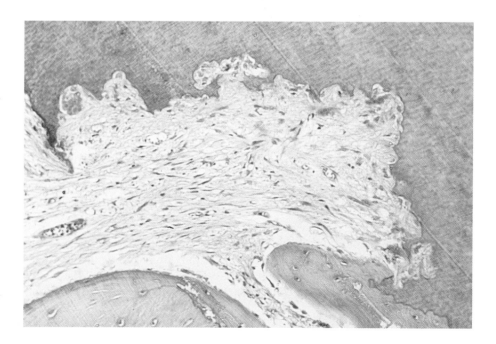

Fig. 3.6 Resorbing dentine surface with resorption lacunae and osteoclast-like cells.

repair by the apposition of cementum or bone and the tooth may occasionally become ankylosed to the surrounding bone. Resorption lacunae are present on the resorbing surface (Fig. 3.6), but as resorption is not a continuous process osteoclasts are not always present.

Pathological resorption starting on the root surface (external resorption) may be associated with:

1. periapical inflammation.
2. mechanical stimulation, for example excessive force in orthodontic treatment.
3. neoplasms or occasionally cysts involving the roots of teeth.
4. teeth that have failed to erupt.
5. transplanted or replanted teeth (Fig. 3.7).
6. idiopathic resorption. A burrowing type of resorption is most commonly seen. A localized area of the root surface is first resorbed, following which the resorption burrows deeply into and ramifies throughout the dentine producing a labyrinthine network of lacunae and channels (Fig. 3.8). The resorbed tissue is replaced by granulation tissue in which varying amounts of calcified repair tissue and/or bone may form and ankylosis may result. The circumpulpal dentine and predentine are generally spared and remain as a narrow shell as the resorption encircles the pulp (Fig. 3.9). This type of resorption frequently starts in the cervical region of the tooth. Rarely an idiopathic, generalized apical resorption may occur, the resorption slowly progressing over a number of years.

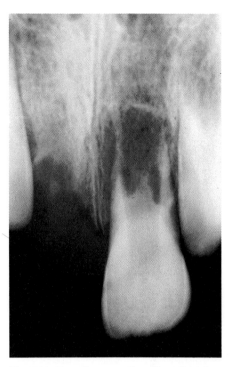

Fig. 3.7 Extensive resorption of a replanted maxillary permanent central incisor.

Pathological resorption starting from the pulpal surface (internal resorption) is usually associated with pulpitis (Fig. 3.10). An idiopathic type of internal resorption also occurs in which there is a well-defined, spherical radiolucent area in the dentine continuous with the pulp chamber or root canal (Fig. 3.11). When the coronal dentine is involved the resorption may present clinically as a pink spot

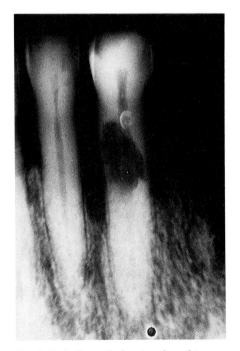

Fig. 3.8 Radiograph showing idiopathic external resorption.

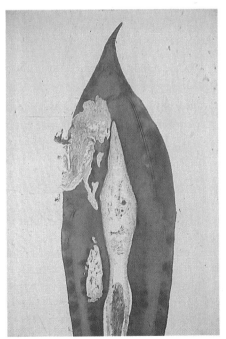

Fig. 3.9 Idiopathic resorption commencing in the cervical region and involving coronal and radicular dentine.

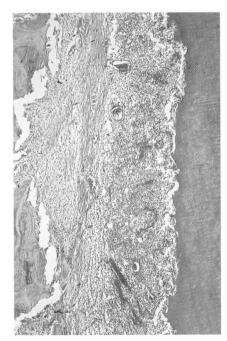

Fig. 3.10 Internal resorption of dentine associated with pulpitis.

due to the vascular pulp tissue being visible through the overlying enamel. Radiological distinction between idiopathic internal and external (burrowing) resorption may be impossible.

External resorption of the crowns of impacted teeth is uncommon. The enamel is normally separated from the surrounding connective tissues by the reduced enamel epithelium which appears to confer protection. If the epithelium is lost, in total or in part, a burrowing type of external resorption may follow. Again, calcified repair tissue resembling cementum and/or bone may be formed and ankylosis may result.

Key points	Pathological resorption of teeth

	• external
	  —secondary to other pathology
	  —idiopathic (burrowing)
	• internal
	  —secondary to pulpitis
	  —idiopathic
	• alternates with repair
	• repair may lead to ankylosis

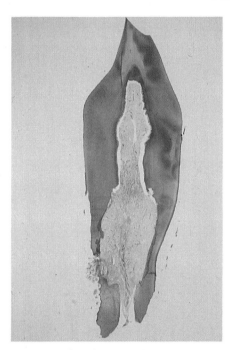

Fig. 3.11 Idiopathic internal resorption involving the root canal.

DISCOLORATION OF TEETH

Normal variation in the colour of teeth must be distinguished from pathological discoloration.

Causes of discoloration

The colour of teeth may be affected by many factors, alone or in combination. The main groups of causes are listed below and examples of each are given in Table 3.1:

(1) surface deposits (extrinsic staining);
(2) changes in the structure or thickness of the dental hard tissues;
(3) diffusion of pigments into the dental hard tissues after their formation;
(4) incorporation of pigments into the dental hard tissues during their formation.

Extrinsic staining

Green, black, brown, or occasionally red or orange deposits may develop on exposed tooth surfaces. The colour may be formed by chromogenic bacteria or be derived from foods, drinks, and topical medicaments used in dentistry, or from tobacco and other habits such as chewing betel nut. Green and black stains produced by chromogenic bacteria are common on the labial surfaces of upper anterior teeth, particularly in children (Fig. 3.12). It has been suggested that there is an inverse relationship between the amount of this black staining and caries for reasons which are not well understood.

Extrinsic staining in adults is seen particularly in individuals who do not use dentifrice abrasives or who have particular dietary or other habits. Staining due to topical medicaments may be seen following the use of chlorhexidine mouth washes and may be associated with protein denaturation of the salivary pellicle on the surface of the teeth which favours the retention of stains.

Table 3.1 Causes of discoloration of teeth

Extrinsic stains:
—substances in the diet
—habitual chewing, betel nut, tobacco
—tobacco smoking
—medicaments
—chromogenic bacteria

Changes in structure or thickness of dental tissues:
—enamel hypoplasias, fluorosis
—amelogenesis imperfecta, hypocalcified, hypomaturation, and hypoplastic types
—enamel opacities
—enamel caries
—dentinogenesis imperfecta
—dentinal dysplasia type II
—age changes in dental tissues

Diffusion of pigments into dental tissues after formation:
—extrinsic stains
—endodontic materials
—products of pulp necrosis

Pigments incorporated during formation of dental tissues:
—bile pigments
—porphyrins
—tetracycline

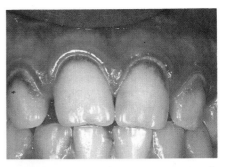

Fig. 3.12 Green extrinsic staining associated with chromogenic bacteria.

Changes in the structure or thickness of dental hard tissues

Abnormally coloured teeth are seen in amelogenesis and dentinogenesis imperfecta, other types of developmentally hypomineralized and hypoplastic enamel, and white spot enamel caries (see Chapters 1 and 2).

Diffusion of pigments into the dental hard tissues after their formation

In addition to discoloration due to intrinsic change in structure, developmentally hypomineralized enamel and carious enamel may take up stains from materials such as food and tobacco and acquire a dark brown colour. Similar stains may diffuse into dentine exposed by caries or tooth wear, and some restorative and root filling materials and their corrosion products may also stain dentine. Pulp necrosis is a common cause of a discoloured tooth. Lysis of necrotic tissue and of red blood cells from areas of haemorrhage leads to pigmented products which diffuse into the dentine. (Fig. 3.13).

Incorporation of pigments into the dental hard tissues during their formation

This occurs in congenital disorders associated with hyperbilirubinaemia, congenital porphyria, and tetracycline pigmentation.

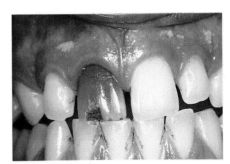

Fig. 3.13 Discoloration following pulp necrosis.

Congenital hyperbilirubinaemia (neonatal jaundice)

Mild transient jaundice is common in neonates but in severe cases, most frequently associated with haemolytic disease of the newborn (rhesus incompatibility), bile pigments may be deposited in the calcifying enamel and dentine of developing teeth, particularly along the neonatal incremental line. The pigment is largely confined to the dentine, the affected teeth being discoloured green to yellowish-brown. Enamel hypoplasia may also occur (see Table 1.2).

Congenital porphyria

This is a rare, recessive autosomal disease in which there is an inborn error of porphyrin metabolism. It is characterized by the excretion of red porphyrin pigments in the urine and circulating porphyrins in the blood which are deposited in many tissues including bone and dental hard tissues. Affected teeth show a pinkish-brown discoloration and a red fluorescence under ultraviolet light. Other prominent clinical features include bullous lesions on the exposed skin and photosensitivity.

Tetracycline pigmentation

Discoloured teeth due to tetracycline have been described since this group of drugs was introduced in 1956. Systemic administration during the period of tooth development results in the deposition of tetracycline in the dental hard tissues as well as in bone. This is subsequently seen in ground sections of affected teeth as a yellow band of pigmentation along the appropriate incremental line in the dentine, the band giving a bright yellow fluorescence under ultraviolet light (Fig. 3.14).

Tetracycline is also deposited in cementum but it is unusual to be able to demonstrate tetracycline bands in enamel. Affected teeth generally are yellowish when they erupt and become darker and browner after exposure to light. The degree of clinical discoloration of the teeth is affected by which particular tetracycline preparation has been taken, the dosage, and the age of the patient at the time of administration of the drug (Fig. 3.15). If the drug is administered when crown formation is already complete, then the tetracycline is confined to the roots and the discoloration will not be clinically discernible. Tetracyclines cross the placenta and the deciduous teeth may be affected if the drug is given any time from 29 weeks to full term. It is particularly important to avoid tetracyclines from 4 months to 6 years of age if severe clinical discoloration of the permanent dentition is to be prevented.

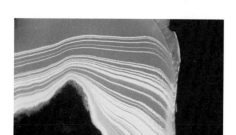

Fig. 3.14 Fluorescent bands of tetracycline along incremental lines of coronal and radicular dentine in a molar tooth.

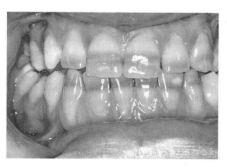

Fig. 3.15 Chronological discoloration of teeth associated with tetracycline.

TRANSPLANTATION AND REIMPLANTATION OF TEETH

Transplanted teeth may be autografts when a tooth from one individual is transplanted to a different site in the same individual, or allografts when a tooth is transplanted from one individual to another of the same species. Reimplantation is an autograft returned to its own socket and usually follows traumatic avulsion.

Autografts do not stimulate an immune response. Experimental studies in animals have shown that following transplantation or reimplantation the pulp and soft tissues attached to the root degenerate due to traumatic severence of the blood supply. In developing teeth with open apices revascularization and repair of the dental papilla may occur and dentinogenesis may resume although the dentine formed may be abnormal. However, continued root growth is rare. The reparative cells are probably derived from residual donor tissue which survives operative trauma. Reattachment of autografts may result from regeneration of the periodontal ligament, the formation of scar-like fibrous tissue running parallel to the root surface, or ankylosis. If ankylosis occurs the alveolar bone may be directly attached to the normal root surface or to resorption concavities (Fig. 3.16). It has been suggested that preservation of the vitality of the periodontal ligament is an important factor in deterring root resorption and ankylosis.

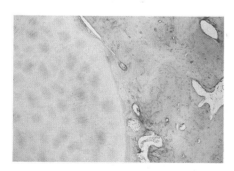

Fig. 3.16 Ankylosis of the root of a transplanted tooth.

Clinical studies of autografts in humans have concentrated mainly on root resorption which is the most commonly encountered complication. Sometimes the resorption is rapid, but more often is slowly progressive and periods of 10–15 years may elapse before resorption causes exfoliation of the transplanted tooth. Root resorption may be extensive before marked tooth mobility occurs and pain is not a feature. Following transplantation and reimplantation there is an early acute traumatic inflammatory reaction which may initiate root resorption and this may be followed by a non-specific chronic inflammatory reaction. Chronic inflammatory resorption of the root is associated with an adjacent area of radiolucency in bone. Long-term replacement resorption may also occur which does not appear to be dependent on an inflammatory reaction in that there is no associated apical radiolucency. In replacement resorption the progressive loss of root substance is matched by bony infilling. Resorption of reimplanted teeth is generally more common and extensive than that seen in transplanted teeth and is largely a function of the length of time the tooth has been out of the jaw.

Although clinically successful allogeneic transplantation of teeth has been reported in humans and laboratory animals, the results are very inconsistent and the possibility of a 'tooth bank' is remote until factors influencing acceptance or rejection are better understood. Allograft rejection involves the immunological response of the host to histocompatibility antigens present in the donor tissues; animal experiments have shown that the pulp and periodontal ligaments are immunogenic. Demineralized dentine and soluble enamel protein are also immunogenic, but whether or not this applies to intact teeth is controversial. Two general observations from experimental studies show that immunological mechanisms are of importance in tooth allograft rejection. First, allogeneic teeth transplanted to immunosuppressed animals behave like autografts and, second, teeth transplanted to animals presensitized to histocompatibility antigens (second-set reactions) show accelerated rejection. However, tooth allografts are more readily accepted than other tissues and it may be that they are of low antigenicity and that there may be fewer histocompatibility loci governing their acceptance.

ROOT FRACTURE

The outcome of an intra-alveolar fracture of a root depends on several factors, which include the presence or absence of infection, the vitality of the pulp, the position of the fragments, the degree of comminution, the location of the fracture, and the mobility of the coronal fragment. If the fracture is sterile, three main patterns of healing may occur similar to those seen in the healing of a fracture of bone:

1. The root fragments become united totally, or in part, by calcified repair tissue resembling bone and/or cementum.
2. The fractured surfaces of each fragment become rounded off and clothed by cementum but are not united by calcified tissue. Fibrous tissue continuous with the periodontal ligament fills the intervening space (analogous to fibrous healing of a bone fracture) (Fig. 3.17).
3. The fracture surfaces become rounded and clothed by cementum as above but the fragments are widely separated. Fibrous tissue continuous with the periodontal ligament covers the fractured ends of the separate fragments and the intervening space is filled by alveolar bone (analogous to non-union of a bone fracture).

The pulp chamber in either fragment may become obliterated by calcified tissue.

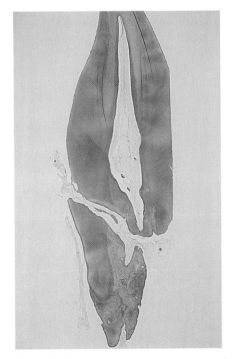

Fig. 3.17 Root fracture showing separation of the remodelled coronal and apical fracture surfaces by fibrous tissue.

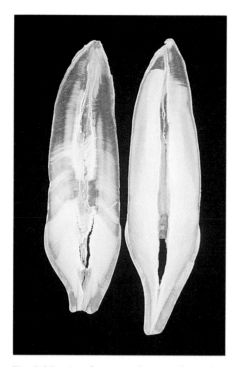

Fig. 3.18 Age changes in dentine. The tooth on the left is from an elderly patient and shows attrition, partial obliteration of the pulp chamber, and prominent sclerosis with increased translucency of radicular dentine compared with the younger tooth on the right.

AGE CHANGES IN TEETH

Age changes in teeth include changes in morphology associated with wear, especially attrition, and changes in structure and composition of the dental hard tissues. Age changes in the dental pulp are discussed in Chapter 4.

Enamel

The enamel tends to become more brittle and less permeable with age, reflecting the ionic exchange which occurs between enamel and the oral environment throughout life. Darkening of the enamel has also been described and may be due to absorption of organic material.

Dentine

The two main age-related changes in dentine are continued formation of secondary dentine resulting in reduction in size and in some cases obliteration of the pulp chamber, and dentinal sclerosis associated with the continued production of peritubular dentine. Both of these processes are also associated with caries and tooth wear. Sclerosis of radicular dentine tends to make the roots brittle and they may fracture during extraction. It is also associated with increasing translucency of the root. This starts at the apex in the peripheral dentine just beneath the cementum and extends inwards and coronally with increasing age. The length of root affected by translucency is used in forensic dentistry as one method of age estimation (Fig. 3.18).

Cementum

Cementum continues to be formed throughout life especially in the apical half of the root resulting in a gradual increase in thickness to compensate for interproximal and occlusal attrition. The amount of secondary cementum at the apex of a tooth is another factor that can be taken into account in forensic dentistry in age estimation, but it is important to distinguish between physiological apposition with age and other causes of hypercementosis.

FURTHER READING

Atkinson, M. E. (1978). Histopathological and immunological aspects of tooth transplantation. *Journal of Oral Pathology*, **7**, 43–61.

Bartlett, D. W., Evans, D. F., Anggiansah, A., and Smith, B. G. N. (1996). A study of the association between gastro-oesophageal reflux and palatal dental erosion. *British Dental Journal*, **181**, 125–32.

Berman, D. S. and Silverstone, L. M. (1975). Natal and neonatal teeth. A clinical and histological study. *British Dental Journal*, **139**, 361–4.

Johanson, G. (1971). Age determination from human teeth. Methods based on structural changes in fully developed and erupted teeth. *Odontologisk Revy*, **22** (Suppl. 21), 40–126.

Kardos, T. B. (1996). The mechanism of tooth eruption. *British Dental Journal*, **181**, 91–5.

Natiella, J. R., Armitage, J. E., and Greene, G. W. (1970). The replantation and transplantation of teeth. A review. *Oral Surgery, Oral Medicine, Oral Pathology*, **29**, 397–419.

Nunn, J., Shaw, L., and Smith A. (1996). Tooth wear—dental erosion. *British Dental Journal*, **180**, 349–52.

Scott, J. and Baum, B. J. (1990). Oral effects of Ageing. In *Oral Manifestations of Systemic Disease* (2nd edn) (ed. J. H. Jones and D. K. Mason), pp. 311–38. W. B. Saunders, London.

Tsukiboshi, M. (1993). Autogenous tooth transplantation: a re-evaluation. *International Journal of Periodontics and Restorative Dentistry*, **13**, 120–49.

Viscardi, D. M., Romberg, E., and Abrams, R. G. (1994). Delayed primary tooth eruption in premature infants: relationship to neonatal factors. *Pediatric Dentistry*, **16**, 23–8.

Winter, G. B. Anomalies of tooth formation and eruption. In *Paediatric dentistry* (ed. R. R. Welbury), pp. 255–280. Oxford University Press, Oxford.

4 Disorders of the dental pulp

4   Disorders of the dental pulp

Inflammation is the single most important disease process affecting the dental pulp and accounts for virtually all pulpal disease of any clinical significance.

PULPITIS

Pulpitis has been classified in the past on either a clinical or pathological basis into a number of different types, such as acute or chronic, partial or total, open or closed, exudative or suppurative. These divisions are somewhat artificial and confusing since inflammation of the pulp presents a continuous spectrum of change and it is seldom possible on clinical or pathological grounds to ascribe an individual case into such a rigid compartmentalization.

Clinical features

Pulpitis presents clinically as pain which the patient may have difficulty in localizing to a particular tooth, the pain often radiating to the adjacent jaw and on some occasions into the face, the ear, or the neck. The pain may be continuous for several days or may occur intermittently over a longer period. A severe throbbing pain, at times lancinating in type, precipitated by hot or cold stimuli or a recumbent position, and commonly keeping the patient awake, is often described clinically as acute pulpitis. The pain generally lasts for about 10–15 minutes but may be more or less continuous. Spontaneous attacks of dull aching pain, lasting for an hour or two, are often described clinically as chronic pulpitis. However, investigations have shown that there is little or no correlation between the clinical features and the type or extent of pulp inflammation as shown by histological examination. An absence of symptoms is not even evidence of a normal pulp as pulp death following pulpitis may occur with no previous history of pain. The critical decision which has to be made clinically is whether pulpitis is reversible or irreversible, as this will determine the management of the affected tooth. This decision is based on factors such as the age of the patient, the size of the carious lesion, the presence or absence of symptoms, pulp vitality tests, radiographic evidence, and direct observation during operative procedures. If pulpitis pain is severe and of short duration, or mild and of long duration, then the terms acute and chronic pupitis, respectively, may be justifiable as clinical diagnoses, but it must be realized that they do not imply any specific histological changes in the pulp.

Aetiology

Dental caries is the commonest cause of pulpitis, but it is also caused by many other irritants reaching the pulp which can be grouped under the following headings.

Microbial

Bacteria generally reach the pulp as a result of dental caries. Inflammation of the pulp starts before the leading organisms in the carious dentine reach the pulp, showing that the initial pulp reactions follow the diffusion of soluble irritants through the dentine. Pulpitis is not usually seen histologically until the leading organisms in the carious dentine are within about 1 mm of the pulp in permanent teeth or twice this distance in deciduous teeth.

Bacteria can also reach the pulp if it is exposed by attrition, abrasion, or traumatic restorative procedures. Bacteria do not normally pass down dentinal tubules which have been exposed during cavity preparation, but they may do so to a limited extent in relation to impression-taking during the preparation of jacket crowns, providing that the preparation has been recently prepared and the dentinal tubules are patent. The importance of marginal leakage of restorations in providing a route for bacterial infection of the pulp has been shown in experiments using animals. A cracked or fractured tooth may also provide a pathway for bacteria to reach the pulp, as may the absent or defective enamel and dentine lining an invaginated odontome. Pulpitis may occasionally follow chronic periodontal disease, the bacteria passing along accessory canals from the exposed root surface to the pulp.

Key point	**Pulpitis** • dental caries is the commonest cause

It is theoretically possible for blood-borne bacteria to lodge within the pulp (anachoretic pulpitis), but experiments suggest that this occurs only if the pulp is already inflamed or damaged.

The enormous importance of bacterial infection in the aetiology of pulpitis has been shown by experiments in germ-free rats in which surgical pulp exposures were not followed by progressive pulpitis even in the presence of gross food impaction.

Chemical

Irritant substances may be directly applied to an exposed pulp, or may diffuse through the dentine after the insertion of a restorative material. The chemical properties of restorative materials play a major role in determining pulpal tissue compatibility. In many instances the pulp may respond by forming reactionary dentine rather than the irritation leading to pulpitis, and the dentinal tubules may become sclerosed.

Thermal

Frictional heat evolved during cavity preparation is a significant pulp irritant and the importance of adequate coolants cannot be overemphasized. Large metallic restorations, particularly where there is inadequate lining material, may also transmit thermal changes to the pulp.

Barotrauma (aerodontalgia)

Dental pain has been described by air crew flying at high altitudes in unpressurized aircraft, and in divers subjected to too rapid decompression following deep-sea diving. This pain has been attributed to the formation of nitrogen bubbles in the pulp tissues or vessels, similar to the decompression syndrome elsewhere in the body. However, gas bubbles are seldom found in decompressed organs and the possibility of fat emboli from altered lipoproteins and platelet thrombi around the fat is suggested by some investigators. Aerodontalgia is really a marker of inadequate pulp protection from the atmosphere and this usually means caries. It is not a direct cause of pulpitis, rather an exacerbating factor.

Histopathology

The inflammatory process in the pulp is basically the same as elsewhere in the body, but the process may be modified by various factors, including the nature and severity of the insult, the efficiency of the host defence mechanisms, and its special anatomical location (Fig. 4.1). The pulp is almost totally surrounded by dentine which limits the ability of the pulp to tolerate oedema. Thus, the pressure rise in the pulp associated with an inflammatory exudate may cause local collapse of the venous part of the microcirculation. This leads to local tissue hypoxia and anoxia, which in turn may lead to localized necrosis. Chemical mediators released from the necrotic tissue lead to further inflammation and oedema, and total necrosis of the pulp may follow the continued spread of local inflammation. Reactionary dentine may continue to form after the onset of pulpitis, providing the pulp has not been irreversibly damaged, and may in time protect the pulp from further injury by increasing the thickness of calcified tissue between the pulp and the irritant in the dentine.

Pulpitis caused by caries always starts as a localized area of inflammation directly related to the carious dentine, the inflammation eventually extending throughout the pulp if the caries is not treated. Carious lesions differ with respect to bacteriology, rates of progression, and pulpodentinal reactions, and so the rate of progression of the inflammation in the pulp will vary from individual to individual and from tooth to tooth. In multi-rooted teeth the inflammation may progress to the apex of one root even before the whole of the pulp chamber is involved.

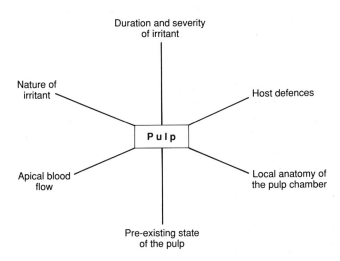

Fig. 4.1 Factors influencing the outcome of inflammation in the dental pulp.

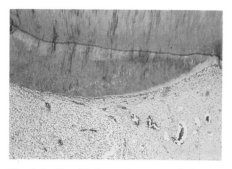

Fig. 4.2 Vasodilation and acute exudative changes in the dental pulp associated with bacterial invasion of reactionary dentine (purple-streaked tubules).

The severity of the irritation to the pulp from dental caries increases as the caries advances pulpwards. The relatively low level of irritation initially leads to an inflammatory response in which there is a diffuse infiltration beneath the odontoblasts by small numbers of lymphocytes, plasma cells, and macrophages. Granulation tissue formation may be seen around the periphery of the area. Acute exudative changes are not prominent at this stage, but as the bacteria in the carious dentine reach the pulp, the vessels in the area become dilated and congested (Fig. 4.2). As the inflammatory exudate develops the local microcirculation may be compromised leading to local death of tissue as previously described. This predisposes to suppuration due to the progressive accumulation of neutrophil leucocytes which release their lysosomal enzymes when they die. Suppuration may be local, forming a pulp abscess (Figs 4.3, 4.4), or may spread diffusely through the pulp depending on the interplay of the variables outlined in Fig. 4.1. Immune reactions in the inflamed tissue may also contribute to the tissue damage.

A pulp abscess may become surrounded by proliferating granulation tissue forming a so-called pyogenic membrane, which in some cases becomes increasingly fibrous and the pus becomes walled off with temporary cessation in the spread of suppuration (Fig. 4.4). In other cases the abscess may continue to expand due to continued tissue damage and massive emigration of neutrophils into the area of suppuration. As bacteria enter the inflamed tissue from the carious dentine most are destroyed by the neutrophil leucocytes and other host defence mechanisms, large numbers of bacteria are not generally seen in the pulp until the late stages of total irreversible pulpitis. If there is cavitation of the overlying carious dentine then the pus may drain into the mouth.

Although the rate of progression of pulpal inflammation is very variable the end result of an untreated pulpitis is total pulp necrosis except in the case of pulp polyp formation (see below).

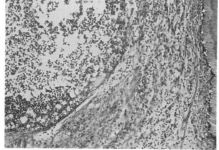

Fig. 4.3 Suppurative inflammation in the dental pulp progressing to abscess formation (top left of field).

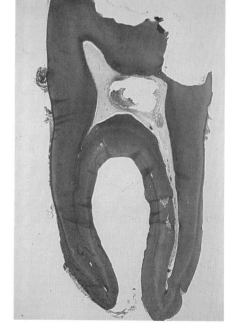

Fig. 4.4 Localized pulpitis with localized pulp abscess.

Pulpitis resulting from irritants other than caries shows essentially similar histological changes, except that in some instances the initial response is an acute exudative inflammation rather than a mononuclear inflammatory cell infiltration as the irritation to the pulp may be much more severe than that provided by caries.

Pulpitis   **Key points**

- histopathological features and rate of progression variable
- outcome depends on interplay of nature and severity of irritant, host defences, and modifying factors
- much of the tissue damage may be the result of the inflammatory reaction

---

Pulp polyp

In deciduous or recently erupted permanent teeth, most often deciduous molars and first permanent molars, with wide-open carious cavities and a good apical blood supply, pulpitis may be associated with a hyperplastic granulation tissue response. The granulation tissue grows out of the boundary of the pulp chamber to form a pulp polyp and such lesions can justifiably be described as chronic hyperplastic pulpitis (Fig. 4.5). The polyp may become epithelialized by the spontaneous grafting of oral epithelial cells present in the saliva (Fig. 4.6). The origin of these epithelial cells is unknown. Most of the desquamated cells in saliva are degenerate superficial squames, incapable of further division. For the polyp to become epithelialized the grafted cells must be capable of division and subsequent differentiation into stratified squamous epithelium. Such cells must come from the region of the basal cell layer and might be released from trauma to the oral mucosa or from the gingival sulcus. Clinically, an ulcerated pulp polyp presents as a dark red, yellow-flecked (because of the fibrinous exudate) fleshy mass protruding from the pulp chamber, which bleeds readily on probing. In contrast, an epithelialized polyp is firmer, pinkish-white in colour, and does not bleed readily. They are both usually devoid of sensation on gentle probing.

Effects of cavity preparation and restorative materials

The speed of instrument rotation, heat, pressure, and coolants may all irritate the pulp tissue and cause pulpitis, particularly with increasing cavity depths. However, the main threat to the pulp is from frictional heat generated during the cutting process. Changes in the dental pulp in association with hard tissue ablation using lasers with water spray have been described as being similar to those associated with a high-speed handpiece with water spray.

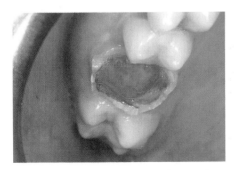

Fig. 4.5 Chronic hyperplastic pulpitis (pulp polyp).

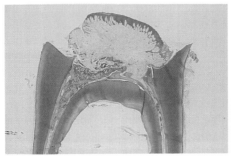

Fig. 4.6 Epithelialized pulp polyp.

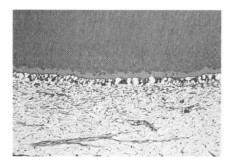

Fig. 4.7   Wheat-sheaving of odontoblasts.

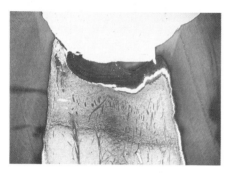

Fig. 4.8   Pulpotomy healing showing richly vascular zone of organization beneath the pulp-capping agent.

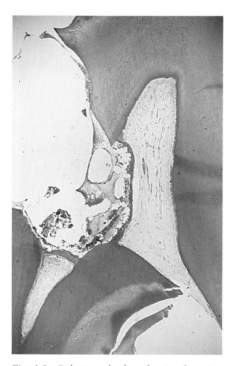

Fig. 4.9   Pulpotomy healing showing formation of calcified barriers bridging the pulpotomy wound.

Additional histological changes often described in pulp reactions to restorative techniques and materials are aspiration or displacement of odontoblasts or their nuclei into the dentinal tubules and a reduction in the number of odontoblasts. Both these changes may be related to inflammatory oedema increasing local tissue pressure, the fluid displacing odontoblasts into dentinal tubules or collecting as vacuoles and compressing groups of odontoblasts together (so-called wheat-sheaving of odontoblasts) (Fig. 4.7). Odontoblast aspiration has also been ascribed to desiccation of dentine during cavity preparation. It must be realized that early pulpitis following dentine caries may be further complicated by the effects of restorative techniques and materials, the response of the pulp being due to the combined effects of the different irritants.

Dental materials vary greatly in their ability to irritate the pulp, the dentine thickness between the pulp and the material often being critical in determining their effect. The nature of the dentine remaining may also affect the response, sclerosed dentine being less permeable than normal primary tubular dentine. A material which has little or no irritant effect when placed at the base of a cavity in the dentine may have a profound effect if it is directly applied to exposed pulp tissue, as in pulp capping.

HEALING OF PULP

Dentine trauma not directly involving the pulp may be followed by the displacement or aspiration of odontoblasts into related dentinal tubules. These aspirated cells may be replaced by new odontoblasts most likely derived from undifferentiated mesenchymal cells in the pulp.

Animal experiments have shown that it is possible for pulpitis to heal if the irritating agents are removed from the dentine. Localized pulp inflammation may resolve even when there is continuing dentinal caries, presumably due to a reduction in permeability of the dentine exposed to the bacterial products as a result of sclerosis and the formation of reactionary dentine.

In a proportion of cases where the pulp is exposed during cavity preparation it is possible to maintain pulp vitality by pulp-capping. Ideally, the capping agent should be non-irritant, should stimulate the formation of a calcific barrier, and have an antibacterial action as most pulp exposures are contaminated by saliva. Various preparations of calcium hydroxide are widely used as pulp-capping agents. Their application to an exposed pulp is followed rapidly by the formation of a necrotic zone next to the calcium hydroxide, and this is separated from the underlying normal tissue by a deeply basophilic zone probably consisting of calcium proteinates. Within 2 weeks (Fig. 4.8) a layer of coarse fibrous tissue develops next to the basophilic zone and beneath this a layer of odontoblast-like cells appears. After a further 2 weeks a calcified barrier with the characteristics of dentine starts to develop beneath the fibrous layer (Fig. 4.9). This calcified barrier or dentine bridge is associated with a palisade of odontoblast cells, probably derived from undifferentiated mesenchymal cells in the pulp. Similar healing occurs under a successful pulpotomy covered with calcium hydroxide.

The mechanism of action of calcium hydroxide in stimulating the formation of a dentine bridge is not understood. It has been shown that the calcium ions in the calcium hydroxide are not incorporated in the adjacent dentine bridge and that calcium hydroxide only induces reparative dentine when it contacts the pulp tissue; it has no such effect when placed at the base of a restoration cavity separated from the pulp by dentine. However, many factors must influence the pulp's response to injury, since other relatively non-irritant lining materials do not apparently promote the formation of a dentine bridge.

PULP CALCIFICATION

Pulp stones (or denticles) are calcified bodies with an organic matrix and occur most frequently in the coronal pulp. True pulp stones contain tubules (albeit scanty and irregular), and may have an outer layer of predentine and adjacent odontoblasts. False pulp stones (Fig. 4.10) are composed of concentric layers of calcified material with no tubular structure. According to their location in the pulp, stones may be described as free, adherent, or interstitial when they have become surrounded by reactionary or secondary dentine. Pulp stones increase in number and size with age and are apparently more numerous after operative procedures on the tooth. When large they may be recognized on radiographs. They do not cause symptoms, although neuralgic pain has sometimes been attributed to their presence.

Dystrophic calcifications in the pulp consist of granules of amorphous calcific material which may be scattered along collagen fibres or aggregated into larger masses. They are most commonly found in the root canals (Fig. 4.11). Dystrophic calcifications and pulp stones may obstruct endodontic therapy.

Pulp obliteration may follow traumatic injury to the apical blood vessels which is not sufficient to cause pulp necrosis. Large quantities of irregular dentine form in the pulp chamber and root canals which become obliterated. Pulp obliteration is also seen in dentinogenesis imperfect and dentinal dysplasia.

PULP NECROSIS

Pulp necrosis may follow either pulpitis or a traumatic injury to the apical blood vessels cutting off the blood supply to the pulp. A coagulative type of necrosis is seen after ischaemia, but if the necrosis follows pulpitis then breakdown of inflammatory cells may lead to a liquefactive type of necrosis which may become infected by putrefactive bacteria from caries. This gangrenous necrosis of the pulp is usually associated with a foul odour when such infected pulps are opened for endodontic treatment.

Pulp necrosis has also been described in patients with sickle cell anaemia, following blockage of the pulp microcirculation by sickled erythrocytes.

AGE CHANGES IN THE PULP

The volume of the pulp gradually decreases with age due to the continued production of secondary dentine. Decreased vascularity, reduction in cellularity, and increase in collagen fibre content have also been reported, and these changes may impair the response of the tissue to injury and its healing potential.

It is generally accepted that the prevalence of pulp stones and diffuse calcification increases with age but the evidence for this is inconclusive.

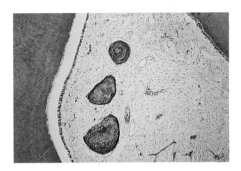

Fig. 4.10 Lamellated (false) pulp stones.

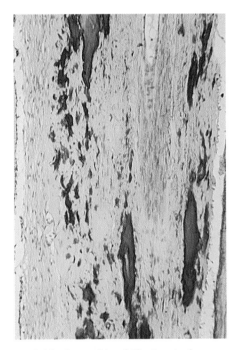

Fig. 4.11 Dystrophic calcifications in the radicular pulp.

FURTHER READING

Baume, L. J. (1970). Dental pulp conditions in relation to carious lesions. *International Dental Journal*, **20**, 309–37.

Bergenholtz, G. (1981). Inflammatory response of the dental pulp to bacterial irritation. *Journal of Endodontics*, **7**, 100–4.

Bernick, S. and Nedelman, C. (1975). Effect of ageing on the human pulp. *Journal of Endodontics*, **1**, 88–94.

Langeland, K. (1981). Management of the inflamed pulp associated with the deep carious lesion. *Journal of Endodontics*, **7**, 169–81.

Pulver, W. H., Taubman, M. A., and Smith, D. J. (1977). Immune components of normal and inflamed human dental pulp. *Archives of Oral Biology*, **22**, 103–11.

Sheehy, E. C. and Roberts, G. J. (1997). Use of calcium hydroxide for apical barrier formation and healing in non-vital immature permanent teeth: a review. *British Dental Journal*, **183**, 241–6.

Shovelton, D. S. (1970). Studies of dentine and pulp in deep caries. *International Dental Journal*, **20**, 283–96.

Torneck, C. D. (1981). A report of studies into changes in the fine structure of the dental pulp in human caries pulpitis. *Journal of Endodontics*, **7**, 8–16.

Trowbridge, H. O. (1981). Pathogenesis of pulpitis resulting from dental caries. *Journal of Endodontics*, **7**, 52–60.

5 Periapical periodontitis

5 Periapical periodontitis

Inflammation in the periapical part of the periodontal ligament is similar to that occurring elsewhere in the body, but, because of the confined space within which the process develops, a particular feature of inflammation in this site is that the adjacent bone, and occasionally the root apex, may resorb. However, the periapical vascular network has a rich collateral circulation, greatly enhancing the ability of the tissue to heal if the cause of the inflammation is removed. This potential for complete periapical healing, providing the source of irritation is removed, is the basis of endodontic treatment. In this respect periapical periodontitis differs markedly from pulpitis where the potential for healing is very limited. The symptoms also differ from pulpits in that they are generally well located by the patient to a particular tooth, stimulation of the proprioceptive nerve endings in the periodontal ligament facilitating this accurate location.

Periapical inflammation   **Key points**

Whether the response to irritation in the periodontal ligament is principally an acute or chronic inflammation depends on factors such as the number and virulence of any microorganisms involved, the type and severity of any mechanical or chemical irritant, and the resistance of the patient. While it is convenient to describe acute and chronic periapical periodontitis as separate conditions, it must be realized that the tissue reaction to irritation is a dynamic response, often vacillating with time between acute and chronic inflammation. The possible changes that may occur around the apex of a non-vital tooth and their inter-relationships are illustrated in Fig. 5.1. The sequelae are determined by the balance between the nature, severity, and duration of the irritant and the integrity of the defence mechanisms of the patient.

AETIOLOGY

The main causes of periapical periodontitis are detailed below.

Pulpitis and pulp necrosis

If pulpitis is untreated bacteria, bacterial toxins, or the products of inflammation will in time extend down the root canal and through the apical foramina to

Fig. 5.1 Changes that may occur around the apex of a non-vital tooth.

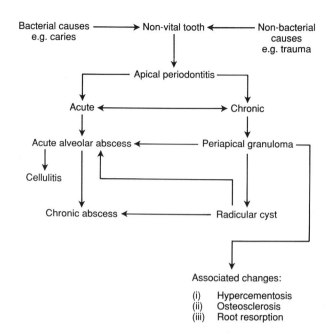

cause periodontitis. When pulp necrosis follows other causes, for example a blow to the tooth damaging the apical vessels, chemical substances released from the necrotic tissue may diffuse through the apex and also cause periodontitis. However, when apical periodontitis is accompanied by bone resorption, bacteria are invariably present in the root canal system.

Trauma

Occlusal trauma, either from a high restoration or less frequently associated with bruxism, may result in periapical periodontitis. Undue pressure during orthodontic treatment, a direct blow on a tooth insufficient to cause pulp necrosis, and biting unexpectedly on a hard body in food may all cause minor damage to the periodontal ligament and localized inflammation.

Endodontic treatment

Mechanical instrumentation through the root apex during endodontic treatment, as well as chemical irritation from root-filling materials, may result in inflammation in the periapical periodontium. Instrumentation of an infected root canal may be followed by periapical inflammation, due to bacterial proliferation in the root canal or to bacteria being inadvertently forced into the periapical tissues. Clinically, this may be mistaken for periodontitis caused by mechanical or chemical irritation and may lead to incorrect treatment.

Key points	**Mnemonic for differential diagnosis of pain of pulpal and periapical origin—LOCATE**
	• Location
	• Other symptoms
	• Character
	• Associations
	• Timing
	• Evaluation of other investigations, e.g. pulp vitality tests

ACUTE PERIAPICAL PERIODONTITIS

This is characterized by vascular dilatation, an exudate of neutrophil leucocytes, and oedema in the periodontal ligament situated in the confined space between the root apex and the alveolar bone. Pain is elicited when external pressure is applied to the tooth because the pressure is transmitted through the fluid exudate to the sensory nerve endings. Even light touch may be sufficient to induce pain. As the fluid is not compressible, the tooth feels elevated in its socket. Hot or cold stimulation of the tooth does not cause pain, as it would in pulpitis. The radiographic appearances are often normal as there is generally insufficient time for bone resorption to occur between the time of injury to the periodontal ligament and the onset of symptoms. If radiological changes are present, they consist of slight widening of the periodontal ligament and the lamina dura around the apex may be less well defined than normal.

The inflammation may be transient if it is due to acute trauma rather than infection and the condition soon resolves. If the irritant persists the inflammation becomes chronic and may be associated with resorption of the surrounding bone. Suppuration may occur if there is severe irritation and tissue necrosis associated with bacterial infection and the continued and massive exudation of neutrophil leucocytes leading to abscess formation. Such an abscess is called an acute periapical or alveolar abscess and, although such abscesses may develop directly from acute apical periodontitis (Fig. 5.1), most arise because of acute exacerbation in an area of chronic inflammation (Fig. 5.2).

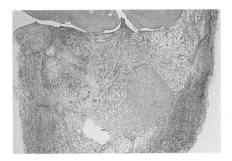

Fig. 5.2 Periapical granuloma with central zone of suppurative inflammation.

CHRONIC PERIAPICAL PERIODONTITIS (PERIAPICAL GRANULOMA)

This is characterized by an inflammatory cell infiltrate rich in lymphocytes, plasma cells, and macrophages, and the production of granulation tissue. Persistence of the inflammation is associated with resorption of the adjacent bone which is replaced by this chronically inflamed granulation tissue to form a periapical granuloma. Deposits of cholesterol and haemosiderin are often present and both are probably derived from the breakdown of extravasated red blood cells. Cholesterol crystals in the granulation tissue are represented in routine histological sections as empty needle-like spaces or clefts, the crystals having dissolved out in the reagents used in section preparation. Multinucleate foreign-body giant cells are grouped around the cholesterol clefts (Fig. 5.3). Foci of lipid-laden macrophages—foam cells—may also be seen (Fig. 5.4). Epithelial cell rests of Malassez frequently become incorporated within the granulation tissue and the chronic inflammatory milieu may, in some way, stimulate their proliferation (Fig. 5.5). The proliferated squamous epithelium forms anastomosing cords, often arranged in loops or arcades, throughout the granulation tissue (Fig. 5.6).

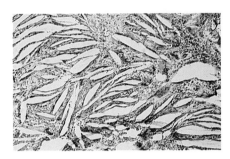

Fig. 5.3 Cholesterol clefts with associated foreign-body giant cells.

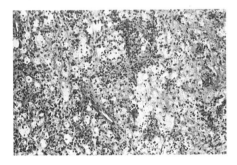

Fig. 5.4 Large, pale lipid-laden macrophages (foam cells) against a background of lymphocytes.

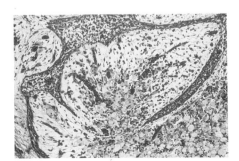

Fig. 5.5

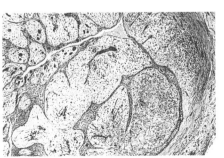

Fig. 5.6

Fig. 5.5 Periapical granuloma containing proliferating strands of squamous epithelium.

Fig. 5.6 Proliferating arcades of squamous epithelium within a periapical granuloma.

Neutrophil leucocytes in varying stages of degeneration are often seen infiltrating the oedematous intercellular spaces of the epithelium.

Collagen fibres may become condensed around the periphery of the lesion, separating the granulation tissue from the surrounding bone. Occasional osteoclasts may be present in areas where bone resorption is in progress.

Although bacteria can seldom be demonstrated histologically in a peripical granuloma, they can be cultured from many of the lesions. Mixed infections are the rule, the organisms present being those generally found in the mouth. Obligate anaerobes such as *Prevotella* species predominate with smaller numbers of facultative anaerobes such as *Streptococcus milleri* and *Streptococcus sanguis*. The importance of the root canal as a continued source of infection in a periapical granuloma is shown by the fact that most periapical lesions heal once the canal is sealed by satisfactory endodontic treatment

Periapical granulomas tend to be asymptomatic, but may be associated with occasional tenderness of the tooth to palpation and percussion. percussion may produce a dull note because of the lack of resonance caused by the granulation tissue around the apex. Radiological examination at first shows a widening of the periodonal ligament space around the apex and later a definite periapical radiolucency may develop. In some instances this radiolucency is well circumscribed and clearly demarcated from the surrounding bone by a corticated margin, while in others the border is poorly defined (Fig. 5.7). These appearances are related to differences in cellular activity around the margins of the lesion. Where there is active bone resorption and expansion of the lesion the margin is ill-defined. Where the lesion is static and a balance is established between the level of irritation and the host defences, the chronic inflammatory stimulus may lead to bone apposition and the formation of a zone of sclerosis around the lesion (see osteosclerosis (point 5) below). Histological evidence of external resorption of the apical cementum and dentine is frequent and is occasionally sufficient to be detected radiographically.

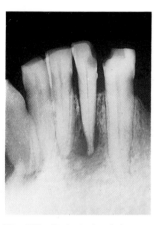

Fig. 5.7 Periapical radiolucency and apical resorption associated with a periapical granuloma.

Key points	**Periapical granuloma**
	• may be symptomless
	• chronically inflamed granulation tissue
	• obligate anaerobes predominate
	• bone resorption
	• proliferation of rests of Malassez

Sequelae (see Fig. 5.1)

1. The granuloma may continue to enlarge and be associated with continued resorption of the bone and/or the root apex, the whole process being symptomless.

2. Although a granuloma is principally a chronic inflammatory lesion, acute exacerbations are common and the patient may present with symptoms of acute periapical periodontitis.

3. Suppuration may occur in the granuloma to form an acute periapical (alveolar) abscess. This may be evidenced clinically by the rapid onset of pain, redness, and swelling of the adjacent soft tissues, tenderness of the affected tooth to percussion and palpation, and tooth mobility. A chronic periapical abscess may also develop, this being a well-circumscribed area of suppuration that shows little tendency to enlarge or to spread and which presents few, if any, clinical features.

4. Proliferation of the epithelial cell rests of Malassez associated with the inflammation may lead to the development of an inflammatory radicular cyst.

5. Low-grade irritation to the apical tissues may result in bone apposition (osteosclerosis) rather than resorption, histologically a mild chronic inflammatory infiltrate being seen in the rather scanty, fibrous marrow. The process is clinically asymptomatic and shows as an opaque area of bone on radiographs. On occasions, the opacity is well-circumscribed while on others it shows no clear line of demarcation from the normal surrounding bone.

6. Low-grade irritation to the apical tissues may also result in the apposition of cementum on the adjacent root surface to produce hypercementosis.

ACUTE PERIAPICAL ABSCESS AND SPREAD OF INFLAMMATION

Aetiology and microbiology

An acute periapical abscess may develop either directly from acute periapical periodontitis or more usually from a chronic periapical granuloma. It is generally the result of a mixed bacterial infection, culture of pus yielding a wide range of different species. Strict anaerobes (for example *Prevotella* and *Porphyromonas* species and anaerobic streptococci) are usually the predominant organisms, but facultative anaerobes are also found. The relative pathogenicities of the bacteria isolated are not known and all isolates have to be regarded as of importance. Synergistic interactions between organisms will increase the severity of the infection.

Routes of spread

If the cause of the abscess is not removed, for example by extraction of the tooth, endodontic treatment, or antibiotic therapy, suppuration will continue and the abscess continues to enlarge. In some cases, a balance may eventually be established between the irritant and the host defences and the abscess becomes chronic and remains localized. More frequently, the increase in hydrostatic pressure within the abscess associated with progressive suppuration causes the pus to track in one of a number of directions (Fig. 5.8). It may drain through the root canal if this is open to the mouth or occasionaly it may track through he periodontal ligament to discharge into the gingival sulcus. More commonly, the pus tends to track through the cancellous bone and eventually perforates the cortex. Most abscesses point buccally (Fig. 5.9) as the root apices lie closer to the buccal than to the lingual or palatal cortical plates. However, abscesses related to the apices of the maxillary teeth, particularly lateral incisors and the palatal roots of the molars and premolars, often track towards and point on the palate. Once the cortical plate is perforated the pus strips up the periosteum and may result in the formation of a subperiosteal abscess. More frequently,it penetrates the periosteum after which it may track in various directions. Although the apices of the roots of the mandibular second and third molars lie close to the lingual cortical plate, the bone in this area is very dense and is rarely penetrated.

After the pus has perforated the cortical plate its subsequent routes of spread are dictated largely by anatomical factors. The relationship of the cortical perforation (which itself is related to the position of the apex of the abscessed root) to the origins of muscles, for example buccinator and mylohyoid, and the strength of the overlying periosteum are important factors.

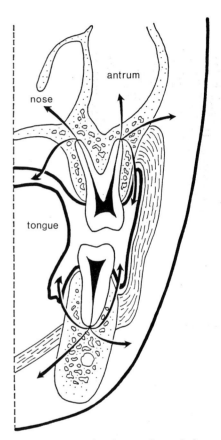

Fig. 5.8 Potential pathways of spread of pus from a periapical abscess.

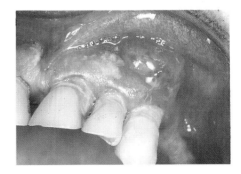

Fig. 5.9 Abscess related to maxillary canine pointing buccally.

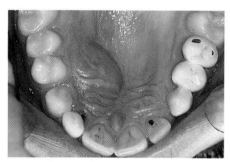

Fig. 5.10   Sinus opening related to abscess associated with maxillary central incisor.

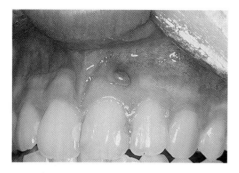

Fig. 5.11   Palatal abscess related to lateral incisor.

Possible outcomes are described below.

1. The pus may discharge directly into the oral cavity through a sinus following local penetration of the overlying periosteum and mucosa. This may occur with little or no pain and only a small swelling may develop on the oral mucosa before the pus breaks through. On other occasions the pus may accumulate beneath the mucosa and the patient may complain of a 'gumboil' before a sinus develops (see Fig. 5.9). A nodule of granulation tissue often forms in response to the irritation by pus and marks the opening of the sinus (Fig. 5.10).

2. The dense palatal mucoperiosteum is resistant to penetration by pus. Pus tracking palatally may spread under the mucoperiosteum posteriorly to the junction of the hard and soft palate and present as a palatal abscess (Fig. 5.11).

3. Abscesses in the molar region of either jaw may penetrate the buccal cortical plate above (in the maxilla) or below (in the mandible) the attachments of the buccinator muscle. In such cases acute inflammatory oedema and suppuration spread into the soft tissues of the face or neck. This may present as a cellulitis (Fig. 5.12) (see later) or less frequently as a localized soft-tissue abscess (Fig. 5.13) depending on the nature of the infection. Such an abscess may track towards the overlying skin to discharge through a sinus on the skin surface. The abscess may then become chronic with the sinus discharging pus periodically, associated with increasing fibrosis, scarring and disfigurement (Fig. 5.14).

4. Abscesses related to anterior maxillary teeth may perforate the labial bone above the attachment of the levator anguli oris muscle. The infection may then pass medially and upwards towards the inner canthus of the eye, obliterating the nasolabial fold, and into the loose connective tissue of the lower eyelid. Alternatively, the infection may pass into the upper lip (Fig. 5.15).

5. Abscesses developing at the root apices of maxillary molars and premolars are very close to the floor of the maxillary sinus and consequently may dis-

Fig. 5.12   Cellulitis associated with spread of inflammation from abscess related to a maxillary molar.

Fig. 5.13   Localized extraoral spread of abscess related to a mandibular molar.

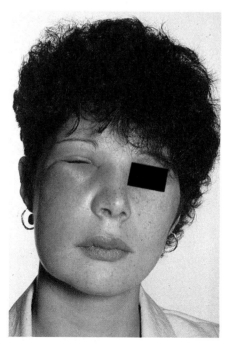

Fig. 5.12

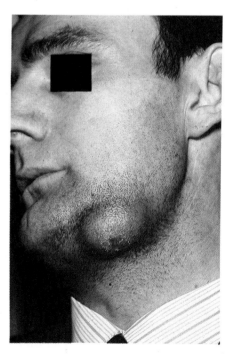

Fig. 5.13

charge into the sinus. Periapical inflammation may account for up to 20 per cent of all cases of sinusitis.

6. An abscess related to a mandibular premolar or molar tooth may perforate the lingual plate of the mandible below the attachment of the mylohyoid muscle to involve the submandibular space. This causes a marked swelling at the lower border of the mandible spreading towards the neck. The submandibular space has communications with the sublingual and lateral pharyngeal spaces, into which the infection may subsequently spread. An abscess in the submandibular region is separated from the skin by the deep fascia of the neck and so tends to track anteroposteriorly under the skin surface.

7. Pus from an abscess associated with a mandibular incisor or canine may track labially and perforate the bone below the insertion of the mentalis muscle and pass downwards to present as a subcutaneous abscess, most often in the midline between the points of attachment of the two mentalis muscles.

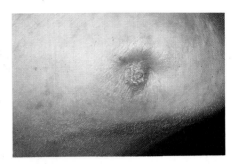

Fig. 5.14 Scarring associated with chronic extraoral sinus.

Cellulitis

Cellulitis is a rapidly spreading inflammation of the soft tissues particularly associated with streptococcal infections. It is not well-localized, in contrast to a circumscribed abscess, and the rapid spread is most likely related to release of large amounts of streptokinase and hyaluronidase which are produced by most strains of streptococci. Clinically, there is diffuse, tense, painful swelling of the involved soft tissues (see Figs 5.12, 5.15) usually associated with malaise and an elevated temperature. Much of the swelling is due to inflammatory oedema; suppuration and abscess formation occur later if treatment is neglected or delayed. Cellulitis associated with maxillary teeth initially involves the upper half of the face. Extension towards the eye is a potentially serious complication because of the risk of cavernous sinus thrombosis as a result of infection involving veins at the inner canthus of the eye which communicate with the cavernous sinus. Cellulitis associated with mandibular teeth initially involves the lower half of the face; extension into the submandibular and cervical tissues may cause respiratory embarrassment. Cellulitis spreading into the deeper surgical spaces usually presents clinically as pain and trismus rather than facial swelling.

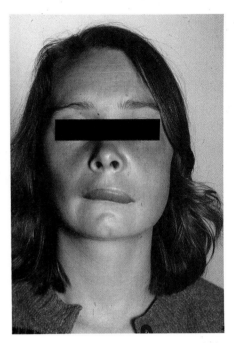

Fig. 5.15 Cellulitis associated with spread of inflammation from abscess related to an anterior maxillary tooth.

Ludwig's angina

Ludwig's angina is severe cellulitis involving the submandibular, sublingual, and submental spaces, usually as a result of initial involvement of the submandibular space. Since the advent of antibiotics it is now rare. The diffuse cellulitis produces a board-like swelling of the floor of the mouth, the tongue being elevated and displaced posteriorly. As a result there is difficulty in eating, swallowing, and breathing. The latter is exacerbated as infection tracks backwards to involve the pharynx and larynx. Oedema of the glottis may occur with risk of death by suffocation.

FURTHER READING

Bergenholtz, G., Lekholm, U., Liljenberg, B., and Lindhe, J. (1983). Morphometric analysis of chronic inflammatory periapical lesions in root filled teeth. *Oral Surgery, Oral Medicine, Oral Pathology*, **55**, 295–301.

Brauner, A. W. and Conrads, G. (1995). Studies into the microbial spectrum of apical periodontitis. *International Endodontic Journal*, **28**, 244–8.

Lewis, M. A. O., MacFarlane, T. W., and McGowan, D. A. (1986). Quantitative bacteriology of acute dentoalveolar abscesses. *Journal of Medical Microbiology*, **21**, 101–4.

Natkin, E., Oswald, R. J., and Carnes, L. I. (1984). The relationship of lesion size to diagnosis, incidence and treatment of periapical cysts and granulomas. *Oral Surgery, Oral Medicine, Oral Pathology*, **57**, 82–94.

Seltzer, S. and Farber, P. A. (1994). Microbiologic factors in endodontology. *Oral Surgery, Oral Medicine, Oral Pathology*, **78**, 634–45.

Tronstad, L. (1992). Recent development in endodontic research. *Scandinavian Journal of Dental Research*, **100**, 52–9.

6 Cysts of the jaws and oral soft tissues

6 Cysts of the jaws and oral soft tissues

A cyst is a pathological cavity having fluid or semi-fluid contents, which has not been created by the accumulation of pus. Cysts of the jaws are more common than in any other bone, and the majority are lined wholly or in part by epithelium. Although the pathogenesis of many of these cysts is poorly understood, they are divided into two main groups depending on the suspected origin of the lining epithelium.

1. *Odontogenic cysts*. The epithelial lining is derived from the epithelial residues of the tooth-forming organ. They can be subdivided into developmental and inflammatory types depending on their aetiology.
2. *Non-odontogenic cysts*. The epithelial lining is derived from sources other than the tooth-forming organ.

This division is supported by studies on the distribution of cytokeratins in cyst epithelium. The cytokeratins are cytoplasmic filaments and are major structural proteins of all epithelial cells. They consist of at least 19 different polypeptides and it appears that all derivatives of odontogenic epithelium are similar in their cytokeratin content.

The classification of jaw cysts used in this chapter is given in Table 6.1. It is based on that recommended by the World Health Organization: the non-epithelialized, primary cysts of bone are appended. Stafne's idiopathic bone cavity is discussed in this chapter since, while it is not a cyst, it may be mistaken for such on a radiograph.

The incidence of each type of jaw cyst varies slightly from series to series and the figures given in Table 6.2 are approximations based on several reports. At least 90 per cent of all jaw cysts are of odontogenic origin.

ODONTOGENIC CYSTS: DEFINITION AND ORIGINS

By definition, the epithelial lining of these cysts originates from residues of the tooth-forming organ. There are three kinds of residue, each primarily responsible for the origin of a particular type of lesion.

1. The epithelial rests or glands of Serres persisting after dissolution of the dental lamina. These give rise to the odontogenic keratocyst. They may also be the origin of some developmental lateral periodontal and gingival cysts.
2. The reduced enamel epithelium which is derived from the enamel organ and covers the fully formed crown of the unerupted tooth. The dentigerous (follicular) and eruption cysts are derived from this tissue, as is the relatively uncommon inflammatory paradental cyst.

Table 6.1   Classification of cysts of the jaws

Epithelial cysts
Odontogenic cysts
Developmental
—Odontogenic keratocyst (primordial cyst)
—Dentigerous (follicular) cyst
—Eruption cyst
—Lateral periodontal cyst
—Gingival cyst
—Glandular odontogenic cyst

Inflammatory
—Radicular cyst (dental cyst)
    (a) apical
    (b) lateral
    (c) residual
—Paradental cyst

Non-odontogenic cysts
—Nasopalatine duct (incisive canal) cyst
—Nasolabial (nasoalveolar) cyst
—Globulomaxillary cyst
—Median cysts

Non-epithelialized primary bone cysts
—Solitary bone cyst (simpe, traumatic, haemorrhagic bone cyst)
—Aneurysmal bone cyst
—Stafne's idiopathic bone cavity

Table 6.2   Incidence of cysts of the jaws

Odontogenic cysts (90%)		Non-odontogenic cysts (10%)	
Radicular cysts	60–75%	Nasopalatine cyst	5 –10%
Dentigerous cyst	10–15%	Other non-odontogenic	
Keratocyst	5–10%	and primary bone cysts	1%
Paradental cyst	3–5%		
Gingival cyst			
Lateral periodontal cyst	< 1%		

3. The rests of Malassez formed by fragmentation of the epithelial root sheath of Hertwig. All radicular cysts originate from these residues.

Radicular cysts

Clinical and radiographic features

Apical radicular cysts are the most common cystic lesions in the jaws and are always associated with the apices of non-vital teeth. They account for about 75 per cent of all radicular cysts. When small they are frequently symptomless and are usually discovered during routine radiological examination. As they enlarge they produce expansion of the alveolar bone and ultimately may discharge through a sinus. However, the majority of radicular cysts do not grow to large dimensions. The expansion of the alveolar bone is due to deposition of successive

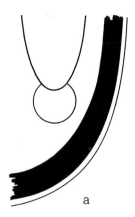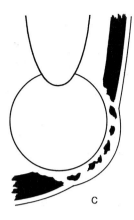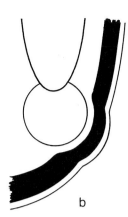

Fig. 6.1 Enlargement of a radicular cyst, a; producing bony expansion, b; and cortical thinning/egg-shell crackling, c.

layers of new bone by the overlying periosteum. As the cyst enlarges and causes bone resorption centrally, increments of new subperiosteal bone are laid down to maintain integrity of the cortex, producing a bony-hard expansion. However, the rate of expansion tends to outstrip the rate of subperiosteal deposition, leading to progressive thinning of the cortex which can be deformed on palpation producing the clinical signs of 'oil-can bottoming' and 'egg-shell crackling' (Fig. 6.1). Eventually, the cyst may perforate the cortex and present as a bluish, fluctuant, submucosal swelling. The rate of expansion of radicular cysts has been estimated at approximately 5 mm in diameter per year.

Radicular cysts   **Key points**

- apical, residual, or lateral
- non-vital tooth
- may be symptomless
- may cause bone expansion

Pain is seldom a feature unless there is an acute exacerbation which may rapidly progress to abscess formation.

The cysts can arise at any age after tooth eruption but are rare in the deciduous dentition. They are most common between the ages of 20 and 60 years. They can occur in relation to any tooth in the arch, although 60 per cent are found in the maxilla where there is a particularly high incidence in anterior teeth. In addition to dental caries, pulp death from trauma and irritant restorative materials is more likely in anterior teeth than at other sites. Pulp death in maxillary lateral incisors may also be associated with an invaginated odontome. In the mandible the majority of cysts occur posterior to the canine tooth.

Radiographically, the apical radicular cyst presents as a round or ovoid radiolucency at the root apex (Fig. 6.2). The lesion is often well circumscribed and may be surrounded by a peripheral radiopaque margin continuous with the lamina dura of the involved tooth. However, whether or not cyst formation has occurred in an apical radiolucency cannot be detected from the radiographic appearances alone.

The other varieties of radicular cyst are less common. The residual cyst is a radicular cyst that has remained in the jaw and failed to resolve following extraction of the involved tooth (Fig. 6.3). About 20 per cent of radicular cysts are of this type. However, it should be noted that most periapical inflammation will resolve after removal of the causative agent. The reasons why some lesions persist as residual cysts are unknown. The lateral type is very uncommon and

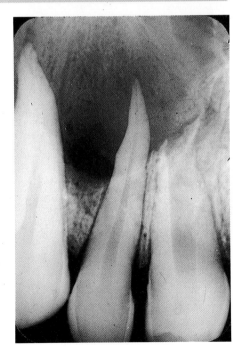

Fig. 6.2 Radicular cyst presenting as a diffuse periapical radiolucency.

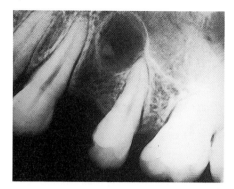

Fig. 6.3 Radiographic appearances of a residual cyst.

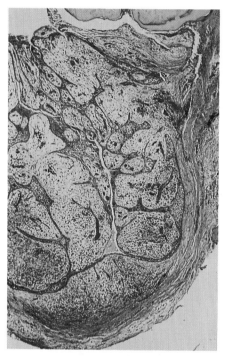

Fig. 6.4 Periapical granuloma containing proliferating arcades of squamous epithelium derived from the rests of Malassez showing early cystic breakdown.

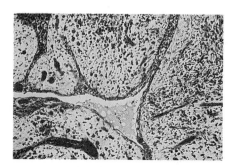

Fig. 6.5 Early (microcyst) formation associated with epithelial breakdown within the lesion shown in Fig. 6.4.

arises as a result of extension of inflammation from the pulp into the lateral periodontium along a lateral root canal.

Pathogenesis

Radicular cysts arise from proliferation of the rests of Malassez within chronic periapical granulomas (Fig. 6.4), but not all granulomas progress to cysts. The factors which determine why cystic transformation occurs in some, and the mechanisms involved in the formation of the cyst are controversial. Persistence of chronic inflammatory stimuli derived from the necrotic pulp appears essential since, as mentioned above, most periapical inflammation will resolve spontaneously once the causative agent has been removed. It is assumed that the environment within the chronically inflamed granuloma, which is likely to be rich in cytokines including growth factors, stimulates the rests of Malassez to proliferate. Strands and sheets of squamous epithelium derived from proliferation of the rests are common findings in periapical granulomas.

The mechanism of formation of an epithelial-lined cyst cavity within the granuloma is unclear. Two main mechanisms have been proposed:

1. Degeneration and death of central cells within a proliferating mass of epithelium. Epithelium is avascular and transport of metabolites and gaseous exchange occur by diffusion. It is argued that when the mass of proliferating epithelium within a granuloma reaches a critical size the central cells (furthest away from the surrounding vascular bed) degenerate and die. The microcyst so formed (Fig. 6.5) then continues to expand.

2. Degeneration and liquefactive necrosis of granulation tissue. It is suggested that areas of granulation tissue within the granuloma may undergo necrosis due to enclavement by proliferating strands of epithelium or to release of toxic products from the dead pulp or from infecting organisms. Epithelial proliferation to surround such an area of necrosis results in the formation of a cyst.

Histopathology

Radicular cysts (Fig. 6.6) are lined wholly or in part by non-keratinized stratified squamous epithelium supported by a chronically inflamed fibrous tissue capsule.

In newly formed cysts the epithelial lining is irregular and may vary considerably in thickness. Hyperplasia is a prominent feature resulting in long anastomosing cords of epithelium (see Fig. 6.4) forming complex arcades extending into the surrounding capsule (Fig. 6.7). The latter is richly vascular and diffusely infiltrated by inflammatory cells; plasma cells often predominate.

In established cysts the epithelial lining is more regular in appearance and of fairly even thickness (Fig. 6.8). Breaks in the lining—epithelial discontinuities— are common (Fig. 6.9). Metaplasia of the epithelial lining may give rise to mucous cells, found in about 40 per cent of radicular cyst linings and, more rarely, ciliated cells and areas of respiratory-type epithelium. In approximately 10 per cent of cases the lining contains hyaline eosinophilic bodies—Rushton bodies—of varying size and shape (Fig. 6.10). They appear to have no clinical or diagnostic significance and their origin is unknown, but they may represent some type of epithelial product.

With time, the connective tissue capsule tends to become more fibrous and less vascular and there is a reduction in the density of the inflammatory cell infiltration. Myofibroblasts in the capsule may help constrain the tendency of the cyst to expand (see below).

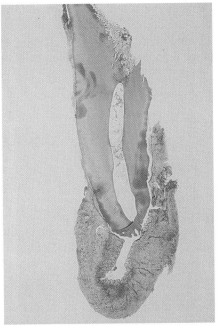

Fig. 6.6

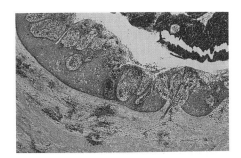

Fig. 6.7

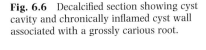

Fig. 6.8

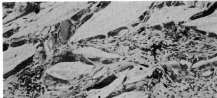

Fig. 6.9

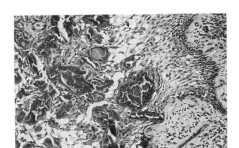

Fig. 6.10

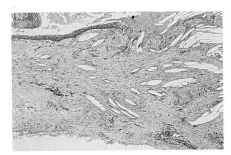

Fig. 6.11

Fig. 6.6 Decalcified section showing cyst cavity and chronically inflamed cyst wall associated with a grossly carious root.

Fig. 6.7 Early radicular cyst showing variation in thickness of the epithelial lining.

Fig. 6.8 Epithelial lining of an established radicular cyst.

Fig. 6.9 Epithelial discontinuity in a radicular cyst associated with a mural cholesterol deposit.

Fig. 6.10 Radicular cyst with numerous Rushton bodies.

Fig. 6.11 Cholesterol clefts and haemosiderin deposits (blue). Perl's reaction.

Deposits of cholesterol crystals are common within the capsules of many radicular cysts. In histological sections cholesterol clefts may be few in number or form large mural nodules, in which case they are often associated with epithelial discontinuities and project into the cyst lumen (see Fig. 6.9). They are the probable origin of cholesterol crystals found in the cyst fluid. Mural cholesterol clefts are associated with foreign-body giant cells. As in periapical granulomas the cholesterol is probably derived from the breakdown of red blood cells as a result of haemorrhage into the cyst capsule, and deposits of haemosiderin are commonly associated with the clefts (Fig. 6.11).

Cyst contents

The cyst contents vary from a watery, straw-coloured fluid through to semi-solid, brownish material of paste-like consistency. Cholesterol crystals impart a shimmering appearance.

The composition of cyst fluid is complex and variable. It is hypertonic compared with serum and contains:

1. Breakdown products of degenerating epithelial and inflammatory cells, and connective tissue components.

2. Serum proteins. All groups of serum proteins are present in cyst fluid and the soluble protein level is 5–11 g/dl. Most are derived as an inflammatory exudate. Compared with serum the fluid contains higher levels of immunoglobulin which probably reflects local production by plasma cells in the capsule.

3. Water and electrolytes.

4. Cholesterol crystals.

Key points	**Radicular cysts**
	• develop within apical granulomas
	• lining derived from rests of Malassez
	• lined by non-keratinizing squamous epithelium
	• supported by a chronically inflamed capsule
	• contents variable but hypertonic

Cyst expansion

Once formed, radicular cysts tend to continue to expand equally in all directions, rather like a balloon. The rate of expansion is governed by the rate of local bone resorption and, as bone is resorbed, the hydrostatic pressure of the contents causes the cyst to enlarge.

It has been demonstrated *in vitro* that explants of cyst lining release bone resorbing factors which stimulate osteoclastic activity, amongst which prostaglandins, especially PGE_2, PGF_2, and PGI, may be particularly important. They are probably derived mainly from fibroblasts in the cyst capsule. Degradation of the bone matrix following demineralization by osteoclasts involves the action of various proteinases, particularly collagenase which may also be synthesized by capsular fibroblasts. Both prostaglandin and collagenase production by fibroblasts are increased by the action of various cytokines which are known to stimulate osteolytic activity and which may be generated locally. Interleukin-1 and interleukin-6 may be particularly important and may be synthesized by the epithelial lining itself as well as by macrophages and other cells within the capsule (Fig. 6.12). (For further discussion of mechanisms involved in pathological resorption of bone see Chapter 7.)

Key points	**Cyst expansion**
	• bone resorption allows —
	• cyst expansion due to —
	• hydrostatic pressure created by —
	• osmotic gradient

Because of the large number of osmotically active molecules in cyst fluid, the cyst contents are hypertonic compared with serum. The cyst wall acts as a semipermeable membrane, freely allowing the passage of water and crystalloids but restraining the passage of colloids. In addition, the cyst contents are virtually separated from the lymphatic drainage system. As a result, osmotically active molecules are retained within the cyst lumen. The high osmolality of the cyst contents and the semipermeable nature of the wall results in the movement of fluid from the tissues into the lumen along the osmotic gradient. This movement of fluid increases the hydrostatic pressure within the cyst causing it to expand in a unicentric ballooning pattern (Fig. 6.13).

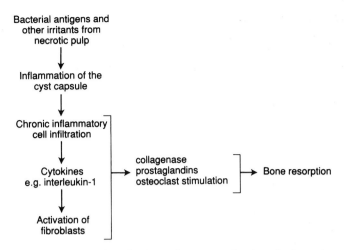

Fig. 6.12 Potential mechanisms of bone resorption in radicular cysts.

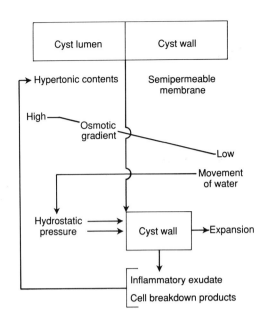

Fig. 6.13 Possible mechanisms involved in cyst expansion.

Dentigerous and eruption cysts

A dentigerous cyst is one which encloses part or all of the crown of an unerupted tooth. It is attached to the amelocemental junction and arises in the follicular tissues covering the fully formed crown of the unerupted tooth (Fig. 6.14). Radiographically, other cysts may present in apparent dentigerous relationship. For example, an odontogenic keratocyst may envelop the crown of an impacted third molar or, rarely, a permanent tooth may erupt into a radicular cyst associated with the deciduous predecessor. These extrafollicular lesions may be difficult to distinguish from true dentigerous cysts.

An eruption cyst is a true dentigerous cyst which arises in an extra-alveolar location.

Clinical and radiographic features

Dentigerous cysts occur over a wide age range and although many are detected in adolescents and young adults there is an increasing prevalence up to the fifth decade. They are about twice as common in males than in females and twice as common in the mandible than in the maxilla. The cysts most frequently involve teeth which are commonly impacted or erupt late. The majority are associated with the mandibular third molar and then, in order of decreasing frequency, the maxillary permanent canines, maxillary third molars, and mandibular premolars. Uncommonly, they are associated with supernumerary teeth or with complex and compound odontomes.

Although a tooth of the permanent series will be missing from the arch (with possible exceptions where a supernumerary or cystic odontome is responsible), a cyst may go undetected until it has enlarged sufficiently to produce expansion of the jaw. Alternatively, a cyst may be detected on routine radiographic examination or on seeking a cause for a retained deciduous tooth. Pain is not a feature unless there is secondary inflammation.

Radiographically, a dentigerous cyst presents as a well-defined unilocular, radiolucency associated in some way with the crown of an unerupted tooth (Fig. 6.15). The latter is often displaced for a considerable distance.

Eruption cysts involve both the deciduous and permanent dentitions. Because they arise in an extra-alveolar location they present as fluctuant swellings on the alveolar mucosa and are often bluish in colour (Fig. 6.16). Haemorrhage into the cyst cavity is common as a result of trauma (Fig. 6.17).

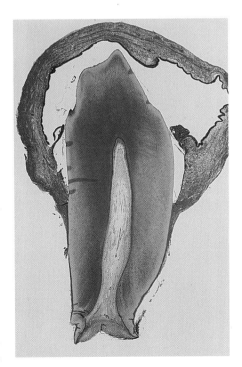

Fig. 6.14 Dentigerous cyst.

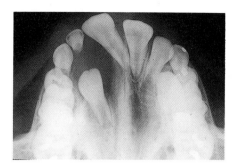

Fig. 6.15 Radiographic appearances of a dentigerous cyst.

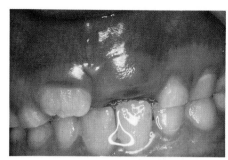

Fig. 6.16 Eruption cyst.

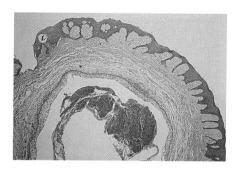

Fig. 6.17 Part of an eruption cyst (removed to expose underlying tooth) showing epithelial-lined cyst cavity beneath the mucosa.

Pathogenesis and expansion

Dentigerous cysts develop from the follicular tissues, but the stimulus is unknown and the mechanism of cyst formation unclear. Although they are associated with unerupted teeth it has been estimated that only about 1 per cent of such teeth develop cysts and other unidentified factors must, therefore, be involved.

The cyst develops between the crown of the unerupted tooth and the reduced enamel epithelium, but the mechanisms of cyst formation are unknown. It has been proposed that compression of the follicle by a potentially erupting, but impacted, tooth obstructs the venous outflow, thereby increasing venous pressure and inducing transudation across capillary walls. The increased hydrostatic pressure of this pooling transudate separates the follicle from the crown resulting in cyst formation.

Alternative hypotheses suggest that the cysts arise by proliferation of the outer layers of the reduced enamel epithelium and subsequent cleft formation within the epithelium, somewhat analogous to changes occurring during tooth eruption, or, in some cases, involve the spread of inflammation from a non-vital deciduous tooth into the follicle of the permanent successor, accumulation of inflammatory exudate leading to cyst formation.

The mechanism of expansion is probably similar to that of radicular cysts and is dependent on bone resorption and hydrostatic pressure. The contents are hypertonic compared with serum and bone resorbing factors, including prostaglandins E_2, F_2, and interleukin-1 are produced by dentigerous cysts.

The rate of cyst expansion in children may be rapid but enlargement is much slower in adults.

Macroscopic features and histopathology

Macroscopic examination of intact specimens reveals a cyst attached to the amelocemental junction. The crown of the associated tooth is related to the cyst in one of three ways.

1. *Central type.* The cyst completely surrounds the crown of the tooth. This is the most common type.
2. *Lateral type.* The cyst projects laterally from the side of the tooth and does not completely enclose the crown.
3. *Circumferential type.* Cystic change occurs in a band around the circumference of the amelocemental junction producing a doughnut-shaped lesion. This type is rare.

The lining of dentigerous cysts is typically a thin, regular layer, some two to five cells thick, of non-keratinized stratified squamous or flattened/low cuboidal epithelium (Fig. 6.18). It resembles the reduced enamel epithelium from which it is derived. Mucous cell metaplasia is common and increases with age, and epithelial discontinuities are frequently observed. The lining is supported by a fibrous connective tissue capsule free from inflammatory cell infiltration, unless there has been secondary inflammation. Cholesterol clefts may be present and islands of odontogenic epithelium are occasionally observed. Occasionally, the lining of an otherwise typical dentigerous (follicular) cyst shows a focal thickening or nodule protruding into the cyst cavity, which, on histological examination, consists of proliferating epithelium resembling a plexiform ameloblastoma. Such lesions are classified as unicystic ameloblastomas and are discussed in Chapter 15.

The cyst contains a proteinaceous, yellowish fluid, and cholesterol crystals are common. The soluble protein content is around 5–7 g/dl.

The lining of eruption cysts may be similar to that described above but is usually modified by chronic inflammation, possibly as a result of trauma. The latter also explains why many contain blood (see Fig. 6.17).

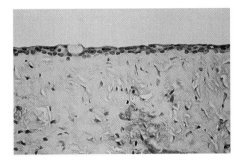

Fig. 6.18 Lining of dentigerous cyst.

Dentigerous cysts   **Key points**

- most frequently involve impacted/ late-erupting teeth
- develop between reduced enamel epithelium and crown
- surround part or all of the involved crown
- lined by non-keratinizing epithelium

Odontogenic keratocyst (primordial cyst)

The odontogenic keratocyst is a relatively uncommon lesion which has aroused much interest because of its unusual growth pattern and tendency to recur. The term 'primordial' was used originally because the lesion was thought to arise by cystic change in the enamel organ (tooth primordium). It is now generally accepted that the cysts most probably arise from remnants of the dental lamina. However, since the dental lamina gives rise to the tooth primordium, cysts derived from that tissue can still justifiably be designated as primordial. Histologically, primordial cysts are odontogenic keratocysts: the two terms are synonymous but odontogenic keratocyst is the preferred term.

Clinical and radiographic features

Odontogenic keratocysts occur over a wide age range, but there is a pronounced peak incidence in the second and third decades with a second smaller peak in the fifth decade. The cysts are more common in males than females, and 70–80 per cent occur in the mandible. The most common site, accounting for at least 50 per cent of all cases, is the third molar region and ascending ramus of the mandible. In both the mandible and maxilla the majority of cysts occur in the region posterior to the first premolar.

Keratocysts give rise to remarkably few symptoms, unless they become secondarily inflamed, and this probably accounts for why some do not present until the fifth decade. Unlike radicular and dentigerous cysts which tend to expand in a unicentric ballooning pattern, keratocysts enlarge predominantly in an antero-posterior direction and can reach large sizes without causing gross bony expansion (Fig. 6.19). They are often discovered fortuitously on routine radiographic examination.

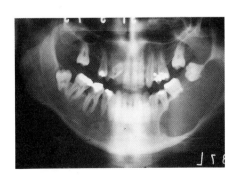

Fig. 6.19 Radiographic appearances of an odontogenic keratocyst.

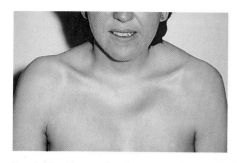

Fig. 6.20 Abnormal neck line associated with cervical ribs in a patient with basal cell naevus syndrome.

Although the majority of keratocysts present as solitary lesions, a small number of patients develop two or more cysts. Multiple cysts are associated with the basal cell naevus syndrome (Gorlin–Goltz syndrome), inherited as an autosomal dominant trait with marked penetrance and variable expressivity. The gene has been mapped to chromosome 9q. It has numerous manifestations but the main signs are:

1. Multiple odontogenic keratocysts. This does not necessarily imply that multiple cysts are present at the same time, but refers to the occurrence of multiple cysts throughout the lifetime of the patient.

2. Multiple naevoid basal cell carcinomas of the skin. Unlike other basal cell carcinomas, which are largely confined to areas of skin exposed to sunlight, the naevi occur anywhere on the body and commonly appear around the age of puberty.

3. Skeletal abnormalities, particularly rib (Fig. 6.20) and vertebral deformities.

4. A characteristic facies with frontal and temporoparietal bossing, hypertelorism, and mild mandibular prognathism.

5. Abnormalities of calcium and phosphate metabolism manifested by calcification in cerebral meninges (falx cerebri) (Fig. 6.21) and lack of phosphate diuresis following administration of parathormone.

Key points	**Odontogenic keratocysts**
	• peak incidence 2nd–3rd decades
	• few symptoms
	• tendency to recur
	• multiple cysts associated with basal cell naevus syndrome

The syndrome is uncommon, but patients with multiple keratocysts alone may be suffering from it in one of its least expressed forms.

An important clinical feature of keratocysts is their tendency to recur after surgical treatment. Recurrence rates vary in different reported series from around 11 per cent to over 60 per cent. It is likely that the rate is decreasing with improved management following recognition of this problem. Possible factors related to recurrence are discussed later.

Radiographically, keratocysts appear as well-defined radiolucencies that may be unilocular or multilocular. Many present in apparent dentigerous relationship associated with unerupted third molars but the crowns of such teeth are usually separated from the cyst cavity, the pericoronal tissues being continuous with the cyst capsule. Keratocysts may also present as developmental lateral periodontal cysts.

Histopathology

The cyst wall is usually thin and often folded and is lined by a regular continuous layer of stratified squamous epithelium some five to ten cells thick (Fig. 6.22). The basal cell layer is well defined and consists of palisaded columnar or occasionally cuboidal cells. The suprabasal cells resemble those of the stratum spinosum of oral epithelium and there is an abrupt transition between these and the surface layers which differentiate towards keratin production (Fig. 6.23). Parakeratosis predominates but areas of orthokeratinization are occasionally seen. The cells desquamate into the cyst lumen. Mitotic activity is higher than in other types of odontogenic cysts and mitotic figures are found in basal and suprabasal cells.

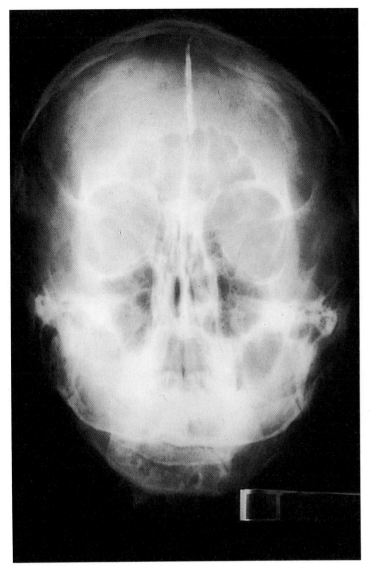

Fig. 6.21

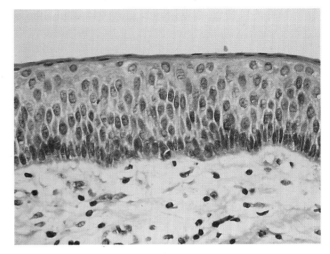

Fig. 6.23

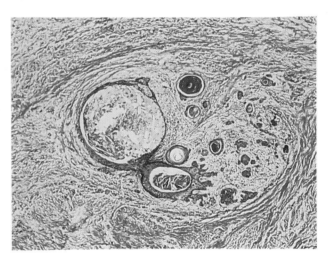

Fig. 6.24

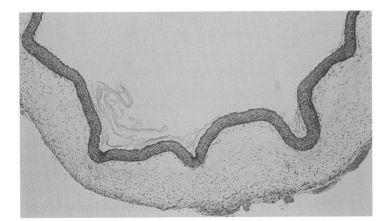

Fig. 6.22

Fig. 6.21 Calcification of falx cerebri in a patient with basal cell naevus syndrome.

Fig. 6.22 Wall of an odontogenic keratocyst showing regular epithelial lining and thin capsule.

Fig. 6.23 Epithelial lining of odontogenic keratocyst showing palisaded basal cells and parakeratinization.

Fig. 6.24 Epithelial residues and satellite cysts associated with odontogenic keratocyst.

The fibrous capsule of the cyst is usually thin and generally free from inflammatory cell infiltration. If the cyst becomes secondarily inflamed the epithelial lining loses its characteristic histology and comes to resemble that of a radicular cyst. Small groups of epithelial cells resembling dental lamina rests are often found in the capsule and these can give rise to independent satellite cysts around the main lesion (Fig. 6.24). Satellite cysts are usually small and often microscopic in size. Epithelial residues and satellite cysts are more common in cysts associated with the basal cell naevus syndrome. Retention of epithelial residues or satellite cysts when the main lesion is enucleated is one of the factors associated with the high recurrence rate of keratocysts. The thinness of the cyst wall and its low tensile and rupture strength compared with radicular cysts make enucleation more difficult and recurrence may thus follow retention of fragments of torn lining.

Keratocysts contain thick, grey/white cheesy material consisting of keratinous debris. There is little free fluid and the contents have a low soluble protein level, less than 4 g/dl, composed predominantly of albumin.

Key points	**Odontogenic keratocyst**
	• thin, easily torn wall
	• lined by an even layer of parakeratinized squamous epithelium
	• palisaded basal cell layer
	• contains keratinous debris
	• satellite cysts in capsule

The term odontogenic keratocyst must not be used to describe any odontogenic cyst producing keratin, it refers to a specific clinicopathological entity. Other jaw cysts such as radicular and dentigerous cysts may, rarely, produce keratin by metaplasia, but the epithelial linings of such cysts are usually orthokeratinized and do not show the regular and ordered epithelial differentiation that characterize the odontogenic keratocyst.

Pathogenesis and expansion

Keratocysts are derived from remnants of the dental lamina, but the stimulus for cystic transformation is unknown. The basal cell naevus syndrome is inherited, but there is no evidence that solitary cysts are genetically determined.

Although hydrostatic forces are probably involved in expansion, other hypotheses have been suggested to account for the peculiar growth pattern of the lesion. Possible factors involved in expansion include:

1. *Hydrostatic forces.* The mechanism is the same as that suggested for radicular cysts. Keratocyst contents are hypertonic when compared with serum and the lining acts as an efficient semipermeable membrane. However, hydrostatic pressure alone would result in a unicentric ballooning pattern of expansion.

2. *Active epithelial growth.* The epithelial lining of keratocysts exhibits greater mitotic activity than other odontogenic cysts. Proliferation of local groups of epithelial cells could account for foldings in the cyst lining and projections of the cyst along cancellous spaces resulting in a multicentric pattern of growth.

3. *Production of bone resorbing factors.* Like the radicular cyst the odontogenic keratocyst releases bone resorbing factors including prostaglandins, collagenase,

and interleukins-1 and -6. However, in comparison to radicular cysts there is less bone resorbing activity per unit surface area. It has been suggested that because keratocysts are relatively poor bone resorbers, they extend preferentially through the less dense cancellous bone.

4. *Accumulation of mural squames.* Variation in the rate of accumulation of squames in different areas of the cyst might result in localized areas of increased pressure resorption of bone.

Gingival cyst

Gingival cysts are of little clinical significance. They are common in neonates when they are often referred to as Bohn's nodules or Epstein's pearls. Most disappear spontaneously by 3 months of age. They arise from remnants of the dental lamina which proliferate to form small keratinizing cysts.

Gingival cysts in adults are rare. It is likely that most represent developmental lateral periodontal cysts (see below) that have arisen in an extra-alveolar location.

Developmental lateral periodontal cyst

The developmental lateral periodontal cyst is an uncommon lesion that must be distinguished from a lateral radicular cyst associated with a non-vital tooth and from an odontogenic keratocyst arising alongside the root of a tooth.

Clinically, the lateral periodontal cyst occurs mainly in the canine and premolar region of the mandible in middle-aged patients. It may present with expansion or be discovered on routine radiographic examination as a well-defined radiolucent area with sclerotic margins.

Histologically, the cyst is lined by thin non-keratinized squamous or cuboidal epithelium resembling reduced enamel epithelium, with focal, plaque-like thickenings. The pathogenesis is uncertain, but it has been suggested that it could arise initially as a lateral dentigerous cyst which, for unknown reasons, is retained in the bone when the tooth erupts.

Occasionally, developmental lateral periodontal cysts are multilocular and may be described by the adjective 'botryoid' because of their resemblance to a bunch of grapes (botryoid odontogenic cyst).

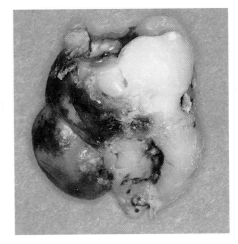

Fig. 6.25 Paradental cyst.

Paradental cyst

This type of cyst arises alongside a partly erupted third molar involved by pericoronitis. The reported cases have occurred in the mandible and most have been buccally or distobuccally placed (Figs 6.25, 6.26). Typically, the teeth associated with these cysts show an enamel spur extending from the buccal cervical margin to the root furcation. Radiographically, they appear as well-defined radiolucencies related to the neck of the tooth and the coronal third of the root.

The cysts are of inflammatory origin but their pathogenesis is uncertain. They could arise as a result of extension of pericoronal inflammation stimulating proliferation and cystic change in the reduced enamel epithelium covering the unerupted part of the crown and buccal enamel spur. Alternatively, cystic expansion of the follicle could be a secondary event following destruction of alveolar bone by extension of pericoronal inflammation into periodontal tissues.

Histologically, paradental cysts resemble inflammatory radicular cysts.

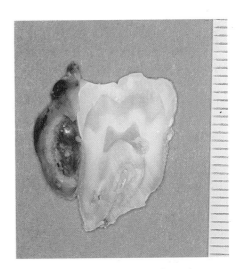

Fig. 6.26 Macroscopic section through cyst shown in Fig. 6.25.

Glandular odontogenic cyst

The glandular odontogenic cyst is a rare and only recently characterized, developmental odontogenic cyst. Almost all the reported cases have occurred in the anterior part of the mandible where they present as a slow-growing, painless unilocular or multilocular radiolucency.

Histologically, the cyst is lined by epithelium of varying thickness with a superficial layer of columnar or cuboidal cells and occasional mucous cells. Crypts or small cyst-like spaces are present within the thickness of the epithelium and the lining has a distinctly glandular structure. The cyst has a potentially aggressive, locally invasive nature and a tendency to recur.

NON-ODONTOGENIC CYSTS

Nasopalatine duct (incisive canal) cyst

The nasopalatine duct cyst is a distinct clinicopathological entity and is the commonest of the non-odontogenic cysts. It is a developmental lesion thought to arise from epithelial remnants of the nasopalatine duct which connects the oral and nasal cavities in the embryo. The stimulus for cystic change is unknown.

Clinical and radiographic features

The cyst presents most commonly in the fifth and sixth decades and occurs more frequently in males than in females. It may be asymptomatic and be discovered on routine radiographic examination, or present as a slowly enlarging swelling in the anterior region of the midline of the palate. Occasionally, it discharges into the mouth when the patient may complain of a salty taste. Pain may occur if the cyst becomes secondarily inflamed. Although cysts may arise at any point along the nasopalatine canal, most originate in the lower part and some arise entirely within the soft tissue of the incisive papilla. Such lesions are often designated cysts of the papilla palatina.

Radiographically, nasopalatine duct cysts present as well-defined round, ovoid, or heart-shaped radiolucencies, often with a sclerotic rim (Fig. 6.27). They are usually symmetrical about the midline but some are displaced to one side. The cyst must be distinguished from the normal incisive fossa and although precise limits cannot be placed on the maximum size of the latter, it is generally accepted that a radiolucency not greater than 6 mm wide may be considered within normal limits. Where there are standing teeth, the lesion must also be differentiated from a radicular cyst.

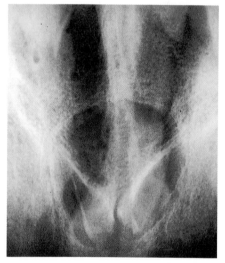

Fig. 6.27 Radiograph of nasopalatine duct cyst.

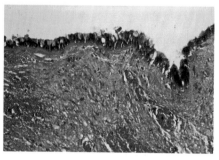

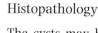

Fig. 6.28 Lining of nasopalatine duct cyst.

Histopathology

The cysts may be lined by a variety of different types of epithelium. Stratified squamous epithelium, pseudostratified ciliated columnar (respiratory) epithelium often containing mucous cells, cuboidal epithelium, or columnar epithelium may be seen alone or in any combination (Fig. 6.28). The epithelium is supported by a connective tissue capsule which usually includes prominent neurovascular bundles from the terminal branches of the long sphenopalatine nerve and vessels. Collections of mucous glands and a scattered chronic inflammatory cell infiltrate are frequently present.

Nasolabial cyst

The nasolabial cyst is a rare lesion which arises in the soft tissue of the upper lip just below the ala of the nose. Although arising in soft tissue, it is traditionally grouped with the jaw cysts previously regarded as fissural lesions.

Clinically, it presents as a slowly enlarging soft-tissue swelling obliterating the nasolabial fold and distorting the nostril. The cyst may arise bilaterally. The majority of cases present in the fourth decade and over 75 per cent occur in women.

The cysts are usually lined by pseudostratified columnar epithelium but stratified squamous epithelium, mucous cells, and ciliated cells may also be present.

The aetiology of the cyst is unknown, but it is thought to be of developmental origin. The fissural hypothesis purports that the lesion arises from epithelium included during fusion of the globular, lateral nasal, and maxillary processes. Alternatively, it has been suggested that the cyst arises from remnants of the lower part of the embryonic nasolacrimal duct.

Globulomaxillary cyst

The so-called globulomaxillary cyst is a rare lesion occurring between the roots of the maxillary permanent lateral incisor and canine teeth. Classically, it presents as an inverted pear-shaped radiolucency. The status of the cyst as a discrete entity is now questioned. It is probable that the majority are of odontogenic origin and represent either a developmental lateral periodontal cyst or even a radicular cyst.

Median cysts

The status of the rare, median cysts that occur in the palate or mandible is uncertain. The median cyst of the palate probably represents a displaced nasopalatine duct cyst. The latter is almost certainly the explanation for lesions that have been described as median alveolar cysts of the maxilla.

Although the aetiology of cysts occurring in the midline of the mandible is unclear it is very likely that they are of odontogenic origin.

NON-EPITHELIALIZED PRIMARY BONE CYSTS

Non-epithelialized bone cysts occur most often in long bones but are occasionally seen in the jaws, almost exclusively in the mandible.

Solitary bone cyst

A variety of terms have been used to designate this lesion including simple bone cyst, traumatic bone cyst, haemorrhagic bone cyst, and unicameral bone cyst.

Clinical and radiographic features

The solitary bone cyst occurs predominantly in children and adolescents with a peak incidence in the second decade. There is no definite sex predilection although some series have shown a slightly higher incidence in males. The cyst arises most frequently in the premolar and molar regions of the mandible. Maxillary lesions are rare. The majority of solitary bone cysts are asymptomatic and are chance radiographic findings; some degree of bony expansion occurs in about 25 per cent of cases.

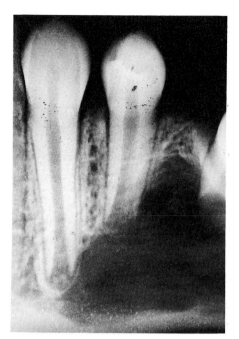

Fig. 6.29 Radiographic appearances of solitary bone cyst.

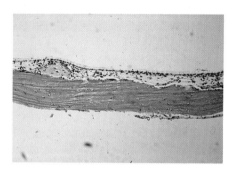

Fig. 6.30 Wall of solitary bone cyst. Loose fibrous tissue covers the bone.

Radiographically, the lesion presents as a radiolucency of variable size and irregular outline. Scalloping is a prominent feature particularly around and between the roots of standing teeth (Fig. 6.29). The margins of the lesion are usually well defined.

Pathological features and pathogenesis

Surgical exploration is undertaken to confirm the clinical diagnosis and characteristically reveals a rough bony-walled cavity devoid of any detectable soft-tissue lining. In many cases the cavity appears empty, but in others there is a little clear or blood-stained fluid. Rapid healing follows surgical exploration but even without surgical intervention the cyst will resolve spontaneously with time.

Microscopic examination of curettings from the lesion shows that the bony walls are covered by a delicate layer of loose, vascular fibrous tissue (Fig. 6.30) containing extravasated red blood cells and deposits of haemosiderin pigment. There is no epithelial lining.

The pathogenesis of the solitary bone cyst is unknown. It is commonly believed that there is a relationship to trauma, but the evidence is not convincing. Although a history of trauma can be elicited in about 50 per cent of cases, the interval between trauma and discovery of the lesion can range from months to years and the apparent relationship may be purely fortuitous. It has been suggested that the solitary bone cyst, aneurysmal bone cyst, and central giant cell granuloma of bone are related lesions reflecting some haemodynamic disturbance in medullary bone. In the case of the solitary bone cyst it has been argued that trauma produces intramedullary haemorrhage which, for unknown reasons, fails to organize and that cavitation occurs by subsequent haemolysis and resorption of the clot.

Aneurysmal bone cyst

The aneurysmal bone cyst is rare in the jaws. Most of the reported cases have arisen in the mandible, usually the posterior part of the body or angle, and have occurred in children or young adults. It presents as a firm painless swelling. Radiographs show a uni- or multilocular radiolucency with a characteristic ballooned-out appearance due to gross cortical expansion (Fig. 6.31).

Microscopically, the lesion consists of numerous, non-endothelial-lined, blood-filled spaces of varying size separated by cellular fibrous tissue. Multinucleated giant cells and evidence of old and recent haemorrhage are common in the fibrous septa (Fig. 6.32).

The pathogenesis of the lesion is unknown, but many aneurysmal bone cysts are preceded by some other primary lesion of bone, such as fibrous dysplasia or central giant-cell granuloma. It is thought that the primary lesion initiates a

Fig. 6.31 Radiographic appearances of an aneurysmal bone cyst showing ballooned-out ascending ramus and multilocular radiolucencies.

Fig. 6.32 Aneurysmal bone cyst with collections of giant cells.

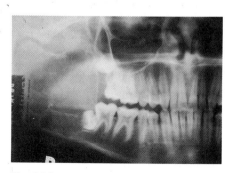

Fig. 6.31

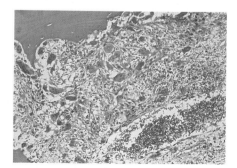

Fig. 6.32

vascular malformation leading to a haemodynamic disturbance resulting in the development of an aneurysmal bone cyst. As with the solitary bone cyst, there may be a history of trauma.

Stafne's idiopathic bone cavity

This is an uncommon developmental anomaly of the mandible that is included here for convenience since it may be mistaken for a cyst on a radiograph. It is a symptomless chance finding which appears as a round or oval, well-demarcated radiolucency between the premolar region and angle of the jaw, and is usually located beneath the inferior dental canal (Fig. 6.33). Occasionally, the anomaly is bilateral.

The radiographic appearances are due to a saucer-shaped depression or concavity of varying depth on the lingual aspect of the mandible, which, in the great majority of cases, contains ectopic salivary tissue in continuity with the submandibular salivary gland. Sialography may be useful in identifying such salivary inclusions.

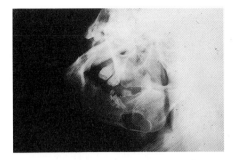

Fig. 6.33 Radiographic appearances of Stafne's idiopathic bone cavity.

CYSTS OF THE SOFT TISSUES

With the exception of the salivary mucoceles, cysts of the oral soft tissues are uncommon. Although strictly speaking gingival and nasolabial cysts are soft-tissue lesions they are traditionally grouped with cysts of the jaws. The main types of soft-tissue cysts, including those occurring in the neck, are listed in Table 6.3.

Salivary mucoceles

Cysts arising in connection with minor salivary glands are common. About 90 per cent of cases are of the mucous extravasation type.

Extravasation mucoceles

Over 70 per cent of all mucous extravasation cysts arise in the lower lip, followed by the cheek and floor of mouth. They are extremely uncommon in the upper lip. (In contrast, salivary tumours occur much more frequently in the upper lip than in the lower lip.) The cyst occurs over a wide age range but most patients are under 30 years of age and there is a peak incidence in the second decade.

Clinically, the lesion presents as a bluish or translucent submucosal swelling (Fig. 6.34) and there may be a history of rupture, collapse, and refilling which may be repeated. It arises as a result of extravasation of mucus from a ruptured duct and a history of trauma can often be elicited from the patient.

Microscopically, the lesion typically consists of a mucin-filled cystic cavity or cavities lined by inflamed granulation tissue (Fig. 6.35). There is no epithelial lining. The extravasated mucus evokes a chronic inflammatory reaction and the wall of the cyst is infiltrated by large numbers of macrophages with vacuolated cytoplasm containing phagocytosed mucin (Fig. 6.36). Similar cells are seen within the cyst lumen. The torn duct may be seen running into the lesion (Fig. 6.37). In some cases the mucus is present as diffuse pools rather than being contained within a more or less discrete cyst-like space.

Retention mucoceles

In contrast to extravasation mucoceles, retention mucoceles occur most frequently in patients over 50 years of age and are almost never found in the lower lip.

Table 6.3 Cysts of the oral soft tissues

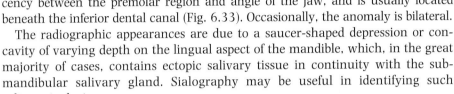

Salivary mucoceles
  (a) mucous extravasation cyst
  (b) mucous retention cyst
Dermoid and epidermoid cysts
Lymphoepithelial cyst
Thyroglossal cyst

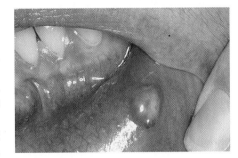

Fig. 6.34 Extravasation mucocele in superficial tissues.

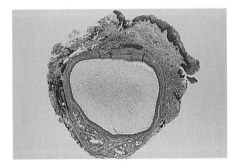

Fig. 6.35 Extravasation mucocele.

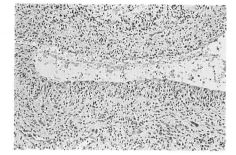

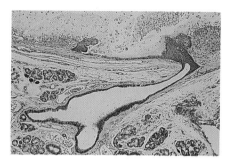

Fig. 6.36 Lining of an extravasation mucocele rich in macrophages (histiocytes).

Fig. 6.37 Ruptured duct running into extravasation mucocele.

Fig. 6.36

Fig. 6.37

They are derived from cystic dilatation of a duct and are lined by epithelium of ductal type (Figs 6.38, 6.39). Because the mucus is still contained within the duct there is no surrounding chronic inflammatory reaction. Their pathogenesis is unknown but progressive ballooning of a partially obstructed duct or even spontaneous cystic change have been suggested.

Ranula

Ranula is a clinical term used to describe a swelling of the floor of the mouth which is said to resemble a frog's belly (Fig. 6.40). It is not a pathological diagnosis. Histologically, most ranulae are mucous extravasation cysts.

Dermoid and epidermoid cysts

Dermoid cysts are relatively uncommon developmental lesions which originate in the midline of the floor of the mouth above the mylohyoid muscle. They may present as intraoral or submental swellings (Fig. 6.41). The cyst is presumed to arise from enclavement of epithelium in the midline as a result of deranged fusion of the mandibular and hyoid branchial arches.

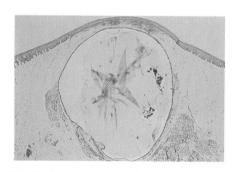

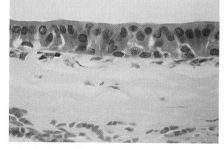

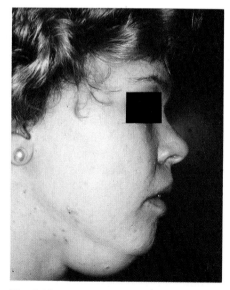

Fig. 6.38

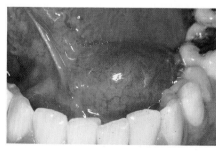

Fig. 6.38 Retention mucocele.

Fig. 6.39 Epithelial lining of a retention mucocele.

Fig. 6.40 Ranula.

Fig. 6.41 Dermoid cyst presenting as submental swelling.

Fig. 6.39

Fig. 6.40

Fig. 6.41

Histologically, the cyst is lined by a regular layer of orthokeratinized stratified squamous epithelium resembling epidermis. The lumen contains keratinous debris. To be designated as dermoid, skin appendages, such as hair follicles, sebaceous and sweat glands, and erector pili muscles, must be identified in the wall of the cyst (Fig. 6.42). In the absence of skin appendages the cysts are designated as epidermoid. Epidermoid cysts occurring elsewhere in the oral soft tissues are acquired rather than developmental lesions. They arise as a result of traumatic implantation of epithelium into the deeper tissues, with subsequent cystic change and expansion.

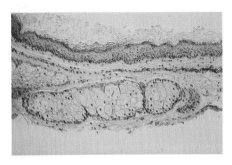

Fig. 6.42 Lining of dermoid cyst showing sebaceous glands.

Lymphoepithelial cyst

Lymphoepithelial cyst is the term now used to describe lesions previously classified as branchial cysts. The majority occur deep to sternomastoid or along its anterior border at the level of the angle of the mandible. It is an unusual lesion in the oral cavity, generally arising in the floor of the mouth. Histologically, the cyst is lined by stratified squamous epithelium and its wall contains well-organized lymphoid tissue (Fig. 6.43).

The cysts are of developmental origin but their pathogenesis is uncertain. The classical explanation that they are derived from remnants of the branchial arches or pharyngeal pouches has been disputed and it is likely that most arise from epithelium, probably of salivary origin, that becomes entrapped by lymphoid tissue. An origin from tonsillar tissue has also been suggested.

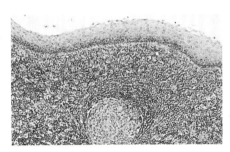

Fig. 6.43 Lining of lymphoepithelial cyst with lymphoid tissue and germinal centre in the wall.

Thyroglossal cyst

The thyroglossal cyst is a developmental lesion derived from residues of the embryonic thyroglossal duct, the vestigeal remains of which are represented by the foramen caecum on the tongue. Intraoral cysts, in the midline of the tongue or floor of the mouth, are very rare. Most thyroglossal cysts arise in the region of the hyoid bone.

It is convenient here to mention that functioning thyroid tissue may also occur in the tongue, although examples are rare. Before excision of ectopic lingual thyroid it is important to establish that the patient has functioning thyroid tissue present in the neck.

FURTHER READING

Ackerman, G., Cohen, M. A., and Altini, M. (1987). The paradental cyst: a clinicopathologic study of 50 cases. *Oral Surgery, Oral Medicine, Oral Pathology*, **64**, 308–12.

Bando, Y., Henderson, B., Meghji, S., Poole, S., and Harris, M. (1993). Immunocytochemical localization of inflammatory cytokines and vascular adhesion receptors in radicular cysts. *Journal of Oral Pathology and Medicine*, **22**, 221–7.

Benn, A. and Altini, M. (1996). Dentigerous cysts of inflammatory origin. A clinicopathological study. *Oral Surgery, Oral Medicine, Oral Pathology, Oral Radiology and Endodontics*, **81**, 203–9.

Browne, R. M. (1972). Metaplasia and degeneration in odontogenic cysts in man. *Journal of Oral Pathology*, **1**, 145–58.

Browne, R. M. (1975). The pathogenesis of odontogenic cysts: a review. *Journal of Oral Pathology*, **4**, 31–46.

Browne, R. M. (1976). Some observations on the fluids of odontogenic cysts. *Journal of Oral Pathology*, **5**, 74–87.

Craig, G. T. (1976). The paradental cyst. A specific inflammatory odontogenic cyst. *British Dental Journal*, **141**, 9–14.

Fanibunda, K. and Soames, J. V. (1995). Malignant and premalignant change in odontogenic cysts. *Journal of Oral and Maxillofacial Surgery*, **53**, 1469–72.

Gao, Z., Mackenzie, I. C., Cruchley, A. T., Williams, D. M., Leigh, I., and Lane, E. B.
(1989). Cytokeratin expression of the odontogenic epithelia in dental follicles and developmental cysts. *Journal of Oral Pathology and Medicine*, **18**, 63–7.

Harrison, J. D. (1975). Salivary mucuceles. *Oral Surgery, Oral Medicine, Oral Pathology*, **39**,
268–78.

Harvey, W., Foo, G-C., Gordon, D., Meghji, S., Evans, A., and Harris, M. (1984). Evidence
for fibroblasts as the major source of prostacyclin and prostaglandin synthesis in dental
cyst in man. *Archives of Oral Biology*, **29**, 223–9.

Hussain, K., Edmondson, H. D., and Browne, R. M. (1995). Glandular odontogenic cysts.
Diagnosis and treatment. *Oral Surgery, Oral Medicine, Oral Pathology, Oral Radiology and
Endodontics*, **79**, 593–602.

Meghji, S., Henderson, B., Bando, Y. and Harris, M. (1992). Interleukin-1: the principal
osteolytic cytokine produced by keratocysts. *Archives of Oral Biology*, **37**, 935–43.

Saito, Y., Hoshina, Y., Nagamine, T., Nakajima, T., Suzuki, M., and Hayashi, T. (1992).
Simple bone cyst. A clinical and histopathologic study of fifteen cases. *Oral Surgery, Oral
Medicine, Oral Pathology*, **74**, 487–91.

Shear, M. (1983). *Cysts of the oral regions*. 2nd edn. John Wright & Sons Ltd, Bristol.

Shear, M. (1994). Developmental odontogenic cysts. An update. *Journal of Oral Pathology
and Medicine*, **23**, 1–11.

Skaug, N. (1977). Soluble proteins in fluid from non-keratinising jaw cysts in man.
International Journal of Oral Surgery, **6**, 107–21.

Woolgar, J. A., Rippin, J. W., and Browne, R. M. (1987). A comparative study of the clinical and histological features of recurrent and non-recurrent odontogenic keratocysts.
Journal of Oral Pathology, **16**, 124–8.

7   Diseases of the periodontium

7 Diseases of the periodontium

Epidemiology

Chronic plaque-associated gingivitis and periodontitis are destructive inflammatory diseases sometimes referred to together simply as chronic periodontal disease, although there is evidence that, at least clinically, several distinct types of chronic destructive periodontal diseases may exist. The term gingivitis is used to designate inflammatory lesions that are confined to the marginal gingiva. Once the lesions extend to include destruction of the connective tissue attachment of the tooth and loss of alveolar bone the disease is designated periodontitis.

Epidemiology of periodontal disease	**Key point**
• advanced periodontal destruction only affects about 10–15 per cent of the population	

Chronic inflammatory periodontal disease of varying severity affects practically all dentate individuals. Gingivitis is common in children, even by the age of 3 years, and early periodontitis may be detected in teenagers; in general, the extent and severity of disease increase with age. This does not imply that all gingivitis progresses unrelentingly to periodontitis and indeed there appears to be a level of inflammation, loosely called 'contained gingivitis', which may remain stable for long periods of time. Nor does it imply that periodontitis is a relentlessly progressive disease. It is likely that periodontal destruction is an intermittent process and that random bursts of active destruction at specific sites alternate with periods of relative inactivity and even with attempts at healing.

Since the adoption of the *Community Periodontal Index of Treatment Needs (CPITN)*, epidemiological data from various parts of the world can be compared. This has confirmed that virtually all adults show evidence of early periodontitis but that advanced disease affects only about 10–15% of the population. Tooth loss as a result of periodontal destruction is uncommon before the age of 50 years.

Most forms of periodontitis in adults are considered to be manifestations of the same disease, but other rarer types occur in younger patients. The main categories of periodontitis that have been described are listed in Table 7.1.

Aetiology

The role of bacteria and dental plaque

There is now overwhelming evidence that dental plaque is the essential aetiological agent in chronic periodontal disease. Detailed discussion of the

Table 7.1   Clinical classification of periodontitis

> *Prepubertal periodontitis*
> A rare form affecting the deciduous dentition that may be localized or generalized. Genetic factors and a variety of medical conditions may be associated.
>
> *Juvenile periodontitis*
> An uncommon form with onset in puberty and adolescence and relatively well-defined clinical features.
>
> *Rapidly progressive periodontitis*
> An uncommon form with onset in late adolescence and early adulthood characterized by episodes of localized or generalized periodontal destruction. Many cases have been associated with defects in leucocyte function.
>
> *Adult type periodontitis*
> The most common form of periodontitis typically seen in adults over the age of 30 years.

evidence is outside the scope of this book, but the main points are summarized below.

1. Epidemiological studies in many parts of the world have demonstrated a strong positive association between dental plaque and the prevalence and severity of periodontal disease.
2. Clinical experiments in man and other animals have demonstrated that withdrawal of oral hygiene in healthy mouths results in the accumulation of dental plaque and that this is paralleled by the onset of gingivitis. Institution of plaque control rapidly restores the tissues to health.
3. A number of topically applied antimicrobial agents have been shown to inhibit plaque formation and prevent the onset of gingivitis.
4. Bacteria isolated from human dental plaque are capable of inducing periodontal disease when introduced into the mouths of gnotobiotic animals.
5. Several species of pathogenic bacteria have been isolated from periodontal pockets that have the capacity to invade tissues and evoke destructive inflammatory changes.

Although there is ample evidence that bacteria in dental plaque play a major role in the aetiology of periodontal disease, it is by no means clear whether their effect is non-specific and dependent primarily on the number of organisms or whether specific bacteria or groups of bacteria are responsible. However, there is increasing evidence that there are differences in the bacterial flora associated with healthy gingival crevices and various stages of disease. A brief summary of some of the differences between so-called pathogenic and non-pathogenic flora is given below and in Table 7.2.

1. Healthy periodontal tissues of humans are associated with a scanty flora located almost entirely supragingivally on the tooth surface. The microbial accumulations are 1–20 cells in thickness and comprise mainly Gram-positive bacteria. *Streptococcus* and *Actinomyces* species predominate, for example *Strep. sanguis, A. naeslundii, A. viscosus.*
2. In developing gingivitis the total mass of plaque is increased and the microbial cell layers often extend to 100–300 cells in thickness. Members of the genus *Actinomyces* predominate, but there is a substantial increase in strict anaerobes and Gram-negative organisms. In long-standing gingivitis, Gram-negative organisms may account for 35 per cent of the flora. The majority are located subgingivally.

Table 7.2 Main differences in plaque microorganisms in health, gingivitis, and periodontitis

Main species	% Aerobic/ anaerobic (facultative anaerobes)	% Gram +ve/ Gram −ve	Motile/non-motile
Healthy gingiva *Streptococcus* *Actinomyces* *Veillonella*	75/25	90/10	Very few motile forms; motile: non-motile, 1 : 40
Chronic gingivitis *Actinomyces* *Streptococcus* *Fusobacterium* *Porphyromonas* *Prevotella* *Capnocytophaga* *Veillonella*	60/40	65/35	Number of motile rods and spirochaetes increases with disease
Chronic periodontitis *Porphyromonas* *Prevotella* *Fusobacterium* *Eikenella* *Campylobacter* *Spirochaetes* *Actinomyces*	20/80	25/75	Abundant motile rods and spirochaetes; motile: non-motile, 1 : 1

Microbiology of periodontal disease **Key points**
- periodontal disease is a polymicrobial infection
- Gram-negative anaerobes increase in number as disease progresses

3. Microbial examination of subgingival plaque in periodontitis has revealed a complex flora rich in Gram-negative rods, motile forms, and spirochaetes. Members of the 'black-pigmented bacteroides' group are the predominant cultivable organisms in most subjects, but this does not imply that these are the most abundant organisms present. This group of bacteria (previously *Bacteroides* species), have been reclassified as *Porphyromonas* or *Prevotella* species, for example *Porphyromonas gingivalis*, *Prevotella melaninogenica*, and *Prevotella intermedia*.

4. The development of gingivitis and periodontitis is associated with sequential colonization and a progressively more complex flora, characterized by an increase in anaerobic, Gram-negative, and motile forms rather than a mere increase in the amount of plaque present.

The role of systemic factors

Dental plaque is the essential aetiological agent in periodontal disease. However, various local factors which may favour plaque accumulation, and systemic factors which may alter the host's response to local irritants, could influence the development and progression of the lesions.

Local factors include the pre-existing anatomy of the teeth, gingiva, and alveolar bone, alignment and occlusal relationships of teeth, and factors such as approximal restorations that may affect the accumulation and growth of plaque or interfere with its removal.

Several systemic factors have been associated with an increased incidence and severity of periodontal disease or with modifying the course of that disease. However, epidemiological studies have shown that over 90 per cent of the variance observed in populations with periodontal disease can be accounted for by age and oral hygiene variables alone.

Diabetes mellitus

The relationship between diabetes and periodontal disease is controversial. Although it is commonly held that periodontal disease is more severe and progresses faster in diabetics than in non-diabetics, the evidence is inconclusive and data from several studies are conflicting. Vascular changes and defects in cellular defence mechanisms have been suggested as possible ways in which diabetes could increase susceptibility of periodontal tissues to irritants from dental plaque.

Pregnancy and sex hormones

Several studies have shown that the severity of a pre-existing gingivitis increases in pregnancy from the second to the eighth month of gestation and then decreases. Areas of healthy gingiva are not affected. Increased levels of circulating hormones are thought to be responsible, but the fact that so-called pregnancy gingivitis can be resolved by adequate plaque control emphasizes that the hormonal changes simply modify the tissue response to dental plaque and do not cause the gingivitis. Increased levels of sex hormones or their metabolites are found in inflamed gingiva, and experimental evidence suggests that the aggravation of gingivitis during pregnancy is related mainly to progesterone which affects the function and permeability of the gingival microvasculature.

Localized gingival hyperplasia also occurs during pregnancy (pregnancy epulis). Increased levels of gingivitis occurring around puberty and in some women taking oral contraceptives may also be related to the concentration of circulating sex hormones.

Nutrition

Results of many studies in nutritionally deficient animals suggest that nutritional factors can modify the course of, but not initiate, periodontal disease. In humans, the relationship between nutrition and periodontal disease is controversial except in rare cases of gross deficiency states.

Advanced periodontal disease has been reported in rural Nigerians who eat a protein-deficient diet and in such children this is an important factor predisposing to cancrum oris.

Severe and prolonged deficiency of vitamin C causes scurvy which may be associated with haemorrhagic gingivitis and generalized oedematous enlargement of the gums, but these are not constant features.

Blood diseases

Acute leukaemia may be accompanied by a generalized enlargement of the gingiva due mainly to infiltration and packing of the tissues by leukaemic cells. Other oral signs of the disease can be related to the associated pancytopenia and include mucosal pallor, necrotizing ulceration (particularly of the oropharynx) petechial haemorrhages, gingival bleeding, and gingival ulceration. Candidosis and recrudescence of herpetic infections are also common. Alveolar bone loss and severe periodontal destruction have also been reported which, in some patients, are caused by leukaemic infiltration.

Severe gingival inflammation, ulceration, and advanced bone destruction may be seen in certain chronic types of neutropenia, such as cyclic neutropenia, and functional disorders of neutrophils have also been implicated in juvenile periodontitis.

Drugs

With the exception of phenytoin, cyclosporin, and nifedipine, which are associated with generalized gingival hyperplasia and are discussed later in this chapter, the evidence that systemic drug therapy can modify the course of periodontal disease is inconclusive. The main drugs which have been reported to affect the periodontium are listed in Table 7.3.

Drugs which affect inflammatory and immune responses, such as immunosuppressants and non-steroidal anti-inflammatory agents, might be expected to influence the course of periodontal disease by modifying the response of the host to products from microbial plaque. However, the evidence is inconclusive, and sometimes contradictory.

Table 7.3 Drugs that can affect periodontal tissues and the activity of periodontal disease

Anti-epileptics	phenytoin	gingival hyperplasia
Immunosuppressants	azathioprine corticosteroids	equivocal reduction in disease activity
	cyclosporin	gingival hyperplasia
Non-steroidal anti-inflammatory drugs	indomethacin ibuprofen	equivocal reduction in disease activity
Calcium channel blockers	nifedipine verapamil	gingival hyperplasia
Sex hormones	oestrogen progesterone	exacerbation of pre-existing gingivitis

Acquired immunodeficiency syndrome (AIDS)

Recent epidemiological studies suggest that the periodontal status of many HIV-positive patients is similar to that of the general population. However, severe and atypical forms of periodontal disease may be seen in some patients, particularly those with AIDS (see Chapter 11).

Smoking

There is a considerable body of evidence that tobacco smoking is an important risk factor for the development and progression of periodontal disease. The mechanism is not fully understood but smoking impairs the phagocytic function of polymorphoneutrophils. It does not appear to be related to differences in the composition of subgingival plaque.

Pathogenesis of periodontal disease

In health a balance exists between the challenge to the tissues from microorganisms in dental plaque and the host defence mechanisms (Fig. 7.1). Disturbances in this host-parasite relationship lead to the development of periodontal disease, but the transition from health to gingivitis is not precisely identifiable. The host

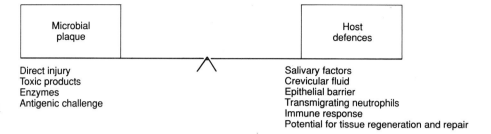

Fig. 7.1 Factors involved in maintaining the host–parasite equilibrium at the plaque–gingival interface.

may be able to adapt to the imbalance in the relationship so that a new equilibrium is established and the disease may become arrested and remain stable over long periods of time. Healing may also occur. Transient imbalances in the host–parasite relationship are likely to occur frequently and yet the natural history of periodontal disease in humans usually spans decades, suggesting that equilibrium is rapidly restored and that for most of the time destruction is not continuous but is episodic in nature.

The histopathological changes occurring in the development of chronic inflammatory periodontal disease are based largely on studies of experimentally induced disease in humans and in various animal models. Although these studies have increased our understanding of the development of periodontal disease under controlled experimental conditions and have focused attention on important pathogenic mechanisms, a degree of caution must be exercised in extrapolating the findings to spontaneous disease occurring in humans for reasons discussed above. In experimental situations a normal, healthy periodontium, free from inflammatory cell infiltration, can be established and maintained by scrupulous plaque control. Under these conditions the histopathogenesis of periodontal disease following withdrawal of oral hygiene procedures and the accumulation of dental plaque has been described as occurring in four stages:

(1) The initial lesion
(2) The early lesion   } Gingivitis
(3) The established lesion
(4) The advanced lesion   Periodontitis

The first three stages occur in the development of gingivitis; the fourth stage corresponds to periodontitis.

The initial lesion

The initial lesion of gingivitis develops within 2–4 days following the onset of plaque accumulation. The changes are histological and cannot be detected clinically. They are summarized in Table 7.4. The lesion is localized to the tissues around the base of the histological sulcus (that is the potential space, approximately 0.5 mm deep, bounded by enamel, sulcular epithelium, and the free surface of the junctional epithelium) and involves portions of the junctional and sulcular epithelia and a microscopic area of underlying gingival connective tissue (Fig. 7.2). It is essentially an acute inflammatory response. Within the inflamed area the vessels become dilated, accompanied by the formation of both a fluid and a cellular exudate. Large numbers of predominantly polymorphonuclear neutrophil leucocytes (PMN) emigrate from the vessels and migrate through the connective tissue to infiltrate the intercellular spaces of the junctional epithelium. They continue to migrate coronally and eventually enter the oral cavity through the base of sulcus. This transmigration of the junctional epithelium by PMN is a response to chemotactic stimuli released into and elaborated within

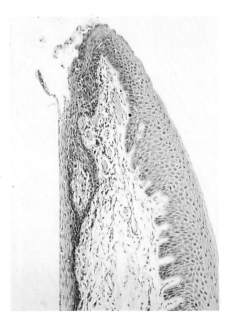

Fig. 7.2 Gingivitis developing around the base of the histological sulcus.

Table 7.4 Pathological features of initial gingivitis

Localized around base of gingival sulcus

Acute inflammatory changes:
 —vasodilation
 —fluid exudation; crevicular fluid
 —cellular exudation; polymorphs (PMN)

Enhanced transmigration of PMN

Disruption of intercellular spaces of junctional epithelium:
 —impairment of barrier function

the sulcular area. The transmigration of PMN causes disruption of the junctional epithelium and widening of the intercellular spaces which impairs the barrier function of this tissue. Although this could allow more ready ingress of antigens and other plaque products into the tissues, thereby potentiating the inflammation and favouring the development of a chronic inflammatory reaction, patients with neutrophil disorders have severe periodontal disease. The weight of evidence indicates that the net effect of the neutrophil response is protective.

Exudation of protein-rich fluid, due to increased vascular permeability, accompanies the cellular exudate. As the disease develops and the volume of fluid exudation increases it manifests as a flow of crevicular fluid. The fluid exudate contains all classes of plasma proteins, notably immunoglobulins and complement which may also play a role in controlling the initial bacterial challenge.

The early lesion

The early lesion develops within 4–7 days following the onset of plaque accumulation and overlaps with and evolves from the initial lesion with no clear-cut dividing line. It develops at the site of the initial lesion, but as it evolves the area of inflamed gingival connective tissue expands laterally and apically, particularly as a narrow band beneath the junctional epithelium, extending towards the amelocemental junction. The infiltrated area still occupies a small fraction of the total gingival connective tissue (Fig. 7.3). The main features are summarized in Table 7.5.

There is persistence and exacerbation of the changes described in the initial lesion. The volume of transmigrating leucocytes increases, which further impairs the integrity of the junctional epithelium and may result in the beginning of the destruction of its attachment to enamel with consequent deepening of the gingival sulcus. This will permit the development of subgingival plaque and the altered environment favours the growth of Gram-negative anaerobes.

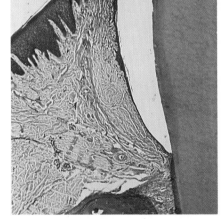

Fig. 7.3 The early lesion of experimental gingivitis.

Table 7.5 Pathological features of early gingivitis

Exacerbation of the features of initial gingivitis

Further impairment of barrier function of junctional epithelium:
 —disruption of intercellular spaces
 —failure to maintain attachment to enamel
 —deepening of gingival sulcus; subgingival plaque

Lymphocytic infiltration

Cytopathic changes in gingival fibroblasts

Loss of collagen

Hyperplasia of junctional epithelium; rete ridge formation

Impairment of the barrier function of the junctional epithelium and the shift to a more complex Gram-negative flora increases the bacterial challenge, and the major feature which distinguishes the early lesion is the formation of a dense infiltration of lymphoid cells within the inflamed gingival connective tissue. The majority are T cells, suggesting that cell-mediated immune reactions may be implicated as the host tries to contain the infection. However, as products from plaque bacteria activate host defences these in turn release a variety of mediators capable of triggering connective tissue breakdown. Possible mechanisms are discussed later. Many fibroblasts within the infiltrated area exhibit structural changes and show extensive damage to cell membranes and organelles, indicative of cellular injury.

As the inflammatory lesion develops, the basal cells of the junctional epithelium begin to proliferate to form small rete ridges.

The established lesion

The established lesion of experimental gingivitis develops within 2–3 weeks of the onset of plaque accumulation and evolves from the early lesion. The experimentally induced lesion develops in a relatively short time in comparison to the natural history of spontaneous periodontal disease in humans. The main features are summarized in Table 7.6.

Histologically, there is accentuation of the features of the initial lesion, but these changes are confined to a narrow band beneath the junctional and pathologically altered epithelium forming the tooth-gingival interface. There is further deepening of the gingival sulcus and further growth of subgingival plaque. The detached and pathologically altered epithelium is referred to as pocket epithelium. The appearance of the pocket epithelium is variable. It may be relatively thick with long anastamosing or arcading rete processes extending into the gingival connective tissue, it may be thinned with perhaps only one or two epithelial cells separating the underlying engorged and inflamed vascular bed from the external environment, or it may show frank ulceration (Fig. 7.4). The engorged and inflamed vascular bed and thinning and/or ulceration of the pocket epithelium are related to the clinical signs of redness and bleeding.

The characteristic feature of the established lesion, which distinguishes it from the early lesion, is the shift in the inflammatory cell population within the infiltrated gingival connective tissue from predominantly lymphocytic (T cell) to predominantly plasma cell (B cell) type. Large amounts of immunoglobulin are present throughout the connective and epithelial tissues. The plasma cell infiltration is not confined to the reaction site around the base of the sulcus but extends along blood vessels and between collagen fibre bundles, into the deeper parts of the gingival connective tissue. There is continuing loss of collagen as the area of inflammation slowly expands.

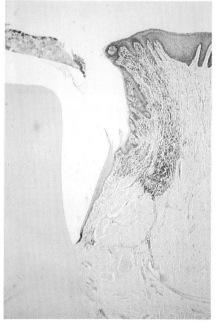

Fig. 7.4 Established gingivitis.

Table 7.6 Pathological features of established gingivitis

Persistence of the features of initial gingivitis
Further disruption and hyperplasia of junctional epithelium
Ulceration of gingival pocket epithelium
Predominance of plasma cells in inflammatory infiltrate: —reduction in relative proportion of lymphocytes
Continued destruction of gingival connective tissue
Expansion of volume of tissue involved
Varying attempts at repair; hyperplastic gingivitis

In areas away from the zone of destruction there may be varying attempts at repair characterized by the formation of fibrous tissue. However, the newly-formed collagen bundles do not simulate the architecture of the previously existing gingival fibres. In some instances, exuberant fibrous tissue formation results in gingival hyperplasia and false pocketing. The destruction of the specifically orientated gingival fibres, fibrosis, and hyperplasia contribute to the loss of normal gingival form seen clinically in chronic gingivitis. Oedematous enlargement, resulting from increased vascular permeability associated with inflammation, is another factor.

Degradation of extracellular matrix

The mechanisms of degradation of the extracellular matrix, especially collagen, in periodontal disease are not well understood, but they are of major importance since destruction of the connective tissue attachment results ultimately in loss of the tooth. In health, normal collagen turnover is reflected in a balance between the relative rates of synthesis and degradation (Fig. 7.5). The loss in disease could, therefore, be the consequence of a decreased rate of synthesis, increased rate of degradation, or a combination of both. Although damage to fibroblasts in the inflamed area would result in decreased synthesis, increased degradation involving enhanced enzyme activity is the major factor.

The destruction of the extracellular matrix may involve the activity of bacterial enzymes from the plaque, but is effected mainly by a family of enzymes, the metalloproteinases, derived from host cells. These enzymes, principally collagenase and stromalysin, are produced mainly by fibroblasts, macrophages, and neutrophil leucocytes and are secreted in a latent form requiring activation before they can degrade matrix proteins. In health, this activity is carefully regulated by mechanisms which are not well understood but which include, for example, the production of tissue inhibitor of metalloproteinase (TIMP) by host cells, probably at the same time as they are synthesizing and secreting metalloproteinases. In periodontal disease, the release of metalloproteinases is increased due to

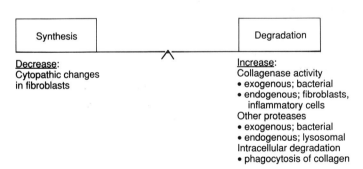

Synthesis

Degradation

Decrease:
Cytopathic changes
in fibroblasts

Increase:
Collagenase activity
• exogenous; bacterial
• endogenous; fibroblasts,
   inflammatory cells
Other proteases
• exogenous; bacterial
• endogenous; lysosomal
Intracellular degradation
• phagocytosis of collagen

Fig. 7.5 Factors involved in loss of collagen and connective tissue destruction in gingivitis.

Gingivitis   **Key points**

• initial lesion—microscopic; acute exudative changes
• early lesion—dominated by T lymphocytes
• established lesion—dominated by plasma cells
• inflammation impairs barrier function of junctional epithelium
• connective tissue destruction involves metalloproteinases
• release of metalloproteinases by host cells increased by inflammatory cytokines

activation of host cells by a variety of cytokines, especially interleukin-1, generated in the inflammatory response to microbial plaque. Increased amounts of both active and latent metalloproteinases are present in inflamed compared with non-inflamed sites.

The advanced lesion—chronic periodontitis

The advanced lesion corresponds to chronic periodontitis, a disease characterized by destruction of the connective tissue attachment of the root of the tooth, loss of alveolar bone, and pocket formation. Although periodontitis is the result of extension of inflammation from the gingiva into the deeper tissues, the natural history of the untreated lesion of established gingivitis is not well understood. Gingivitis in some patients may remain stable for years, in others it either progresses slowly to periodontitis or, in a minority of patients, there may be rapid progression and advanced bone-loss occurring at an early age. Factors governing the rate of progression remain largely unknown.

The earliest histological evidence of the progression of gingivitis to periodontitis is the extension of inflammation beneath the base of the junctional epithelium into the supra-alveolar connective tissue. Plasma cells dominate the infiltrate at all stages of the advanced lesion, although lymphocytes and macrophages are also present. As the area and density of the infiltrate increase there is destruction of collagen in the supra-alveolar connective tissue and the fibres lose their attachment to cementum (Fig. 7.6). This is accompanied by apical migration of the junctional epithelium to cover the denuded root surface resulting in early true pocket formation (Fig. 7.7). As the disease extends into the supporting tissues there is progressive destruction of the fibres of the periodontal ligament accompanied by osteoclastic resorption of the alveolar bone. The junctional epithelium continues to migrate apically, resulting in progressive deepening of the pockets. As the junctional epithelium migrates apically the more coronal and inflamed tissue loses its specialized attachment and is converted into pocket epithelium. The width of the zone of attachment of the junctional epithelium at the base of the pocket remains fairly constant throughout the course of the disease.

Key points

Periodontitis
- extension of inflammation into alveolar bone and periodontal ligament
- destruction of the connective tissue attachment
  —collagen degradation
  —bone resorption
  —pocket formation

The pathway of spread of inflammation into the supporting tissues influences the pattern of bone destruction and morphology of the pockets. In general, the spread of inflammation follows the course of blood vessels. In the interdental areas the infiltrate extends mainly along the rich anastomotic supply running from beneath the interdental col towards the midpoint of the crest of the interdental septa and into underlying marrow spaces (Fig. 7.8). Osteoclastic resorption results in interdental cratering. In marginal areas, inflammation follows the course of supraperiosteal vessels, enters the marrow spaces along vessels penetrating the outer cortical plates, and progresses inwards towards the root of the tooth. These pathways of spread, which follow the main vascular supplies, tend

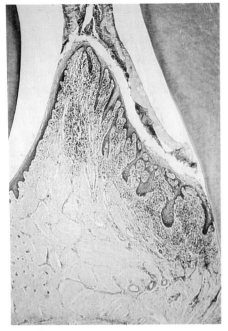

Fig. 7.6

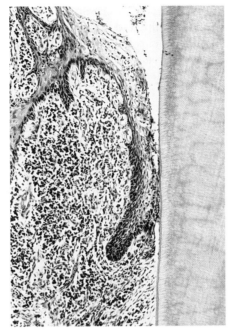

Fig. 7.7

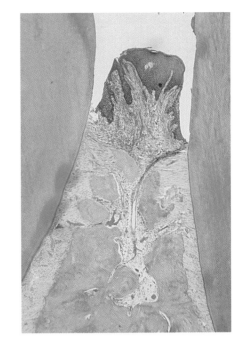

Fig. 7.8

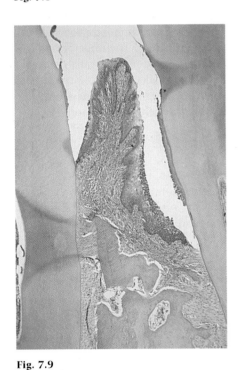

Fig. 7.9

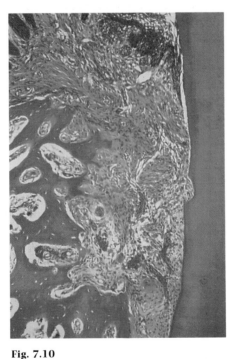

Fig. 7.10

Fig. 7.6 Early periodontitis showing extension of inflammation into supra-alveolar tissues and early loss of attachment.

Fig. 7.7 High-power view of Fig. 7.6 showing apical migration of the junctional epithelium over the denuded root surface at the base of the developing pocket.

Fig. 7.8 Spread of inflammation towards the midpoint of the interdental septum.

Fig. 7.9 Chronic periodontitis with infrabony pocket.

Fig. 7.10 Spread of inflammation into periodontal ligament associated with resorption of bone at the base of an infrabony pocket.

to result in a horizontal pattern of bone loss and suprabony pockets. However, various factors can modify these pathways and may divert the spread of inflammation towards and directly into the periodontal ligament resulting in vertical patterns of bone loss and infrabony pockets (Figs 7.9, 7.10). These factors include the previously existing bone morphology, the morphology and alignment of teeth, occlusal trauma, and plaque retentive factors such as overhanging restorations. Thus, in any one patient the pattern of bone loss can be affected by many factors. Both horizontal and vertical defects may occur in different areas of the same mouth and in different areas around a single tooth.

Although chronic periodontal disease is characterized by destruction of the connective tissue attachment of the teeth, the rate of progression of the lesions is not constant and phases of tissue destruction and bone resorption may alternate with periods of remission. Current hypotheses suggest that loss of attachment occurs as brief bursts of destructive activity at random time intervals throughout an individual's life. During periods of remission there may be attempts at healing. For example, as the pockets deepen, there are continuous attempts to re-form the transeptal, and to some extent the dentogingival and dentoperiosteal, fibres at progressively more apical levels. Also, the bony wall of a pocket may show osteoblastic activity in addition to osteoclastic resorption, although the extent of this bony healing in untreated disease appears limited to the microscopic infilling of some of the resorptive lacunae.

The main features of the advanced lesion are summarized in Table 7.7. Histological examination of an established periodontal pocket (Fig. 7.11) shows the following features. The pocket is bounded on one side by denuded root surface and on the other by pocket epithelium. At the base of the pocket a narrow zone of junctional epithelium mediates the soft-tissue attachment to the root. The pocket contains subgingival calculus and plaque and inflammatory exudate comprising fluid and cells, mainly PMN. The pocket epithelium varies in quality and thickness. Areas of irregular hyperplasia and rete ridge formation alternate with areas of thinning and even frank ulceration. The vessels in the subjacent connective tissue are markedly dilated and there is emigration of large numbers of PMN which transmigrate the pocket epithelium. The underlying connective tissue is densely infiltrated by inflammatory cells; plasma cells predominate. The inflammatory infiltrate may extend into adjacent marrow spaces. In actively progressing disease, osteoclasts may be seen along the bone front and within marrow spaces, but they are infrequent in relatively stable lesions.

Bone resorption in periodontal disease

Mechanisms involved in bone loss in periodontitis are still unclear, but involve factors which stimulate the proliferation, differentiation, and activation of osteoclasts. In normal remodelling of bone, osteoblastic and osteoclastic activity are tightly coupled, after a wave of osteoclastic resorption osteoblastic deposition

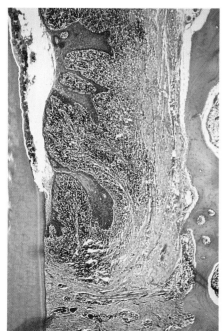

Fig. 7.11   Deep, established infrabony pocket.

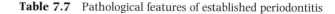

Table 7.7   Pathological features of established periodontitis

Persistence of the features of established gingivitis

Apical extension of destructive inflammation:
—into supra-alveolar connective tissues
—into alveolar bone
—into periodontal ligament

Predominance of plasma cells

Loss of connective tissue attachment:
—destruction of collagen
—apical migration of junctional epithelium
—pocket formation

Destruction of alveolar bone

Periods of quiescence/stability; episodes of destruction:
—attempts at healing

occurs. The control of this process involves the activities of a number of cytokines which stimulate or inhibit either osteoclastic or osteoblastic activity. In pathological processes associated with bone destruction this coupling is disturbed and the balance is shifted, resulting in loss of bone.

Several local mediators capable of stimulating osteoclastic activity have now been identified. They fall into three main categories: cytokines, prostaglandins, and growth factors influencing osteoblastic and osteoclastic interactions (Table 7.8). Interleukin-1, interleukin-6, and tumour necrosis factor (TNF) are the main cytokines which stimulate bone resorption and they probably mediate their activity through prostaglandin synthesis, especially PGE_2, which enhances osteoclastic activity. Interleukin-1 is probably the most potent stimulator of bone resorption known and many pathways exist for its generation, and that of other cytokines, in periodontal inflammation, some of which are illustrated in Figs 7.12, 7.13.

In addition to the stimulation of osteoclast activity by inflammatory cytokines, the development of osteoclasts is also enhanced by cytokines and growth factors released by bone matrix and bone cells during resorption. These include interleukin-6 and an osteogenic inductive factor.

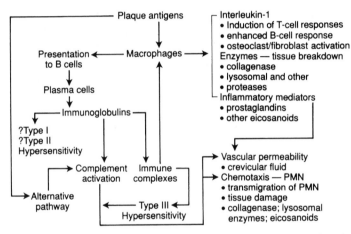

Fig. 7.12 Possible humoral immune mechanisms involved in periodontal disease.

Table 7.8 Local mediators affecting bone resorption

Cytokines:	interleukin-1
	interleukin-6
	tumour necrosis factors
Prostaglandins:	especially PGE_2
Growth factors:	e.g. factors from osteoblasts which regulate osteoclast recruitment

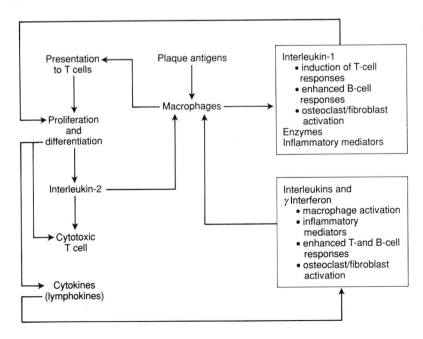

Fig. 7.13 Possible cell-mediated immune mechanisms involved in periodontal disease.

Pathogenic mechanisms in chronic periodontal disease

Substances from plaque initiate an inflammatory and immune response which is designed to resist the challenge to the integrity of the tissues posed by infection by periodontopathic bacteria. In meeting this challenge a complex array of inflammatory and immune mediators are generated which, whilst being essential for defence, are capable of activating host mechanisms of connective tissue breakdown. Most of the tissue destruction in periodontal disease is thought to be due to inappropriate activation of tissue degradation systems triggered by the host response to microbial plaque. The outcome of the challenge from the plaque depends, therefore, on the balance between the protective and destructive aspects of the host response. This will vary from individual to individual and from site to site, as well as with time and with plaque composition.

Fluctuation in the host–parasite relationship upset the balance between the protective and destructive aspects of the host response, and in most patients periodontal destruction occurs as random bursts of activity separated by periods of stability. Thus, following infection by periodontopathic bacteria there may be a period of active destruction before the host response is sufficiently protective to restore equilibrium to the host–parasite relationship. This new equilibrium will remain stable until at some unpredictable time in the future either the sudden overgrowth of a pathogen or some change in immunoregulation of the host response triggers another burst of tissue destruction. This will continue until balance is restored and a new equilibrium is established, and so on, at random intervals throughout life.

When this hypothesis is compared with the histopathological features seen in the development of periodontal disease the following points can be noted which relate to protective aspects of the host response:

1. Enhanced transmigration of the junctional and pocket epithelium by polymorphoneutrophils occurs at all stages. Comment has already been made of the importance of these cells in the local defence of the gingival sulcus. They accumulate in response to chemotactic factors generated in the sulcus, amongst which complement activation products present in crevicular fluid may be important.
2. The early lesion of experimental gingivitis is characterized by a T-cell response. Spontaneous gingivitis in children is also a lymphocyte dominated lesion which tends to remain stable or contained for long periods. Healthy children rarely develop periodontitis.
3. Established gingivitis and periodontitis are dominated by plasma cells, although T cells are well represented. Patients with periodontal disease have antibodies to periodontopathic bacteria in serum and in crevicular fluid. Some of the latter could be produced locally. It is likely that antibodies play an important role in combating periodontal pathogens.

Possible humoral and cell-mediated immune mechanisms involved in the pathogenesis of periodontal disease are summarized in Figs 7.12, 7.13. Although many of these are protective it will be noted that there are many pathways which could lead to the enhanced synthesis and secretion of a wide variety of potentially damaging cytokines and inflammatory mediators. Interleukin-1 is highlighted because of its potential importance in stimulating both degradation of the extracellular matrix and bone resorption, as discussed previously. Other mediators that are thought to play key roles in periodontal breakdown include interleukin-6 and prostaglandin E_2 (IL-1, IL-6, and PGE_2 are also thought to play an important role in bone resorption associated with cyst expansion—see p. 78). It is likely also that tumour necrosis factors (TNF-α, TNF-β) which share similar activities to IL-1 may also be involved, but the evidence is less strong than that for the mediators above.

Many of these cytokines and inflammatory mediators can be detected in crevicular fluid, along with products of tissue degradation and catabolic enzymes released by inflammatory and host tissue cells. Differences exist between disease active and inactive sites and it is likely that as understanding of the mechanisms of periodontal breakdown increases, diagnostic markers will be defined in crevicular fluid which identify patients and sites at risk of progressive disease.

Key points

Pathogenesis of periodontal disease
- disturbance in host–parasite relationship, leading to:
- activation of host inflammatory and immune response, leading to:
- enhanced synthesis of inflammatory mediators/cytokines, leading to:
- burst of breakdown of connective tissue/bone resorption, leading to:
- new equilibrium in host–parasite relationship as host response contains the challenge from plaque bacteria

Clinical forms of periodontitis

Four main categories of periodontitis have been described which can be distinguished by their clinical and, to some extent, pathological features (see Table 7.1). The main features of each type are described below, but for more detailed discussion the reader should consult texts in periodontology.

Prepubertal periodontitis

Prepubertal periodontitis is a rare form of periodontitis presenting in childhood and involving the deciduous and subsequently the permanent dentition. It is characterized by extensive destruction of alveolar bone and is associated with a variety of uncommon systemic disease (Table 7.9). Most involve abnormalities in number and/or function of PMN. Because of the deficient or defective neutrophils such patients are prone to severe systemic infections. The Papillon-Lefèvre syndrome is characterized by skin lesions of palmar-plantar hyperkeratosis and severe periodontal destruction involving both the deciduous and permanent dentitions. It is probably transmitted as an autosomal recessive, but the mechanisms underlying the oral changes are uncertain, although a neutrophil abnormality has been reported.

Table 7.9 Causes of prepubertal periodontitis

Diseases associated with major abnormalities of neutrophils:
—agranulocytosis
—cyclic neutropenia
—Chediak–Higashi syndrome
—Job syndrome

Diseases in which there may be associated neutrophil dysfunction:
—Papillon–Lefèvre syndrome
—Down syndrome
—juvenile onset diabetes mellitus

Other systemic diseases:
—hypophosphatasia
—Langerhans cell histiocytosis (histiocytosis-X group)
—Ehlers–Danlos syndrome (Type VIII)

Juvenile periodontitis

Juvenile periodontitis is a rare from of periodontitis which commences in young people and is clinically distinct from the usual form of periodontitis seen in adults. It commences around puberty and there is a higher incidence in females. The disease is characterized by rapid destruction of alveolar bone with vertical bone loss resulting in deep infrabony pockets. Initially, the permanent first molars and/or maxillary incisor teeth are affected, usually symmetrically, but the number of teeth involved increases with age. The pattern of involvement tends to follow the sequence of eruption.

The aetiolgy and pathogenesis of the condition remain obscure. The lesions are inflammatory and bacterial plaque is the prime aetiological factor, but the degree of destruction is not commensurate with the generally small amounts of plaque present. However, the subgingival flora in juvenile periodontitis differs significantly from that in adult periodontitis and is dominated by Gram-negative anaerobic rods, particularly *Actinobacillus actinomycetemcomitans*. *Capnocytophaga* species and *Eikenella corrodens* may also be of aetiological significance. In addition to a unique flora, host factors have also been implicated. In particular, a familial pattern has been found in several cases and there is increasing support for the suggestion that genetic factors are involved. Abnormalities in cell-mediated immunity and in PMN function have also been demonstrated.

Rapidly progressive periodontitis

Less common than juvenile periodontitis, rapidly progressive periodontitis has an onset between puberty and 30 years of age but lacks well-defined characteristics. The periodontal lesions are severe and generalized with evidence of rapid bone destruction occurring within a few weeks or months. The gingivae may appear acutely inflamed or relatively normal, and the amounts of microbial deposits are highly variable. Almost the entire dentition is usually affected and the disease may either progress without remission to tooth loss or subside and become quiescent. Vertical or angular bone loss occurs with marked differences in attachment loss between adjacent teeth or on different surfaces of the same tooth. The aetiology and pathogenesis are ill understood. Some patients have associated malaise or weight loss while many have associated defects in leucocyte function.

Adult type periodontitis

Adult type periodontitis is by far the most common form of chronic periodontal disease and is characterized by its chronicity. The onset of disease is in early adult life (or even before), but in the majority of patients does not progress to tooth loss until after 50 years of age. A generally regular pattern of predominantly horizontal bone loss is seen with suprabony pocketing. The entire dentition is usually involved, with the lower incisors and molars tending to show the most advanced bone loss.

GINGIVAL ENLARGEMENT

Chronic hyperplastic gingivitis and drug-associated hyperplasias

As discussed previously, chronic hyperplastic gingivitis represents a variation in host tissue response to the accumulation of dental plaque. In most cases the factors predisposing to the hyperplastic reaction are unknown, but it is well established that some degree of gingival enlargement can occur in epileptics and other patients taking the anticonvulsant drug phenytoin (Fig. 7.14). The percentage of patients affected varies from less than 10 per cent to over 60 per cent in different series. Dental plaque is an essential aetiological factor; the drug modifies a previously existing chronic gingivitis and good oral hygiene can prevent the gingival hyperplasia. The mechanisms by which the drug or its metabolites induce the hyperplasia are unknown, but certain gingival fibroblasts can metabolize phenytoin and this may be accompanied by an increased production of collagen. The distribution and activity of such a subpopulation of fibroblasts could be a factor determining the different susceptibilities of patients to gingival hyperplasia.

Clinically, the hyperplasia may be more or less generalized but primarily involves the interdental tissues, particularly around the labial surfaces of anterior teeth. The enlargement manifests as firm, pink, often lobulated fibrous masses that may obscure the crowns of the teeth. In patients where the marginal gingiva is relatively uninvolved, deep clefts separate adjacent bulbous interdental papillae. Histologically, the overgrowth consists mainly of bundles of collagen fibres but fibroblasts are common and there is a scattered chronic inflammatory cell infiltration. The surface epithelium is also often markedly hyperplastic and shows long slender rete processes extending into the underlying connective tissue.

A similar hyperplastic gingivitis may also occur in patients taking the immunosuppressive drug cyclosporin, following transplant procedures, and in those taking calcium channel blocking agents or calcium antagonists, such as nifedipine (Fig. 7.15) and verapamil, for cardiovascular disorders. The mechanisms are unclear but genetic predisposition, related to fibroblast susceptibility, and variations in the pharmacokinetics of drug metabolism are possible factors in addition to pre-existing gingivitis.

Gingival fibromatosis

Gingival fibromatosis is an uncommon hereditary condition transmitted through an autosomal dominant gene, although sporadic cases occur. It is probably the result of a developmental abnormality of fibroblast function. Clinically, the condition manifests as a generalized, or occasionally localized, fibrous enlargement of the gingiva. The enlargement usually appears in young children but may present from birth or may not be noticed until adult life. Occasionally, the condition is associated with hypertrichosis, epilepsy, and mental retardation. Microscopically, the fibrous tissue consists mainly of coarse bundles of collagen fibres, but mucoid

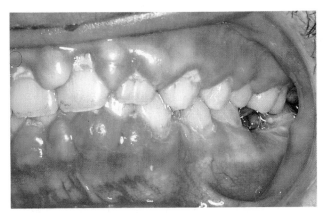

Fig. 7.14 Phenytoin-associated hyperplastic gingivitis.

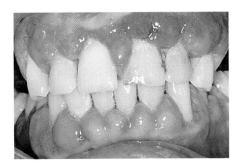

Fig. 7.15 Nifedipine-associated hyperplastic gingivitis.

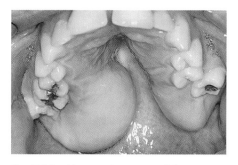

Fig. 7.16 Fibrous enlargement of the maxillary tuberosities.

change, due to the accumulation of ground substance, is common. The covering epithelium is often hyperplastic. Recurrence is likely following surgical excision.

Symmetrical fibrous enlargements may also occur in the maxillary tuberosity region (Fig. 7.16) and it is possible that some cases are related to gingival fibromatosis.

Other causes of gingival enlargement

In addition to fibrous overgrowth, generalized enlargement of the gingiva may be caused by oedema, by leukaemic infiltration in acute leukaemia, and may be a feature of other systemic diseases (Table 7.10). Localized enlargements (epulides) are discussed in Chapter 8.

DESQUAMATIVE GINGIVITIS

Desquamative gingivitis is not a disease entity but a clinical term applied to the gingival manifestation of several different diseases.

Clinically, the gingiva are red, oedematous, and glazed, and show areas of superficial ulceration or desquamation of varying extent. Vesicles, bullae, white flecks or striae may also be seen depending on the underlying aetiology. The involvement is patchy but the buccal and labial gingiva are more commonly affected than lingual or palatal tissues. The condition is more common in females than males and most cases occur after 30 years of age.

Key points	**Desquamative gingivitis**
	• the common clinical manifestation of a variety of different diseases
	• involves full width of attached gingiva

Correct identification of the underlying aetiolgy is important and the dermatoses, particularly mucous membrane pemphigoid and lichen planus (Fig. 7.17), account for most cases. Other cases may represent local hypersensitivity reactions to various substances, for example toothpastes, cosmetics (Fig. 7.18), chewing-gum, and cinnamon, used as a flavouring in some of the previous examples, and may occur alone or as part of an orofacial granulomatosis (see Chapter 13). The gingival reaction associated with chewing-gum hypersensitivity

Table 7.10 Causes of generalized enlargement of the gingiva

Fibrous overgrowths:	Gingival fibromatosis
	Chronic hyperplastic gingivitis
	Drug-associated hyperplasias
	—epanutin
	—cyclosporin
	—nifedipine and verapamil
Oedematous enlargement:	Oedematous gingivitis
	—puberty
	—pregnancy
	—oral contraceptives
	—scurvy
Systemic disease:	Acute leukaemias
	Wegener's granulomatosis

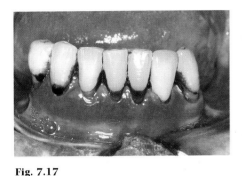

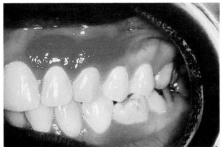

Fig. 7.17

Fig. 7.18

Fig. 7.17 Desquamative gingivitis associated with lichen planus.

Fig. 7.18 Desquamative gingivitis associated with hypersensitivity to lipstick localized to where the cosmetic contacted the gingiva.

has also been referred to as 'plasma-cell gingivitis' because of the widespread distribution of large numbers of plasma cells throughout the gingiva. Several other uncommon aetiological factors have also been suggested, which include hormonal disturbances in menopausal females, unusual manifestations of chronic infections, and abnormal responses to dental plaque. Dental plaque will exacerbate the inflammation from whatever cause and maintenance of adequate oral hygiene is important in management, but may be difficult because of soreness and bleeding associated with erosions.

LATERAL PERIODONTAL ABSCESS

The lateral periodontal abscess is a localized area of suppurative inflammation arising within the periodontal tissues alongside a tooth and is distinct from the more common periapical abscess. Most arise in patients with pre-existing advanced periodontitis, and may occur either as a direct result of an increase in virulence and toxic factors released by plaque organisms or secondary to reduction in host resistance. Obstruction to the drainage of exudate from a pocket predisposes to abscess formation. This may occur particularly in infrabony pockets pursuing a tortuous course around the root, or where fibrosis or oedema in the superficial parts of the pocket cause tight approximation of the soft-tissue wall to the neck of the tooth. Impaction of foreign material, such as food debris, into a pocket may also lead to abscess formation. In the absence of pocketing, periodontal abscesses may follow traumatic injury to a tooth, lateral perforation of the root in endodontic therapy, or stab infections. The latter arise when a foreign object, such as a toothbrush bristle or fish bone, penetrates the tissue introducing infection into the periodontal ligament. If there is only superficial penetration the abscess will be located in the gingiva.

Clinically, periodontal abscesses may be acute or chronic. An acute abscess develops rapidly and is accompanied by throbbing pain and redness, swelling, and tenderness of the overlying mucosa. The affected tooth is usually tender to percussion but most are vital. The abscess may discharge spontaneously through the mouth of a pocket, but in deep-seated lesions or where drainage is obstructed, it may track and present with a sinus opening on the mucosa somewhere along the length of the root (Fig. 7.19). Discharge of pus relieves the acute symptoms and the lesion may heal or become chronic with intermittent discharge. The chronic abscess may be asymptomatic or give rise to episodes of dull pain. Acute exacerbations are common.

Radiographic appearances are very variable and are influenced by the extent of previously existing bone destruction, the stage of the abscess, and its location. There is often extensive pocketing and abscess formation may be accompanied by rapid deepening of such defects, but in the early stages of an acute lesion there

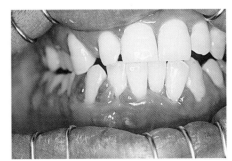

Fig. 7.19 Pointing lateral periodontal abscesses.

may be no associated radiographic changes. In deep-seated lesions there may be a discrete radiolucent area along the lateral aspect of the root.

PERICORONITIS

Pericoronitis is inflammation of the soft tissues around the crown of a partially erupted tooth and is seen commonly in association with mandibular third molars. The space between the crown of the tooth and the overlying gum flap is an ideal area for the accumulation of bacterial plaque and food debris, leading to inflammation. Inflammatory oedema leads to swelling of the flap which predisposes to trauma from the opposing teeth and exacerbation of the inflammation. The usual symptoms are pain, tenderness in the gum flap, and a bad taste which is associated with persistent oozing of pus from beneath the flap. Limitation of opening and discomfort on swallowing may also be present. In severe cases, an acute pericoronal abscess may develop which can remain localized or be associated with cellulitis and extension of infection into adjacent surgical spaces.

AGE CHANGES IN THE PERIODONTIUM

Although epidemiological studies have shown that the prevalence and severity of periodontal disease increases with age, this is most likely the result of repeated attacks of active destruction occurring with time rather than an intrinsic change associated with the ageing process itself. Gingival recession has been considered as an age change, but is now thought to be part of the clinical spectrum of periodontitis in which plaque and mechanical trauma are aetiological factors. There is no evidence that the elderly are particularly susceptible to periodontal disease, although this might be expected because of the decreased efficiency of both host defence systems and healing which are associated with ageing.

Several histological changes associated with ageing have been reported but it is likely that they are of little clinical significance. They include increased apposition of cementum, decreased cellularity of periodontal tissues, and disordered insertions of periodontal ligament fibres into bone and cementum.

FURTHER READING

Beck, J. D. and Slade, G. D. (1996). Epidemiology of periodontal diseases. *Current Opinion in Periodontology*, **3**, 3–9.

Birkedal-Hansen, H. (1993). Role of metalloproteinases in human periodontal diseases. *Journal of Periodontology*, **64**, 474–84.

Birkedal-Hansen, H. (1993). Role of cytokines and inflammatory mediators in tissue destruction. *Journal of Periodontal Research*, **28**, 500–10.

Brown, R. S., Beaver, W. T., and Bottomley (1991). On the mechanism of drug-induced gingival hyperplasia. *Journal of Oral Pathology and Medicine*, **20**, 201–9.

Cutress, T. W. (1986). Periodontal health and periodontal disease in young people: global epidemiology. *International Dental Journal*, **36**, 146–51.

Dahlen, G. (1993). Role of suspected periodontopathogens in microbiological monitoring of periodontitis. *Advances in Dental Research*, **7**, 163–74.

Embery, G. and Waddington, R. (1994). Gingival crevicular fluid: biomarkers of periodontal tissue activity. *Advances in Dental Research*, **8**, 329–36.

Genco, R. J. (1992). Host responses in periodontal diseases: current concepts. *Journal of Periodontology*, **63**, 338–55.

Genco, R. J., Christersson, L. A., and Zambon, J. J. (1986). Juvenile periodontitis. *International Dental Journal*, **36**, 168–76.

Hardie, J. M. (1992). Oral microbiology: current concepts in the microbiology of dental caries and periodontal disease. *British Dental Journal*, **172**, 271–8.

Kinane, D. F. and Davies, R. M. (1990). Periodontal manifestations of systemic disease. In *Oral manifestations of systemic disease* (2nd edn) (ed. J. H. Jones and D. K. Mason), pp. 512–36. W. B. Saunders, London.

Page, R. C. (1986). Gingivitis. *Journal of Clinical Periodontology*, **13**, 345–55.

Page, R. C. (1986). Current understanding of the aetiology and progression of periodontal disease. *International Dental Journal*, **36**, 153–61.

Page, R. (1991). The role of inflammatory mediators in the pathogenesis of periodontal disease. *Journal of Periodontal Research*, **26**, 230–42.

Saxen, L. (1980). Juvenile periodontitis. *Journal of Clinical Periodontology*, **7**, 1–19.

Seymour, R. A., Thomason, J. M., and Ellis, J. E. (1996). The pathogenesis of drug-induced gingival overgrowth. *Journal of Clinical Periodontology*, **23**, 165–75.

Socransky, S. S. and Haffajee, A. D. (1992). The bacterial etiology of destructive periodontal disease: current concepts. *Journal of Periodontology*, **63**, 322–31.

Van Dyke, T. E., Lester, M. A., and Shapira, L. (1993). The role of the host response in periodontal disease progression: implications for future treatment strategies. *Journal of Periodontology*, **64**, 792–806.

8 Connective tissue hyperplasia, neoplasia, and related disorders of oral mucosa

8 Connective tissue hyperplasia, neoplasia, and related disorders of oral mucosa

CONNECTIVE TISSUE HYPERPLASIA

Localized hyperplastic lesions of the oral mucosa are common and are usually responses to chronic inflammation. An essential feature of chronic inflammation is that the processes of inflammation and repair occur simultaneously and the production of granulation tissue is one of the hallmarks of the disease process. Most connective tissue hyperplasias of the oral mucosa represent exuberant production of granulation tissue in chronic inflammatory reactions. Although several named lesions are distinguished either on clinical or histological grounds, it is important to appreciate that many are variations of the same basic disease process. Histologically, there is a spectrum of change varying from chronically inflamed, richly cellular granulation tissue to relatively non-inflamed and avascular masses of dense collagen.

Connective tissue hyperplasias can originate anywhere in the oral cavity, but those arising from the gingiva usually receive the designation 'epulis'. Although the term is non-specific and literally means 'on the gum', by common usage it implies a localized chronic inflammatory hyperplasia of the gingiva. The exception is the rare congenital epulis of the newborn (see Chapter 10).

The common, localized connective tissue hyperplasias of oral mucosa are listed in Table 8.1.

Epulides

Epulides are common. They present as localized tumour-like gingival enlargements but are hyperplastic and not neoplastic lesions. Most arise from the interdental tissues. Trauma and chronic irritation, particularly from subgingival plaque and calculus, are considered to be the main aetiological factors.

Table 8.1 Localized connective tissue hyperplasias of the oral mucosa

Epulides
  —fibrous epulis
  —pyogenic granuloma
  —pregnancy epulis   } Vascular epulides
  —peripheral giant-cell granuloma (giant-cell epulis)

Pyogenic granuloma

Fibroepithelial polyp

Denture irritation hyperplasia

Papillary hyperplasia of the palate

Many terms have been applied to these lesions, which makes analysis of their incidence difficult. In one study of 200 consecutive cases, 65 per cent were of fibrous type, 28 per cent vascular, and 7 per cent were peripheral giant-cell granulomas. The lesions share several common clinical features. They are all more common in females than males, particularly so in the case of vascular lesions, and about 80 per cent occur anterior to the molar teeth. Over half of the lesions present in the intercanine area and they are slightly more common in the maxilla than the mandible. They have a tendency to recur, and from the same survey of 200 cases the recurrence rates were about 2 per cent for fibrous epulides, 14 per cent for vascular epulides, and 36 per cent for the peripheral giant-cell granuloma. However, recurrence rates differ considerably between series. Attempts to relate recurrence to histological features have largely been unsuccessful, and in most cases failure to identify and remove local precipitating factors and/or failure to completely excise the lesion in the first instance are the main factors.

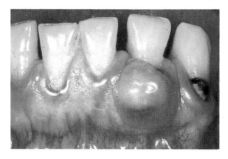

Fig. 8.1   Fibrous epulis.

Fibrous epulis

The fibrous epulis presents as a pedunculated or sessile mass which is usually of firm consistency and of similar colour to the adjacent gingiva (Fig. 8.1), although this will depend on the degree of vascularity and inflammation within the lesion. The surface may be ulcerated, in which case it will be covered by a yellowish fibrinous exudate. The epulis occurs over a wide age range but most arise between 11 and 40 years of age.

Histologically, the lesion comprises varying amounts of richly cellular fibroblastic granulation tissue and interlacing bundles of mature collagen fibres. There is a variable inflammatory cell infiltration, predominantly of plasma cells. Amorphous deposits of calcification and/or trabeculae of metaplastic bone are found within the fibroblastic tissue in about one-third of cases (Fig. 8.2), particularly if there is ulceration of the covering stratified squamous epithelium. However, there is no reason for regarding such epulides as a distinct entity and the presence or absence of calcification does not affect their clinical behaviour.

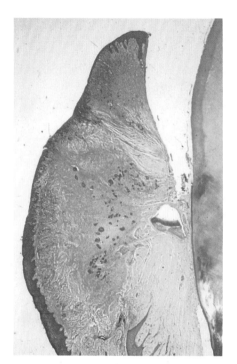

Fig. 8.2   Fibrous epulis with foci of calcification.

Vascular epulides

The pyogenic granuloma and pregnancy epulis present as rather soft, deep reddish-purple swellings (Fig. 8.3) which are often extensively ulcerated. Haemorrhage may occur either spontaneously or on minor trauma. The distinction between the lesions is purely clinical. Histologically, they are identical and the pregnancy epulis is regarded as a pyogenic granuloma occurring in a pregnant female. The lesions occur over a wide age range but, as might be expected, there is a peak incidence in females of child-bearing age. Lesions occurring in pregnancy can arise at any time from the first to the ninth month, although onset is usually around the end of the first trimester. They gradually increase in size, but after delivery may regress spontaneously or decrease in size and assume the clinical and histological features of a fibrous epulis. Control of haemorrhage may be difficult after excision of a pregnancy epulis but fibrosis of the lesion, following birth of the child, reduces the problem. Lesions excised during pregnancy also frequently recur and for these reasons it may be preferred to delay surgical treatment until after the birth of the child.

Histologically, the pyogenic granuloma and pregnancy epulis are characterized by vascular proliferation, which may take the form of rather solid sheets of endothelial cells with little evidence of canalization (Fig. 8.4) or of numerous small vessels and large, dilated, thin-walled vascular spaces (Fig. 8.5). Both patterns may

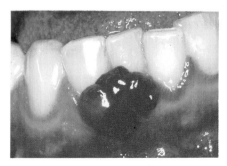

Fig. 8.3   Pyogenic granuloma (vascular epulis).

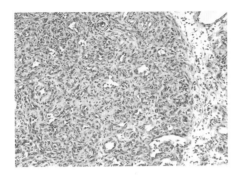

Fig. 8.4

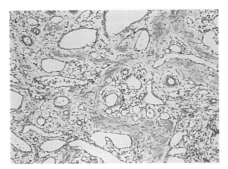

Fig. 8.5

Fig. 8.4 Pyogenic granuloma showing sheets of endothelial cells.

Fig. 8.5 Pyogenic granuloma showing numerous dilated capillary vessels.

coexist in different parts of the same lesion. The vascular element is supported by a delicate and often oedematous cellular fibrous stroma. Inflammatory cell infiltration is variable but seldom prominent except beneath areas of ulceration.

The term pyogenic granuloma is historical. It was originally applied because the identical lesion on skin was thought to be a reaction to infection by pyogenic organisms. Although this is no longer accepted, the term is now firmly entrenched in the dermatological and dental literature.

Peripheral giant-cell granuloma (giant-cell epulis)

The peripheral giant-cell granuloma has characteristics which separate it from the fibrous and vascular epulides. It occurs over a wide age range but the peak incidence in males is in the second decade compared to the fifth decade for females. The lesion can arise anywhere on the gingival or alveolar mucosa in dentate or edentate patients but most occur anterior to the molar teeth. Females are affected about twice as frequently as males, and slightly more occur in the mandible than in the maxilla. It presents as a pedunculated or sessile swelling of varying size which is typically dark red in colour and commonly ulcerated. In dentate areas of the jaws the lesion usually arises interdentally and may have an hour-glass shape with buccal and lingual swellings joined by a narrow waist between the teeth (Fig. 8.6). Radiographs may reveal superficial erosion of the crest of the interdental bone or, in edentulous areas, of the alveolar bone margin but these are not constant features. However, radiographs are essential for diagnosis since a central giant cell lesion which has perforated the cortex will present as a peripheral swelling.

Microscopically, the peripheral giant-cell granuloma consists essentially of focal collections of multinucleated osteoclast-like giant cells lying in a richly vascular and cellular stroma (Figs 8.7, 8.8). The collections of giant cells are separated by fibrous septa. A narrow zone of fibrous tissue, often containing dilated

Fig. 8.6 Peripheral giant-cell granuloma arising interdentally.

Fig. 8.7 Peripheral giant-cell granuloma with ulcerated surface showing focal collections of giant cells in a vascular, cellular stroma.

Fig. 8.8 Multinucleated giant cells in a peripheral giant-cell granuloma.

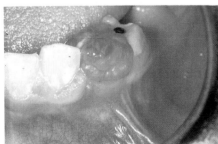

Fig. 8.6

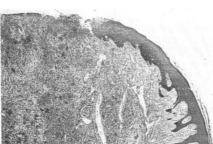

Fig. 8.7

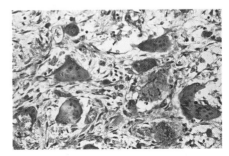

Fig. 8.8

blood vessels, also separates the core of the lesion from the covering stratified squamous epithelium.

The giant cells are numerous and show considerable variation in size, shape, staining reaction, and number of nuclei. Their cytoplasmic boundaries may be distinct or may appear to blend with each other or with the surrounding mononuclear stromal cells. Large numbers of vascular channels of varying diameter are found throughout, and occasionally giant cells may appear to protrude into or to be located within these channels. Extravasated red blood cells and deposits of haemosiderin are also common. The mononuclear stromal cells are ovoid or spindle-shaped and ultrastructural studies have identified fibroblasts, macrophages, osteoblasts, and undifferentiated cell types. Some macrophages contain phagocytosed haemosiderin. Occasionally, a few trabeculae of bone or osteoid may be found within the lesion.

Key points	Epulides
	• localized gingival hyperplasias
	• reactive to local irritation/trauma
	• may recur unless predisposing factors removed
	• exuberant granulation/fibrous tissue
	• vascular type may mature to fibrous type
	• giant-cell type clinically and histologically distinct

The pathogenesis of the peripheral giant-cell granuloma is unknown, but it is generally accepted that it is a reactive hyperplasia and, like other hyperplastic conditions of the oral mucosa, trauma may be an important aetiological factor. An origin from periosteum rather than gingiva has been suggested since the lesion can cause superficial erosion of bone and occurs in edentate as well as dentate areas of the jaws. The origin of the giant cells is not fully resolved. They are probably derived from mononuclear precursors in the surrounding stroma possibly as a result of fusion of macrophages. Similarities to osteoclasts have also been reported.

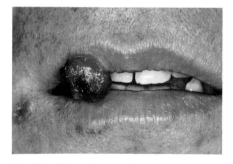

Fig. 8.9 Pyogenic granuloma.

Pyogenic granuloma

Although the majority of pyogenic granulomas in the oral cavity arise on the gingiva, the lesion can occur at other sites, for example the tongue, and buccal and labial mucosa (Fig. 8.9) as a result of trauma. The clinical appearances and histology are the same as for the gingival lesion.

Fibroepithelial polyp

The fibroepithelial polyp is a common lesion occurring over a wide age range. It arises mainly in the cheeks, particularly along the occlusal line, lips, and tongue and presents as a firm, pink, painless pedunculated or sessile polypoid swelling which varies in size from a few millimetres to a centimetre or more in diameter (Fig. 8.10). When the lesion occurs in the palate under a denture it becomes flattened and leaf-like and is commonly referred to as a leaf fibroma (Fig. 8.11). This is a misnomer since the lesion is not a benign neoplasm. Once established, the fibroepithelial polyp does not appear to increase significantly in size with time, and some patients may have been aware of a lump in the mouth for many years. Minor trauma is thought to be an important initiating factor and occasionally the surface is whitish due to mild frictional keratosis. Ulceration is not a feature unless the patient has bitten into the polyp.

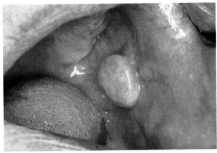

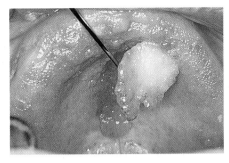

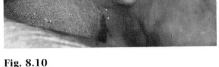

Fig. 8.10

Fig. 8.11

Fig. 8.10   Fibroepithelial polyp.

Fig. 8.11   Leaf fibroma (fibroepithelial polyp).

Histologically, the lesion comprises a core of dense, relatively avascular and acellular fibrous tissue, which has a scar-like quality (Fig. 8.12). Thick interlacing bundles of collagen fibres are the dominant feature and they blend with those of the adjacent normal tissue through the base of the lesion. Fibroblasts are scanty although plump, angular, and occasionally multinucleate forms are sometimes observed, particularly in the subepithelial zone, and such lesions are referred to by some authors as giant-cell fibromas (see later). The surface is covered by stratified squamous epithelium which may vary in thickness and show areas of hyperkeratosis in response to frictional irritation. Typically, there is little or no inflammatory cell infiltration and the lesion can be regarded as an exuberance of reparative scar tissue.

Denture irritation hyperplasia

The term denture irritation hyperplasia is applied to hyperplastic mucosa related to the periphery of an ill-fitting denture. The lesions may be single or multiple and present most frequently as one or several broad-based, leaf-like folds of tissue embracing the over-extended flange of the denture (Figs 8.13, 8.14). They usually arise in the depths of the vestibular and lingual sulci but can involve the inner surfaces of the lips and cheeks, and the palate along the posterior edge of an upper denture. They occur more frequently in relation to lower than upper dentures, and more often in females than males. Most of the patients have worn ill-fitting dentures for many years. Clinically, the hyperplastic tissue is usually firm in consistency and not grossly inflamed, but there may be ulceration at the base into which the flange of the denture fits.

Papillary hyperplasia of the palate

The aetiology of this condition is not fully understood, but minor trauma, related to rocking and rotation of ill-fitting dentures, and poor denture hygiene are

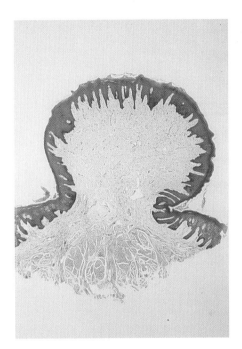

Fig. 8.12   Fibroepithelial polyp.

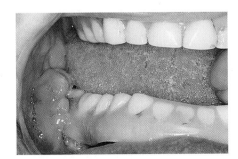

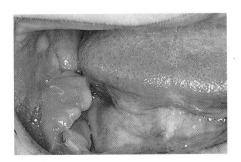

Fig. 8.13

Fig. 8.14

Fig. 8.13   Denture irritation hyperplasia.

Fig. 8.14   Folds of hyperplastic tissue associated with the ill-fitting denture in Fig. 8.13.

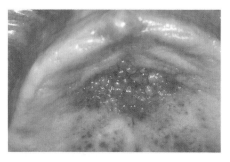

Fig. 8.15 Papillary hyperplasia of the palate.

factors in most cases. The patient may give a history of sleeping with dentures in and often there is a chronic atrophic candidosis (see Chapter 11) which may be a contributing factor. Clinically, the condition presents as numerous, small, tightly packed papillary projections over part or all of the denture-bearing area which gives the hard palate a pebbled appearance (Fig. 8.15). The mucosa is often red and oedematous particularly if there is an accompanying candidosis.

Microscopically, the lesion shows numerous papillary projections each comprising a core of hyperplastic, chronically inflamed granulation and fibrous tissue. The covering stratified squamous epithelium is also hyperplastic, and in some cases this may be so prominent that the unwary pathologist may mistake it initially for a squamous cell carcinoma. This appearance may be referred to as pseudo-epitheliomatous hyperplasia and is characterized by irregular proliferation and branching of rete ridges which extend for considerable distances into the underlying connective tissue, suggesting invasion. Keratin pearl formation may also occur within the hyperplastic epithelium, but there are no atypical cytological features.

CONNECTIVE TISSUE NEOPLASMS AND ALLIED CONDITIONS

A great variety of benign and malignant connective tissue tumours and tumour-like lesions have been reported from the oral cavity but, with few exceptions, they are all rare. Clinically, most of the benign connective tissue tumours present as swellings which may be indistinguishable from hyperplastic lesions. Histologically, oral connective tissue tumours resemble their counterparts occurring at other sites in the body. The various lesions will be discussed under their tissues of origin.

Tumours of fibrous tissue

In comparison to hyperplastic lesions, neoplasms and other causes of fibrous overgrowth (Table 8.2) are rare in the mouth.

True fibromas, if they exist at all, are very rare and seldom diagnosed. Clinically and histologically they may be indistinguishable from fibroepithelial polyps. However, where there is a clear zone of distinction between the fibrous

Table 8.2 Localized fibrous overgrowths of the oral mucosa. (Causes of generalized fibrous overgrowth of the gingiva are discussed in chapter 7)

Hyperplastic lesions
—epulides (fibrous, vascular, giant cell)
—pyogenic granuloma
—fibroepithelial polyp
—denture irritation and papillary hyperplasia

Neoplastic and neoplastic-like lesions
—fibroma
—giant-cell fibroma
—fibrous histiocytoma
—malignant fibrous histiocytoma
—fibrosarcoma

Fibromatoses
—nodular fasciitis
—gingival fibromatosis

tissue of the lesion and that of the surrounding normal tissues such lesions have been designated as fibromas.

The status of the so-called giant-cell fibroma is also doubtful. Although it has fairly distinct histopathological features it is most likely a variant of the fibro-epithelial polyp. The lesion occurs anywhere on the oral mucosa but is com-monest on the gingiva and presents as a polypoid growth. Most develop within the first three decades. Histologically, it consists of interlacing bundles of colla-gen (resembling a fibroepithelial polyp) amongst which multinucleated and angular giant cells of fibroblastic origin are scattered (Fig. 8.16). The giant cells are quite different in appearance from the osteoclast-like giant cells seen in giant-cell granulomas.

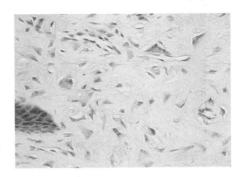

Fig. 8.16   Giant-cell fibroma.

The fibrous histiocytoma is a rare tumour in the oral cavity and is derived from cells which show varying degrees of fibroblastic and histiocytic differentia-tion. It can present a range of histopathological appearances, but typically is richly cellular and consists of short, interwoven bundles of spindle cells which on section produce a characteristic cartwheel or storiform pattern. Multinucleated giant cells of varying appearances may be scattered amongst the spindle cells. The tumour is of unpredictable but aggressive behaviour. There is no clear-cut distinction between benign and malignant lesions, but malignant fibrous histio-cytomas are more pleomorphic and some contain large numbers of multinucle-ated giant cells.

Fibrosarcoma of the oral soft tissues is rare but appears to have a good progno-sis with reported 5-year survival rates of about 70 per cent.

It is convenient to mention here that overgrowths of fibrous tissue may occur not only as inflammatory hyperplasias and true neoplasms but also as a wide range of dysplastic lesions which have none of the features of unequivocal neo-plasia nor of an inflammatory response. These lesions are grouped together as fibromatoses. Some have an infiltrative capacity which mimics fibrosarcoma but metastases do not occur. Histologically, they may resemble fibrosarcoma or malignant fibrous histiocytoma, but a differential diagnosis is essential since they do not require the radical excision necessitated by malignant neoplasms. They are rare in the orofacial region but sporadic cases of nodular fasciitis have been reported. This lesion, which is a relatively common subcutaneous growth else-where, arises as a solitary nodule from the superficial fascia and extends into underlying fat and muscle. It is locally infiltrative and has a pseudosarcomatous appearance.

Gingival fibromatosis (see Chapter 7) can also be considered as one of the fibro-matoses, but its characteristic clinical features and bland histological appearances distinguish it. It has none of the pseudosarcomatous features that other members of the group may show.

Tumours of adipose tissue

The lipoma presents as a soft, elastic, yellowish-coloured swelling which in the mouth occurs most commonly in the cheek and tongue (Fig. 8.17). Microscopically, the tumour consists of a circumscribed mass of mature adipose tissue supported by a fibrous stroma (Fig. 8.18). The amount of stroma varies considerably and in some tumours forms a significant part of the lesion. Such lesions are usually described as fibrolipomas. A typical feature of a lipoma is that the tumour floats in the fixative solution when dropped into a specimen bottle.

Liposarcomas are uncommon neoplasms in the orofacial region. The majority of those reported have been of the well-differentiated, myxoid type which responds well to local excision. Most of the intraoral lesions arise in the cheek or floor of the mouth/base of tongue.

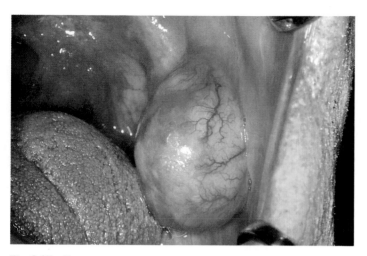

Fig. 8.17 Lipoma.

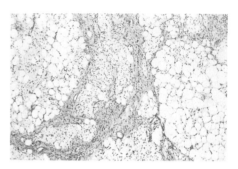

Fig. 8.18 Lipoma.

It should be remembered that in infants and very young children ulcerated tumour-like masses of partly necrotic fat may occasionally be seen protruding through the mucosa of the cheek as a result of traumatic herniation of the buccal pad of fat.

Tumours of vascular tissue

Haemangioma

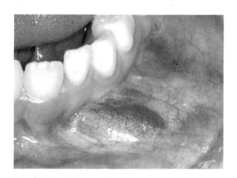

Fig. 8.19 Haemangioma.

Haemangiomas are common tumours which are generally accepted to be hamartomatous rather than truly neoplastic. They occur more commonly in the head and neck region than in any other part of the body, and most are present at birth or arise in early childhood, although some may not be noticed until old age. Oral lesions occur most commonly in the lips, tongue, cheeks, or palate and vary considerably in size and shape. They are characteristically dark reddish-purple in colour (Fig. 8.19), of soft consistency, and may present as a smooth, flat or raised, sometimes globular lesion of the mucosa. Typically, they blanch on pressure. Some may have a nodular consistency on palpation as a result of thrombosis and calcification, in which case the phleboliths may be detected radiographically. The lesions are usually symptomless although trauma may give rise to haemorrhage. A history of recent increase in size may be due to haemorrhage, thrombosis, or inflammation. Haemangiomas are usually solitary, although multiple lesions may occur and, rarely, these may be part of a generalized angiomatous syndrome.

Histologically, haemangiomas are usually divided into capillary and cavernous types depending on the size of the vascular spaces, although mixed types are common (Figs 8.20, 8.21). The spaces are lined by endothelium and contain red blood cells. Thrombosis, organization, and calcification may occur Some lesions, particularly in infants, may be more solid and extremely cellular and consist of sheets of endothelial cells with little evidence of canalization. These may represent an immature stage of the capillary or cavernous type and differentiation from a pyogenic granuloma may be difficult. Angiomatous malformation may also involve arteries and veins and some lesions consist almost entirely of thick-walled vessels. They may be referred to as racemose or cirsoid haemangiomas.

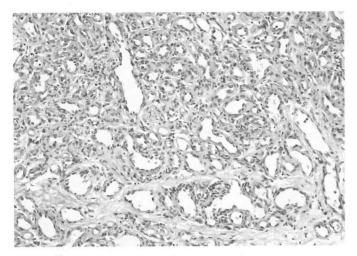

Fig. 8.20 Capillary haemangioma.

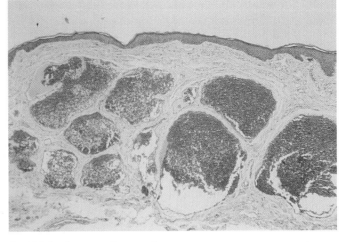

Fig. 8.21 Cavernous haemangioma.

Haemangiomas **Key points**

- common, hamartomatous lesions
- various clinical/histological subtypes
- may be part of an angiomatous syndrome

In addition to the mucosa, oral haemangiomas may also involve muscle, bone, and the major salivary glands. Although the latter are infrequent, the juvenile haemangioma is the commonest tumour occurring in the salivary glands during infancy and childhood. It occurs more frequently in females than in males.

Other vascular anomalies seen in oral mucosa are sublingual varicosities affecting the ranine veins, and haemangiomatous lesions on the vermilion border of the lips. Both of these conditions increase in frequency with age.

Malignant vascular tumours are rare, but the lesions of Kaposi's sarcoma are commonly found in the mouth of patients with the Acquired Immunodeficiency Syndrome (AIDS). It is discussed in more detail in Chapter 11.

Generalized angiomatous syndromes that may have oral lesions include:

Sturge–Weber syndrome

This congenital disorder is characterized by the combination of haemangiomatous lesions of the face over one or more branches of the trigeminal nerve (Fig. 8.22), ipsilateral haemangiomas and calcifications of the leptomeninges over the cerebral cortex, and convulsions affecting the limbs on the opposite side of the body. Haemangiomas may also occur in the oral mucosa.

Hereditary haemorrhagic telangiectasia

This disorder is transmitted as an autosomal dominant and is characterized by multiple knots of dilated malformed capillaries (telangiectases) in skin, mucous membranes (Fig. 8.23), and internal organs. Frequent nose-bleeding is the commonest presenting symptom.

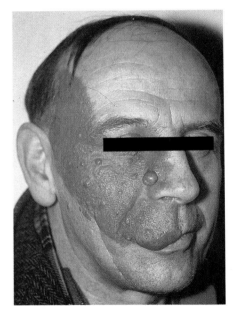

Fig. 8.22 Haemangiomatous malformation related to maxillary division of the trigeminal nerve in Sturge–Weber syndrome.

Lymphangioma

Lymphangiomas are less common than haemangiomas but like the latter are considered to be hamartomatous rather than neoplastic lesions. They are usually present at birth or arise in early childhood, and although they can occur anywhere

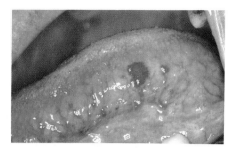

Fig. 8.23

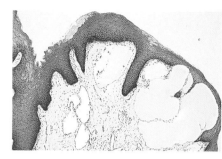

Fig. 8.25

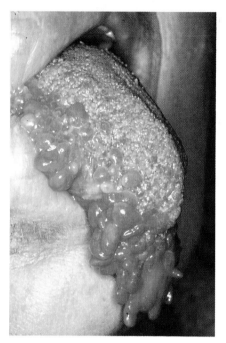

Fig. 8.24

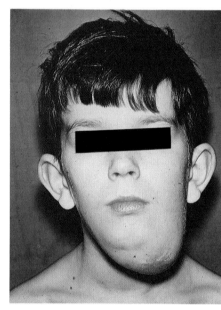

Fig. 8.26

Fig. 8.23 Hereditary haemorrhagic telangiectasia.

Fig. 8.24 Lymphangioma with macroglossia.

Fig. 8.25 Lymphangioma of the tongue.

Fig. 8.26 Cystic hygroma.

in the oral mucosa they are seen most frequently in the tongue and are a well-recognized cause of macroglossia (Fig. 8.24). Trauma to a lymphangioma may give rise to inflammation, calcification, or a sudden increase in size.

Histologically, the lesion consists of capillary or more commonly cavernous, endothelial-lined spaces containing lymph. A rather typical feature of superficially located lesions is that the lymphatic spaces extend close up to the overlying epithelium which they may cause to bulge (Fig. 8.25). Clinically, the surface of such lesions manifests numerous papillary projections or small nodular masses.

The cystic hygroma (Fig. 8.26) is a lymphangiomatous malformation which occurs early in the development of the lymphatic system and most frequently affects the head and particularly neck region. Most are detected at birth and present as large, fluctuant swellings often up to 10 cm in diameter. They may extend to involve the base of tongue, floor of mouth and, less commonly, buccal mucosa.

Tumours of peripheral nerves

The main tumours of peripheral nerves, which arise in connection with the nerve sheath, are the neurofibroma and neurilemmoma. Traumatic neuromas which are non-neoplastic, tumour-like masses also occur.

Tumours of peripheral nerves

- neurofibroma
  —solitary
  —multiple (neurofibromatosis)
- neurilemmoma (Schwannoma)
- multiple mucosal neuromas
- traumatic neuroma

The neurofibroma may present as a solitary lesion or occur as multiple tumours associated with neurofibromatosis (von Recklinghausen's disease of nerves). Neurofibromatosis is a developmental disorder of nerve sheaths characterized by multiple hamartomatous tumour-like masses which can occur either anywhere in the body (type 1) or more rarely only involve the central nervous system (type 2). About half of the patients with type 1 give a family history of the disorder which is transmitted as an autosomal dominant characteristic. This disorder is associated with abnormality in the neurofibromatosis-1 gene, a tumour suppressor gene on chromosome 17. The cutaneous nerves (Fig. 8.27) are usually involved and large tumour-like masses can cause considerable disfigurement—elephantiasis neuromatosa. The skin may also show melanic pigmentation described as *café-au-lait* spots, which precede the neural lesions. Oral lesions occur in about 7 per cent of cases as mucosal swellings (Fig. 8.28) involving most frequently the tongue and gingiva or, more rarely, as intraosseous growths. The latter are more common in the mandible than the maxilla and arise in association with the inferior dental and mental nerves.

Malignant change in neurofibromas is a well-recognized complication in patients with neurofibromatosis, occurring in about 5–15 per cent of cases. Malignant change in solitary lesions is very rare.

Histologically, neurofibromas show considerable variation, but consist basically of a mixture of Schwann cells and fibroblasts with varying amounts of collagen and mucoid ground substance. A few nerve fibres run through the lesion which may be circumscribed or diffuse (Fig. 8.29). Lesions arising within or around the nerve trunk consist of a mass of convoluted nerves surrounded by a proliferation of Schwann cells and fibroblasts. This pattern is referred to as a plexiform neurofibroma and is characteristic of neurofibromatosis.

The neurilemmoma (Schwannoma) is a well-demarcated or encapsulated tumour (Fig. 8.30) consisting either of parallel arrays of collagen fibres and spindle-cells with palisaded nuclei (Antoni type A pattern) (Fig. 8.31) or of disorderly arranged cells and collagen fibres in a mucinous, microcystic stroma (Antoni type B). Unlike the neurofibroma, nerve fibres do not run through the lesion but may be splayed over the capsule.

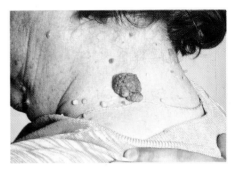

Fig. 8.27 Neurofibromatosis involving cutaneous nerves.

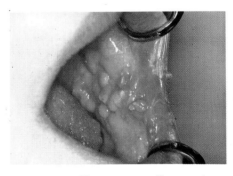

Fig. 8.28 Oral lesions in neurofibromatosis.

Fig. 8.29 Neurofibroma showing nerve fibres surrounded by proliferated Schwann cells and fibroblasts.

Fig. 8.30 Neurilemmoma showing encapsulation.

Fig. 8.31 Palisading of nuclei in neurilemmoma.

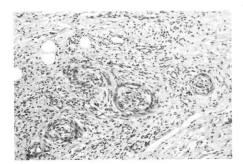

Fig. 8.29

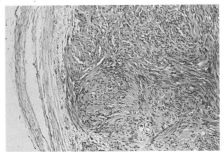

Fig. 8.30

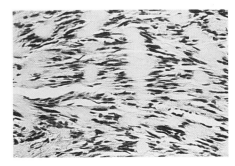

Fig. 8.31

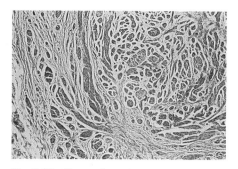

Fig. 8.32   Traumatic neuroma.

Multiple tumour-like malformations (neuromas) of peripheral nerves in oral mucosa, particularly along the lateral margins of the tongue, are an important feature of the multiple endocrine neoplasia syndrome Type 3 (MEN-3) which is also known as MEN 2b. The other main features of the syndrome are medullary carcinoma of the thyroid (developing in childhood or adolescence) and phaeochromocytoma. It is important to recognize multiple neuromas as they may precede the thyroid carcinoma by several years. Their presence indicates the need for urgent endocrine evaluation, particularly measurement of plasma calcitonin.

The traumatic neuroma is a non-neoplastic disorganized overgrowth of nerve fibres, Schwann cells, and scar tissue occurring at the proximal end of a severed nerve (Fig. 8.32). It represents an exaggeration of the normal process of nerve regeneration and usually presents as a small nodule which can give rise to considerable pain on pressure. It is uncommon in the oral cavity, which is surprising considering the frequency with which nerves are severed as a consequence of tooth extraction and other common minor surgical procedures.

Tumours of muscle

Tumours of either voluntary or smooth muscle are rare in the oral cavity.

Leiomyomas are smooth muscle tumours and in the mouth most arise from the walls of blood vessels (angiomyomas). The tongue, hard palate, and buccal mucosa are the most frequent sites. The majority are asymptomatic but they sometimes present as tender or painful nodules. Leiomyomatous hamartomas have also been reported but are very rare.

Rhabdomyosarcoma in the head and neck region is primarily a disease of the first decade of life. Although it is the most common soft-tissue sarcoma of the head and neck, it is still a rare neoplasm and relatively few arise in the oral and oropharyngeal soft tissues. Of these, most occur in the soft palate, presenting as a rapidly growing fleshy painless mass. In some cases, the tumour presents as a cluster of multiple polypoid swellings resembling a bunch of grapes, referred to as botryoid rhabdomyosarcoma.

Leiomyosarcoma is exceedingly rare.

The granular cell tumour

It is convenient here to describe the granular cell tumour which was commonly referred to in the past as the granular cell myoblastoma, although a myoblastic origin is now disputed. Numerous other theories on the histogenesis of the lesion have been reported but most evidence now supports a neural origin, probably from Schwann cells or their precursors.

Clinically, the granular cell tumour presents as a painless, slow-growing swelling which arises most commonly in the tongue. It occurs over a wide age range and although it is generally stated that there is no sex predilection, there is some evidence of an increased incidence in females. Multiple tumours may occur.

Histologically, the lesion is non-encapsulated and consists of sheets and strands of large cells with an extremely granular, eosinophilic cytoplasm (Fig. 8.33). Striated muscle fibres lying between the granular cells may give the impression of invasion. but the lesion is entirely benign. Apparent transition between muscle fibres and granular cells may also be noted. However, ultrastructural studies have shown that in most cases groups of granular cells are surrounded by a basal lamina which separates them from adjacent muscle cells. The granules represent lysosomes, autophagic vacuoles, and residual bodies.

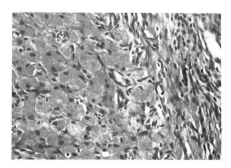

Fig. 8.33   Granular cell tumour.

The covering stratified squamous epithelium commonly shows pseudo-epitheliomatous hyperplasia (epithelial hyperplasia that may be mistaken for carcinoma). (Fig. 8.34).

Malignant lymphomas

Malignant lymphomas may be defined as neoplastic proliferations of the cells of the lymphoreticular system. Numerous classifications have been devised and are still evolving as more information regarding clinical behaviour and recognition of the cell types involved in different lymphomas becomes available. However, most schemes divide lymphomas into two major categories:

(1) Hodgkin's disease (Fig. 8.35);

(2) non-Hodgkin's lymphomas.

Hodgkin's disease accounts for about 30 per cent of all malignant lymphomas and is predominantly a disease of young adults, with peak incidence in the third decade. A second smaller peak occurs around the seventh decade. It presents clinically with progressive, usually painless enlargement of lymph nodes, most frequently the cervical nodes. Subsequently, adjacent nodal groups, distant nodes, or extranodal sites may be involved.

Histological diagnosis depends on identification of Reed-Sternberg cells (or their variants) which are regarded as the neoplastic component (Fig. 8.35). The classic Reed-Sternberg cell is a large cell with either a double or bilobed nucleus, the two nuclei lying side-by-side to produce a 'mirror image' effect.

The aetiology of the disease is unknown, but genetic factors and viral infection, particularly Epstein-Barr virus infection, have been suggested. Prognosis depends on clinical staging and histological type, the prognosis decreasing from lymphocyte-predominant to lymphocyte-depleted types, but with modern chemotherapy overall survival rates of 50–70 per cent are reported.

The non-Hodgkin's lymphomas are classified further according to their cell of origin, cytological features, and histological pattern. With regard to the cell of origin, immunocytochemistry has shown that the majority of lymphomas arise from the neoplastic proliferation of B lymphocytes and their precursors found in the follicles of normal lymph nodes (follicular centre cells; centrocytes and centroblasts) (Figs 8.36, 8.37). Neoplastic proliferation of these cells at different stages of development accounts, to a large extent, for the variation in cytological

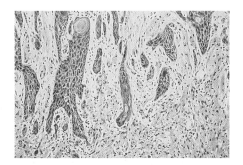

Fig. 8.34 High-power view of pseudoepitheliomatous hyperplasia associated with granular cell tumour.

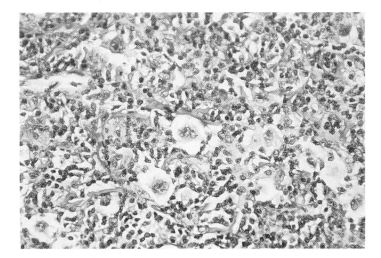

Fig. 8.35 Hodgkin's disease showing Reed–Sternberg cells.

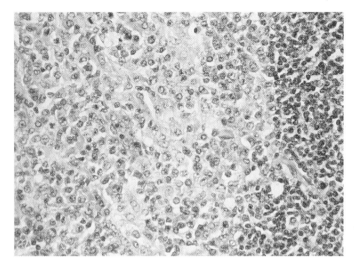

Fig. 8.36 Non-Hodgkin's malignant lymphoma. The malignant lymphoid cells (large pale cells) are replacing part of a lymph node (small dark lymphocytes).

Table 8.3 Modified (and simplified) Kiel classification of non-Hodgkin's malignant lymphomas

I   Low-grade malignancy (mainly small-cell types)
    Follicular
        —lymphocytic
        —centrocytic
        —centroblastic/centrocytic

II High-grade malignancy (mainly large-cell types)
    Diffuse
        —centroblastic
        —lymphoblastic
        —immunoblastic

Fig. 8.37 Corresponding field to that in Fig. 8.36. Immunohistochemical reaction (brown) using a monoclonal antibody to detect a B-cell antigen in malignant lymphoid cells.

appearances between different lymphomas. With regard to the histological pattern, the neoplastic cells may be in focal aggregates resembling the follicles of normal lymphoid tissue (follicular lymphomas) or in diffuse sheets (diffuse malignant lymphomas). Follicular lymphomas have a better prognosis than their diffuse counterparts. Despite the complexities of some classifications, histologically most non-Hodgkin's lymphomas can be divided into either high-grade or low-grade malignant types, the expected behaviour of a tumour being related to its histological typing. A modified and simplified classification is given in Table 8.3.

Malignant lymphomas in the head and neck region are relatively uncommon but may occur as part of widely disseminated disease or as a primary lesion. Their frequency is difficult to assess but Burkitt's lymphoma is of particular interest since this type, which is endemic in parts of Africa, commonly presents as a jaw tumour. It is discussed in more detail later.

The majority of malignant lymphomas in the head and neck arise in lymphoid tissue, the cervical lymph nodes are most often affected followed by the lymphoid structures of Waldeyer's ring. Almost all types of Hodgkin's and of non-Hodgkin's lymphomas have been reported. Hodgkin's disease is almost invariably nodal in distribution and part of disseminated malignancy.

Non-Hodgkin's lymphomas arising in tissues other than lymph nodes (extranodal lymphomas) are much less common than nodal tumours, but may arise in the oral soft tissues, salivary glands, and jaw bones as primary tumours which may remain as solitary lesions or progress to disseminated disease.

The lymphoid tissue associated with mucosa (including the salivary glands) forms part of a system specifically designed for mucosal defence, known as mucosa-associated lymphoid tissue or MALT. There is a tendency for lymphomas derived from MALT to remain localized for long periods and to disseminate only late in the course of the disease. When they do so, they tend to spread to other sites containing MALT rather than widely throughout the lymphoid system. For both of these reasons MALT lymphomas have a better prognosis than nodal types. Mucosal lesions present as soft, fleshy often ulcerated swellings. With regard to the salivary glands malignant lymphomas may arise from lymphoid aggregates within these tissues or as malignant transformation in a myoepithelial sialadenitis (lymphoepithelial lesion) and Sjögren syndrome. The majority arise in the parotid gland.

An increased incidence of non-Hodgkin's malignant lymphomas is seen in patients with AIDS (see Chapter 11).

Malignant lymphomas   **Key points**
- divided into Hodgkin's and non-Hodgkin's types
- can present as nodal or extranodal lesions
- MALT lymphomas have a better prognosis than nodal types
- jaw bone lesions are a major feature of Burkitt's lymphoma

Burkitt's lymphoma

Burkitt's lymphoma is endemic in tropical equatorial Africa where it occurs mainly between the ages of 2 and 14 years and accounts for about 50 per cent of all malignant disease in children. Since the original reports from Africa, sporadic cases have subsequently been recorded from many countries throughout the world.

The disease is usually multifocal but in the endemic areas of Africa a jaw tumour is the presenting symptom in over half the cases. Other sites of involvement include abdominal and/or pelvic viscera, retroperitoneal soft tissues, other facial and/or long bones, thyroid gland, salivary glands, and central nervous system. Retroperitoneal masses and nodular involvement of abdominal/pelvic viscera are found in virtually all cases, even when jaw tumours are the dominant feature. Lymph node involvement is inconspicuous. In non-African cases, abdominal lesions predominate and jaw lesions are relatively uncommon.

In the jaws, the lesions usually arise posteriorly and are more frequent in the maxilla than mandible, but more than one quadrant may be involved. The tumours are rapidly growing and are often of massive size, producing gross facial disfigurement. In the maxilla, the tumours may extend into the sinuses, nose, nasopharynx, and orbit. Teeth in the area are loosened, displaced, and may be exfoliated.

Histologically, the tumour consists of sheets of undifferentiated, small, round, lymphoid cells derived from B lymphocytes. In the Kiel classification Burkitt's lymphoma is categorized as a lymphoblastic lymphoma. Numerous large, pale macrophages are scattered amongst the darkly-staining lymphoid cells producing a characteristic, but not specific, 'starry sky' pattern.

Burkitt's lymphoma is a good example of a human neoplasm for which there is strong evidence that a virus is a causal factor, a clear association having been established between endemic Burkitt's lymphoma in Africa and the Epstein–Barr virus (EBV). EBV infection is ubiquitous in human populations, the main reservoir after initial infection being B lymphocytes. However, endemic Burkitt's lymphoma has a strict geographical distribution which also corresponds with that of hyperendemic malaria, suggesting that malaria is a cofactor. During acute attacks of malaria there is marked impairment in the ability of EBV-specific T lymphocytes to control EBV infection, and it is suggested that in some individuals repeated attacks of malaria over several years favour the unrestrained growth of EBV-carrying B lymphocytes.

A chromosome abnormality has been detected in tumour cells of Burkitt's lymphoma which involves a reciprocal translocation of part of chromosome 8 with chromosome 14 or, more rarely, with chromosome 2 or chromosome 22. The c-*myc* oncogene is located on chromosome 8 near the point of translocation, and it is probable that its activation following translocation to chromosome 14 (2 or 22) is associated with malignant transformation. It has been demonstrated that EBV can produce similar chromosomal abnormalities in infected B lymphocytes.

In contrast to Burkitt's lymphoma from endemic areas, the majority of sporadic cases occurring elsewhere in the world are not associated with EBV infection. Nevertheless, the tumour cells show similar chromosomal abnormalities to those described above.

Without treatment Burkitt's lymphoma is a rapidly fatal condition, but with chemotherapy dramatic remissions are obtained in the great majority of patients.

Nasal T-cell lymphomas

A variety of terms has been applied in the past to destructive lesions of the midface including midline (lethal) granuloma, Stewart's granuloma and polymorphic reticulosis. Evidence now suggests that these are all examples of the same distinctive type of T-cell malignant lymphoma which occurs within the nose and paranasal sinuses. The lymphoma has characteristic histological features in that the malignant cells cluster around blood vessels—an angiocentric pattern.

Angiocentric T-cell lymphoma of the nose presents most frequently with nasal obstruction, nasal discharge, and pain or numbness in the nose. As the destructive lesion spreads, adjacent structures such as the palate and face become involved. In addition to its distinctive clinicopathological features, the neoplastic cells contain Epstein–Barr virus (EBV) proteins suggesting that the virus plays a role in the pathogenesis of the disease.

FURTHER READING

Carney, J. A., Sizemore, G. W., and Lovestedt (1976). Mucosal ganglioneuromatosis, medullary thyroid carcinoma and pheochromocytoma: Multiple endocrine neoplasia type 2B. *Oral Surgery, Oral Medicine, Oral Pathology*, **41**, 739–52.

Eisenbud, L., Sciubba, J., Mir, R., and Sachs, S. A. (1983). Oral presentations in non-Hodgkin's lymphoma: A review of thirty-one cases. *Oral Surgery, Oral Medicine, Oral Pathology*, **56**, 151–6.

Fowler, C. B., Hartman, K. S., and Brannon, R. B. (1994). Fibromatosis of the oral cavity and paraoral region. *Oral Surgery, Oral Medicine, Oral Pathology*, **77**, 373–86.

Isaacson, P. G. (1990). Lymphoma of mucosa associated lymphoid tissue (MALT). *Histopathology*, **16**, 617–19.

Lucas, R. B. (1984). Pathology of tumours of the oral tissues (4th edn). Churchill Livingstone, Edinburgh.

Macleod, R. I. and Soames, J. V. (1987). Epulides: a clinicopathological study of a series of 200 consecutive lesions. *British Dental Journal*, **163**, 51–3.

Magnusson, B. C. and Rasmusson, L. G. (1995). The giant cell fibroma. A review of 103 cases with immunohistochemical findings. *Acta Odontologica Scandinavica*, **53**, 293–6.

Matthews, J. B. and Basu, M. K. (1983). Primary extranodal lymphoma of the oral cavity: an immunohistochemical study. *British Journal of Oral Surgery*, **21**, 159–70.

Mighell, A. J., Robinson, P. A., and Hume, W. J. (1995). Peripheral giant cell granuloma: a clinical study of 77 cases from 62 patients, and literature review. *Oral Diseases*, **1**, 12–19.

Natiella, J. R., Neiders, M. E., and Greene, G. W. (1982). Oral leiomyoma. *Journal of Oral Pathology*, **11**, 353–65.

Ramsay, A. D. and Rooney, N. (1993). Lymphomas of the head and neck. 1: Nasofacial T-cell lymphoma. *Oral Oncology, European Journal of Cancer*, **29B**, 99–102.

Ramsay, A. D. and Rooney, N. (1994). Lymphomas of the head and neck. 2: The B-cell lymphomas. *Oral Oncology, European Journal of Cancer*, **30B**, 155–9.

Stewart, C. M., Watson, R. E., Eversole, L. R., Fischlschweiger, W., and Leider, A. S. (1988). Oral granular cell tumours. A clinicopathologic and immunocytochemical study. *Oral Surgery, Oral Medicine, Oral Pathology*, **65**, 427–35.

Werning, J. T. (1979). Nodular fasciitis of the orofacial region. *Oral Surgery, Oral Medicine, Oral Pathology*, **48**, 441–6.

Williams, H. K. and Williams, D. M. (1997). Oral granular cell tumours: a histological and immunocytochemical study. *Journal of Oral Pathology and Medicine*, **26**, 164–9.

Wright, B. A. and Jackson, D. (1980). Neural tumours of the oral cavity. *Oral Surgery, Oral Medicine, Oral Pathology*, **49**, 509–22.

9 Keratoses and related disorders of oral mucosa

9 Keratoses and related disorders of oral mucosa

The colour of normal oral mucosa depends on the interplay between four factors—vascularity, melanin pigmentation, epithelial thickness, and keratinization. The term 'white patch' is often used clinically to describe the appearance of lesions presenting as white areas on the oral mucosa, and as many such lesions are associated with abnormal or increased keratin production, they are often described as keratoses. Oral keratoses appear white because the thickened or abnormal keratin becomes hydrated as a result of being bathed by saliva, and then evenly reflects light. A similar reaction is seen in areas of the skin, for example palms and soles, following prolonged soaking or bathing in water.

Other factors such as accumulation of keratinous debris on the surface of the epithelium may also produce a white patch. For example, a furred tongue associated with febrile illness appears white due to the retention of desquamated epithelial cells on the surface resulting from the lack of mechanical stimulation from the diet and decreased salivary flow associated with fever. However, the loosely attached cells are readily removed by wiping or gently scraping.

Keratoses   **Key points**
- increased and/or abnormal keratin production
- not removed by scraping
- classified on basis of aetiology

White patches can be grouped in a number of ways. Clinically, they can be separated depending on whether or not the lesion can be wiped away. In general, lesions which can be wiped away are due to accumulation of epithelial debris or an inflammatory exudate on the surface, as opposed to the keratoses which are resistant. Histologically, they can be divided into those which show epithelial dysplasia and those which do not (see later). They can also be grouped depending on their aetiology, and this forms the basis of their clinical differential diagnosis (Table 9.1). Carcinoma-*in-situ* and squamous cell carcinoma are described in Chapter 10, and white lesions of infective origin are discussed in Chapter 11.

Although the word 'leukoplakia' means 'white patch' this term is now only used to describe lesions defined by the World Health Organization as: 'A white patch or plaque that cannot be characterised clinically or histopathologically as any other disease'. In 1984, an International Symposium modified the definition of leukoplakia to 'a whitish patch or plaque, which cannot be characterised clinically or pathologically as any other disease, and is not associated with any physical or chemical agent except the use of tobacco'. Leukoplakia is, therefore, a clinical

Table 9.1 Aetiological classification of white lesions of the oral mucosa

Hereditary	oral epithelial naevus
	pachyonychia congenita
	dyskeratosis congenita
	tylosis
	hereditary benign intraepithelial dyskeratosis
	follicular keratosis (Darier's disease)
	leukoedema
Traumatic	mechanical (frictional keratosis)
	chemical
	thermal
Infective	candidosis
	—acute pseudomembranous
	—chronic hyperplastic
	—chronic mucocutaneous
	syphilitic leukoplakia
	hairy leukoplakia
Idiopathic	leukoplakia
Dermatological	lichen planus
	lupus erythematosus
Neoplastic	carcinoma-*in-situ*
	squamous cell carcinoma

diagnosis arrived at by exclusion, and what is included under the term is determined by what current opinion accepts as a diagnosable disease. For example, a traumatic keratosis should not be regarded as leukoplakia since a local cause of trauma must have been identified to enable the diagnosis to be made. The classification of such lesions should then be linked to the cause, for example, frictional keratosis. On removal of the cause the keratosis should resolve with time.

At the second International Symposium in 1994 it was accepted that, whilst tobacco usage was an aetiological factor in leukoplakia, some white patches could be linked directly to the local effects of tobacco usage since they resolved when the tobacco was withdrawn. As discussed above, the classification of such lesions should be linked to the cause and described as, for example, smokers' keratosis. This has led to some confusion and created difficulties in applying the previous definition, and for this reason the Symposium recommended a revised definition. Oral leukoplakia is now defined as 'a predominantly white lesion of the oral mucosa that cannot be characterized as any other definable lesion'.

DEFINITION OF HISTOPATHOLOGICAL TERMS

The following terms are used in this chapter to describe some of the histological changes which may occur in squamous epithelium, particularly in relation to white patches.

Orthokeratosis	—the superficial cell layers (squames) of the epithelium are flattened, anucleate, and have homogeneous, acidophilic cytoplasm.
Parakeratosis	—the superficial cell layers of the epithelium are again flattened and acidophilic, but contain pyknotic nuclei.
Hyperkeratosis	—increased thickness of the keratin layer.

Hyperparakeratosis	—increased thickness of the parakeratin
Keratosis	—keratinization of epithelium that is not normally keratinized.
Acanthosis	—a type of epithelial hyperplasia in which the increased thickness is due to an increased number of cells in the prickle cell layers, producing broadening and lengthening of the rete ridges.
Atrophy	—the thickness of the epithelium is decreased and usually associated with loss of the rete ridges, the epithelium being of roughly equal thickness throughout.
Cellular atypia	—a group of cellular changes which cytologically characterize malignant and premalignant lesions.
Epithelial dysplasia	—a term applied to describe epithelium when features of cellular atypia are present. Atypia refers to cells; dysplasia is used when referring to the tissue.

HEREDITARY CONDITIONS

A number of hereditary disorders of skin and of mucosae covered by squamous epithelium are characterized by disturbances of keratinization. Hereditary patterns are well established in most of these diseases which are sometimes termed 'genokeratoses' or 'genodermatoses'. In general, they are rare and oral involvement in some may be absent or inconspicuous. The oral epithelial naevus is the main disorder affecting oral mucosa. Other examples are discussed briefly, but the list in Table 9.1 is not meant to be comprehensive.

Oral epithelial naevus (white sponge naevus)

This hereditary disorder is transmitted as an autosomal dominant but with incomplete penetrance and variable expressivity. Any part of the oral mucosa may be involved (Fig. 9.1), and clinically the edges of the lesion are not well defined but gradually merge with the normal mucosa. The superficial layers of the epithelium are soft and of uneven thickness producing a shaggy or folded surface. Other mucosal surfaces, for example the nose, oesophagus, and anogenital region, may also be involved. The oral mucosal lesions may be apparent in infancy or early childhood, or may not become evident until adolescence. Histologically, the epithelium is acanthotic and the surface shows marked hyperparakeratosis (Fig. 9.2). A characteristic feature is marked intracellular oedema of the prickle and parakeratinized cell layers. Only the cell walls and the pyknotic nuclei in the centres of the cells are visible, thus giving a so-called basketweave appearance. There are no inflammatory changes in the lamina propria and there is no evidence that this disorder undergoes malignant transformation.

Mutations in the genes coding for keratins 4 and 13 (the pair of keratins expressed by epithelial cells in the mucosae affected by the disorder) have been identified, suggesting the disorder is due to keratin defects. The heaping-up of the cells on the surface also suggests the possibility of some abnormality of the normal desquamation process.

Pachyonychia congenita

In this autosomal dominant hereditary condition, gross thickening of the nails (pachyonychia) is noticed at or soon after birth and may be associated with palmoplantar keratosis and hyperhidrosis. Oral lesions consist of white opaque

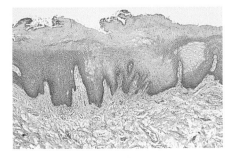

Fig. 9.1 Oral epithelial naevus affecting buccal mucosa. The other cheek was similarly affected.

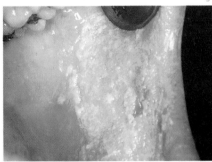

Fig. 9.2 Oral epithelial naevus.

patches on the dorsum or lateral borders of the tongue or the cheeks which histologically resemble the oral epithelial naevus.

Dyskeratosis congenita

This rare disorder mainly affects males but the mode of inheritance is unclear. It is characterized by abnormal pigmentation of the skin, dystrophic nails, and hyperkeratosis of mucous membranes including the oral mucosa. Severe gingivitis and periodontal destruction resembling juvenile periodontitis have been reported.

Tylosis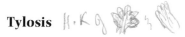

This is a rare disorder inherited as an autosomal dominant trait, and is characterized by congenital hyperkeratosis of the palms and soles (tylosis) and the development in later life of oesophageal carcinoma. In some patients hyperkeratotic plaques may be seen on the oral mucosa.

Hereditary benign intraepithelial dyskeratosis

This is a rare, autosomal dominant hereditary condition occurring mainly in a particular racial isolate in North Carolina. Oral lesions consist of asymptomatic, soft white folds of spongy mucosa. Histological examination shows thickened, oedematous epithelium with enlarged, eosinophilic cells that have undergone premature keratinization (dyskeratotic cells).

Follicular keratosis (Darier's disease)

This rare condition has an autosomal dominant mode of inheritance, but sporadic cases also occur. The characteristic skin lesions consist of multiple, heavily keratinized papules which coalesce, become secondarily infected, and foul smelling. The forehead, scalp, and ears are common sites. The oral mucosa is affected in approximately half the cases and lesions present as whitish, coalescing papules (Fig. 9.3) most commonly affecting the hard palate and gingiva.

Key points	Genodermatoses
	• rare
	• oral epithelial naevus is main disease involving oral mucosa
	• oral involvement may occur in several other conditions as incidental findings

Histological examination of skin and mucosal lesions (Fig. 9.4) shows hyperkeratosis and suprabasal clefts containing acantholytic cells. Large, abnormally keratinized squamous cells (corps ronds) and smaller flattened cells with hyperchromatic nuclei (grains) are seen in the roof of the cleft and overlying epithelium.

Leukoedema

This condition is particularly evident in persons with racial pigmentation of the oral mucosa, and presents as a translucent, milky whiteness of the surface of the mucosa with a slightly folded appearance. Histologically, the epithelium is thicker than normal with broad rete ridges, and the cells in the superficial part of the prickle cell layer appear vacuolated and contain considerable quantities of glycogen. Local irritation has been suggested, but ethnic and racial clustering suggest hereditary factors, and leukoedema is best regarded as a variation of normal.

TRAUMATIC KERATOSES

Mechanical

The oral mucosa reacts to friction in one of two ways. An acute frictional response leads to a blister and ulceration, while a chronic frictional response leads to epithelial thickening and hyperkeratinization. Irritants such as a sharp tooth, cheek biting, and the prolonged wearing of often ill-fitting dentures are examples of causes of chronic friction. The lesions produced are referred to as frictional keratoses and may in time become dense and white, and show a roughened surface (Figs 9.5, 9.6). To diagnose frictional keratosis a source of chronic irritation must be identified which fits the size and shape of the lesion, and the lesion must resolve when the source of irritation is removed (cf. chronic traumatic ulcer). Histologically, frictional keratoses show hyperkeratosis which may be accompanied by some acanthosis but there is no dysplasia (Fig. 9.7). The lesion is innocent and is analogous to the callus on the hand of a manual worker.

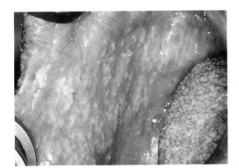

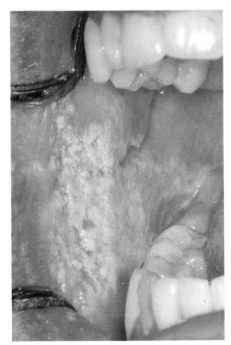

Fig. 9.3

Fig. 9.5

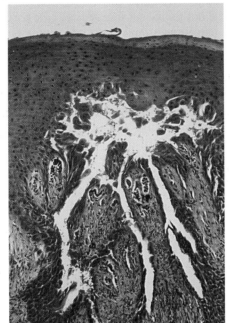

Fig. 9.4

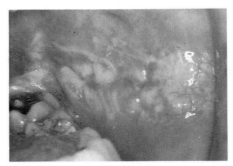

Fig. 9.6

Fig. 9.3 Oral lesions in Darier's disease.

Fig. 9.4 Darier's disease.

Fig. 9.5 Hyperkeratosis associated with habitual cheek chewing.

Fig. 9.6 Frictional keratosis related to the occlusal line.

Fig. 9.7 Frictional keratosis showing hyperkeratosis and acanthosis.

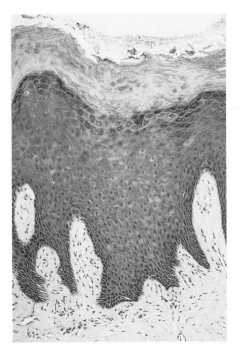

Fig. 9.7

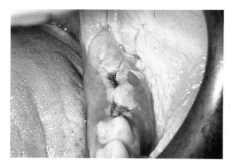

Fig. 9.8 Aspirin burn showing a range of mucosal reactions from oedema to necrosis and sloughing.

Chemical

Chemical insult to the oral mucosa may produce a variety of reactions depending on the severity of the insult and its duration. A severe insult such as that produced by the topical use of aspirin (aspirin burn) is likely to produce epithelial necrosis, sloughing, and ulceration (Fig. 9.8), while a low-grade, chronic insult may result in hyperkeratosis.

Chronic chemical insult to the mucosa is seen in patients who use tobacco, whether it is smoked, chewed, or used as snuff, and in those with other chewing habits such as betel nut. These habits produce epithelial thickening and hyperkeratosis in a similar manner to chronic friction.

Thermal

Regular smokers of cigarettes, cigars, and pipes often develop white plaques on their oral mucosa, particularly the anterior parts of the buccal mucosa, tongue, and palate. It is likely that both thermal and chemical factors are involved in the development of these hyperkeratotic lesions. Smokers who constantly dangle a cigarette from the lips may develop a localized keratosis at that site, and similar lesions may occur in pipe smokers on the dorsum of the tongue or palate where the hot smoke constantly impinges, particularly if the pipe has a favoured position.

Nicotinic stomatitis of the palate is a characteristic clinical condition which may develop in association with any type of smoking, but particularly in pipe smokers. In early lesions the palatal mucosa is greyish-white with scattered red spots representing the orifices of minor salivary gland ducts. In more advanced lesions there are tessellated patches of rough white epithelium with red, umbilicated duct orifices (Fig. 9.9). Histological examination shows hyperkeratosis and acanthosis of the palatal epithelium and keratin plugs in some of the duct orifices associated with mild periductal chronic inflammation. The condition is usually reversible if smoking is stopped and is not considered to be a precancerous lesion. However, the condition does indicate that potential carcinogens are operating in the mouth and the whole of the mucosa must be carefully examined. In general, a patient with a white patch anywhere on the oral mucosa has a much greater risk of developing oral cancer than a patient without such a lesion, but this does not imply that the malignant disease always develops within the initial white patch.

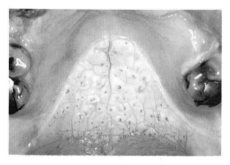

Fig. 9.9 Stomatitis nicotina of the palate in a partial denture wearer.

Key points	Traumatic keratoses
	• reaction to local causes
	• reversible if cause removed

LEUKOPLAKIA

As mentioned previously, leukoplakia is now defined as a predominantly white lesion of the oral mucosa that cannot be characterized as any other definable lesion. This rather negative definition highlights the fact that the diagnosis of leukoplakia is one of exclusion. The definition may well be further revised and refined in the future as new knowledge accumulates.

Although leukoplakia is a clinical diagnosis which implies no particular histological change or behaviour, there is no doubt that a small percentage of leukoplakias are premalignant and some may be invasive carcinomas at presentation. It is impossible to predict which lesions are likely to become malignant, but certain clinical and histological features are recognized as being associated with an increased risk. The behaviour of a leukoplakia may also be related to the aetiological factors (if any) which are thought to be involved in a particular patient. In the evaluation of a leukoplakic lesion all of these factors must be taken into consideration.

Incidence

The reported prevalence of oral leukoplakia in unselected populations in different parts of the world varies from 0.2 to 4 per cent, but difficulties in the standardization of diagnostic criteria make comparison of the prevalence in different areas somewhat problematical. Studies in Western Europe and North America some years ago showed that oral leukoplakia occurred predominantly in men, but recent studies show that now almost as many women in these countries are affected. This probably reflects changes in smoking habits. Leukoplakia is generally described as occurring in older people, but recent studies show that the incidence in younger adults is increasing. Leukoplakia may occur anywhere on the oral mucosa, but in Western Europe and North America, the floor of the mouth and buccal mucosa are now regarded as being the most common sites affected. However, marked variations in the incidence, sex, and age-group affected and site of leukoplakia occur between different ethnic and cultural groups, reflecting variations in possible aetiological factors such as smoking and chewing habits. Leukoplakias involving the ventral tongue and/or floor of the mouth (sublingual keratosis) have a higher risk of malignant transformation than lesions at other sites.

Clinical features

Leukoplakia may vary from a quite small and circumscribed plaque to an extensive lesion involving a large area of mucosa. Lesions may be white, whitish-yellow, or grey and may have a homogeneous or non-homogeneous surface. Homogeneous leukoplakias are usually plaque-like but some variation in the surface is allowed. Some are smooth but others may be wrinkled or the surface may be criss-crossed by small cracks or fissures producing a tessellated appearance. In contrast, non-homogeneous leukoplakias may show areas of redness, producing a speckled appearance, ulceration, nodular thickening, or heaping-up of the surface (Figs 9.10, 9.11). In some cases the lesions may take on a distinctly warty appearance, described as verrucous leukoplakia. Speckling is due to the association of leukoplakia with erythroplakia.

Clinical features of leukoplakia   **Key points**
- homogeneous
- non-homogeneous (including speckled)
- non-homogeneous have a worse prognosis

Erythroplakia is defined as a bright-red velvety plaque on the oral mucosa which cannot be categorized clinically or pathologically as being due to any other condition (Fig. 9.12). Erythroplakic lesions may be homogeneous with a well-defined but irregular outline, or may be intermingled with patches of leukoplakia—such lesions are often called speckled leukoplakias. Histologically, erythroplakia may represent carcinoma-*in-situ* or even invasive carcinoma (see Chapter 10). Its development in a previously uniform white lesion is, therefore, an important clinical sign that may indicate sinister change. Fixation, induration,

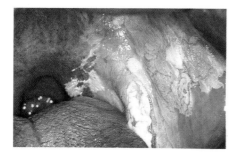
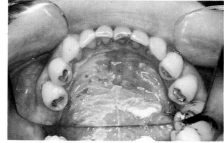
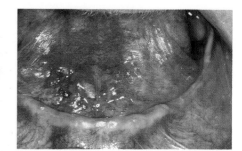

Figs 9.10 and 9.11   Non-homogeneous leukoplakias.

Fig. 9.12   Erythroplakia of the right floor of mouth.

ulceration, lymphadenopathy, and bone destruction if the lesion overlies bone are other clinical features that may indicate malignant change in a leukoplakic or erythroplakic patch.

Aetiological factors

The aetiology of idiopathic oral leukoplakia is by definition unknown, but in some patients predisposing factors can be identified that are associated with the development of other white lesions or in the aetiology of squamous cell carcinoma (see Chapter 10). However, that does not imply that they are causative. The following factors may be important.

Tobacco

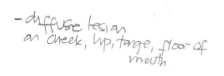

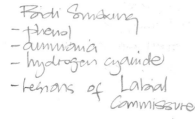

Tobacco usage is probably the most common aetiological factor in patients with leukoplakia, the tobacco being either smoked or chewed. Any part of the mucosa may be involved and the distribution of the lesions may vary with the particular type of habit. In cigarette smokers the lesion may be diffuse and seen on the cheeks, lips, tongue, and less frequently the floor of the mouth. In India, bidi smoking is associated with leukoplakia in up to 16 per cent of *habitués*, a bidi being a cheap type of cigarette made by rolling a rectangular piece of leaf with a locally grown tobacco and securing the roll with a thread. Bidi smoke has a high content of several toxic agents such as ammonia, hydrogen cyanide, and phenol when compared with other tobacco smoke. Bidi smoking typically produces lesions at the labial commissure. Reverse smoking, in which the glowing end of the cigarette is held inside the mouth, is practised in some parts of the world and is associated with diverse changes including white patches, red areas, and ulceration.

In many parts of the world the use of smokeless tobacco is also prevalent and is associated with oral keratosis. Tobacco chewing is widely practised in Asia, where it is frequently combined with betel nut and lime and wrapped in a betel leaf to form a small parcel, a pan (see Chapter 10). This is usually kept in the area of the lower mucobuccal fold close to the molars and produces lesions on the buccal mucosa. Tobacco chewing is also practised by coal miners as a substitute for smoking in the underground conditions where smoking would be dangerous.

Snuff dipping is a similar habit seen particularly in Scandinavia and parts of the USA and involves the use of a wet snuff which is placed in the buccal sulcus. In some countries snuff may also be purchased in small sachets designed to be held in the mouth.

In the majority of patients tobacco-associated keratosis regresses on cessation of the habit and such lesions would not be classified as leukoplakia.

2 Alcohol

There is no clear evidence to show the importance of alcohol in the aetiology of leukoplakia (cf. oral squamous cell carcinoma), but it is likely that it does have some part to play. Many heavy smokers are also heavy drinkers.

3 Candida

As discussed in Chapter 11, candidal hyphae can be demonstrated in biopsies of chronic hyperplastic candidosis (candidal leukoplakia), but are occasionally found in association with idiopathic leukoplakia. Doubts still remain as to whether such candidal infection is a cause of leukoplakia or a superimposed infection. Although candida plays a causal role in chronic hyperplastic candidosis, the organism thrives particularly well in altered tissues and this may be why it is occasionally seen in other keratoses.

Oral leukoplakia   **Key points**
- aetiology likely to be multifactorial
- tobacco use is a major factor

---

4 Viruses

It has been clearly demonstrated that hairy leukoplakia in HIV-positive and some other immunosuppressed patients is associated with infection with the Epstein-Barr virus (see Chapter 11). It has also been suggested that human papillomaviruses (HPV) may be involved in the aetiology of some leukoplakias. HPV 16 is the most commonly isolated type, but since the virus may be found in a proportion of healthy oral mucosa its role in the pathogenesis of leukoplakia is uncertain.

5 Oral epithelial atrophy

There is a tendency for leukoplakia to develop in atrophic epithelium. Conditions which predispose to epithelial atrophy and leukoplakia include iron deficiency, oral submucous fibrosis, tertiary syphilis, and possibly some vitamin deficiencies. Sideropenic dysphagia (Patterson-Kelly or Plummer-Vinson syndrome) is associated particularly with postcricoid carcinoma but may also be associated with oral leukoplakia and oral squamous cell carcinoma.

6 Tumour suppressor genes—p53

Tumour suppressor genes are involved in regulation of the normal cell-proliferation cycle. One of the best known is the p53 gene located on chromosome 17p. Mutation of the gene can result in inactivation of the normal suppressor activity of the p53 protein leading to uncontrolled cell proliferation. Abnormalities of the p53 gene have been identified in a wide range of malignancies, including oral cancer (see Chapter 10) and in some leukoplakias, particularly those showing dysplasia (see below) and those associated with heavy smoking and drinking. This suggests that, in some patients, alteration of the p53 gene is an early event in the development of oral cancer.

Pathology, epithelial dysplasia

There is a wide range in the histological appearances of oral leukoplakia which reflect varying degrees of keratosis, epithelial thickness, epithelial dysplasia, and

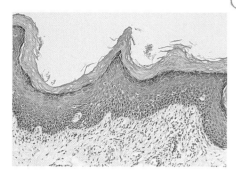

Fig. 9.13 Hyperorthokeratosis with chevron pattern often related to tobacco smoking.

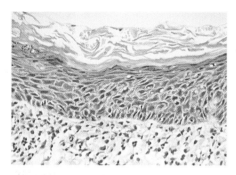

Fig. 9.14 Atrophic hyperkeratotic and dysplastic epithelium.

ORTHOKERATOSIS

St. corneum
(w/ no nuclei)
|
St. granulosum
(well defined)
|
St spinosum
|
St. basale

PARAKERATOSIS

St corneum
(pyknotic nuclei)
|
St spinosum
|
St basale

NON KERATINIZED

St Spinosum
|
St basale

④

chronic inflammatory cell infiltration in the lamina propria. However, it must be appreciated that leukoplakia is a clinical diagnosis arrived at after the exclusion of other diseases and is not based on any specific histopathological features. The term leukoplakia has no histological connotation.

The hyperkeratosis may be due to orthokeratosis, parakeratosis, or a mixture of both, and may vary in thickness. Orthokeratin is generally associated with a prominent granular cell layer (Fig. 9.13). The epithelium may be hyperplastic or atrophic (Fig. 9.14), areas of erythroplakia often being associated with epithelial atrophy. The junction between the abnormal and normal epithelium at the edge of the lesion may be abrupt, or there may be a gradual transition from one to the other. In some cases, melanin pigment may be present both in the basal epithelial cells and in macrophages in the lamina propria as a result of leakage of melanin from basal cells (melanin incontinence). Melanin pigmentation accounts for the grey colour of some leukoplakias.

In some cases, the keratosis and change in thickness are the only abnormal epithelial features but others show features of epithelial dysplasia (Figs 9.15–9.18). The individual cellular changes (cellular atypia) seen in dysplastic epithelium reflect abnormalities in proliferation, maturation, and differentiation of epithelial cells. The features of epithelial dysplasia are:

1. Nuclear and cellular pleomorphism. Nuclei and cells are of different size and shape.
2. Alteration (invariably an increase) is seen in the nuclear/cytoplasmic ratio by either area or volume.
3. Nuclear hyperchromatism. Nuclear staining which is abnormally intense.
4. Prominent nucleoli are present.
5. Increased and abnormal mitoses. Mitoses may be increased in number, occur higher up in the epithelium than is usual (i.e. away from the basal layer—suprabasal mitoses), or have an abnormal form (for example triradiate mitosis).
6. Disturbed polarity of the basal cells or loss of cellular orientation. The cells in the basal layer have no definable long axis and the nuclei have no regular polarity.
7. Basal cell hyperplasia. The presence of several layers of cells of basaloid appearance. It is often associated with drop-shaped rete pegs.
8. Drop-shaped rete pegs. The rete pegs are wider at their deeper part than they are more superficially.
9. Irregular epithelial stratification or disturbed maturation. The cells no longer show a proper sequence of morphological and maturational changes as they pass from the basal layer to the surface.
10. Abnormal keratinization. Keratinization occurring below the normal keratin layer, either as individual cell keratinization within the stratum spinosum or as disturbed maturation of groups of cells resulting in the formation of intraepithelial keratin pearls.

Key points	**Leukoplakia**
	• is a clinical diagnosis
	• has no histological connotation
	• epithelial dysplasia may or may not be present
	• non-homogeneous types are more likely to be dysplastic
	• the severity of dysplasia is assessed subjectively

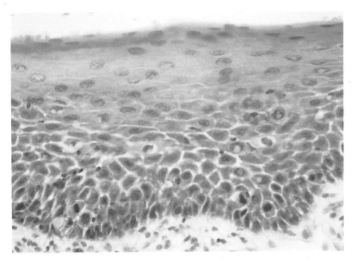

Fig. 9.15 Epithelial dysplasia involving the lower third of the epithelium showing pleomorphism, suprabasal mitoses, and loss of ordered stratification.

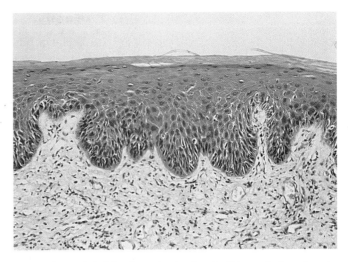

Fig. 9.16 Epithelial dysplasia showing basal cell hyperplasia and drop-shaped rete pegs.

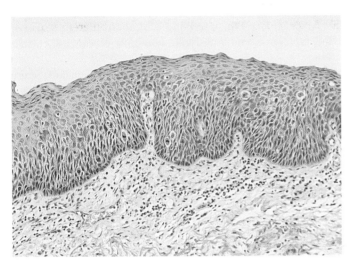

Fig. 9.17 Moderate/severe epithelial dysplasia involving about two-thirds of the epithelium.

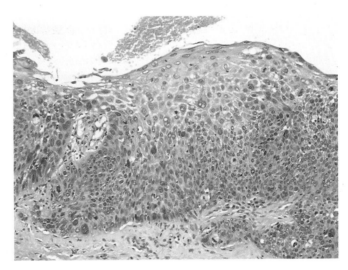

Fig. 9.18 Severe epithelial dysplasia showing marked cellular atypia and disturbed maturation of the epithelium.

11. Loss or reduction of intercellular adhesion (or cohesion). This may be difficult to distinguish from intercellular oedema.

Not all these changes are necessarily seen in any one case, and epithelial dysplasia of a minor degree may be seen in some inflammatory conditions such as lichen planus and candidosis. Although it is not possible to predict the presence and severity of dysplasia from the clinical appearances of the lesion, erythroplakias and non-homogeneous leukoplakias are much more likely to be dysplastic (or even invasive carcinoma) than homogeneous leukoplakias. Several studies have demonstrated that only about 10 per cent of homogeneous leukoplakias are dysplastic as opposed to 50 per cent or more of non-homogeneous types. Attempts to give a numerical score to the severity of dysplasia in the hope that it would correlate with prognosis have proven unsuccessful, and so the degree of dysplasia is usually subjectively assessed using terms such as mild, moderate, and severe.

Prognosis

Leukoplakia has an unpredictable tendency to undergo malignant transformation. There is a marked variation in the reported malignant transformation rates in studies from different areas of the world, ranging in most cases from 0.3 per cent to 18 per cent over prolonged periods. This wide range is likely to be due to many factors including differences in diagnostic criteria and in aetiological factors, such as smoking, other habits, and nutritional status, between different countries and also between different cultural groups within a country. Despite these problems, by combining the results from several studies, a rate of about 14 per cent over a period of up 20 years has been reported. A malignant transformation rate in Western Europe of 4 per cent over 10 years is likely to be a reasonable estimate. In Denmark, an annual incidence of malignant transformation of 0.75 per cent has been reported which is consistent with the long-term transformation rate.

Although the rate of malignant transformation is variable, the ventral tongue, floor of the mouth, and the lingual aspect of the lower alveolar mucosa are high-risk sites. Lesions in these areas are often designated as sublingual keratosis to draw attention to the importance of site. Studies in the United Kingdom and in America have shown about 25 per cent of such lesions are invasive squamous cell carcinoma when first biopsied (see Fig. 10.8) and that about a further 25 per cent will subsequently develop carcinoma when followed-up over varying periods of time.

It is generally accepted that a leukoplakia showing epithelial dysplasia is more likely to become malignant than one not showing epithelial dysplasia, and that the more severe the features of epithelial dysplasia, the greater the risk of malignant transformation. Transformation rates for dysplastic leukoplakias range from less than 10 per cent to over 30 per cent in different studies. However, several series have shown that the majority of dysplastic leukoplakias remain unchanged during the observation period and that a proportion (about 18 per cent) will improve or regress. There is no clear correlation, therefore, between histological appearances and clinical behaviour. This is particularly relevant to sublingual keratoses where importance must be attached to even mild dysplasia. Speckled and other non-homogeneous types of leukoplakia also have an increased rate of malignant transformation compared to homogeneous lesions, which presumably reflects the higher incidence of dysplasia in non-homogeneous leukoplakias. Speckled leukoplakias associated with candidal infection (candidal leukoplakias, see Chapter 11) also have a high incidence of dysplasia and about 30 per cent of patients with such lesions may develop oral carcinoma on follow-up.

Key points	**Prognosis of oral leukoplakia**
	• a proportion undergo malignant transformation
	• transformation times vary from one to several years
	• dysplastic lesions carry an increased risk of malignant transformation
	• the potential for malignant transformation is greater in high-risk sites

As discussed previously, erythroplakia, whether as part of a speckled leukoplakia or as a separate lesion, is an important and serious condition and one of the most common manifestations of early malignant change. Biopsy studies have shown that about half of such lesions are invasive carcinoma or carcinoma-*in-situ* on initial biopsy and that the great majority of those remaining show severe dysplasia.

Although it is assumed that the risk of developing carcinoma increases as the severity of dysplasia increases, there are no reliable methods to predict the behaviour of premalignant lesions. Considerable research is currently directed towards the identification of prognostic markers, involving study of genetic alterations, oncogene and tumour suppressor gene activities, and abnormalities in the control of the cell cycle. However, at present, most of these techniques are research tools and no reliable indicator of malignant transformation has yet been identified. In assessing the overall risk of malignant change in leukoplakia, it is appropriate to consider the size, the site, and the clinical appearance of the lesion, together with an assessment (albeit subjective) of the degree of dysplasia on histological examination.

DERMATOLOGICAL CAUSES OF WHITE PATCHES

A number of primarily dermatological diseases in addition to the genodermatoses have oral lesions which may present as white patches. Lichen planus is by far the commonest, but it is convenient here to include lupus erythematosus since, clinically and histologically, the chronic discoid type may mimic lichen planus. The other diseases are very rare and beyond the scope of this book.

Lichen planus

This relatively common disease, the prevalence of which varies from about 0.5 to 1.9 per cent in the general population, has a world-wide distribution and involves the skin and mucous membranes. The majority of patients are between 30 and 50 years of age and about 60 per cent are women. Oral lesions can be detected in approximately 50 per cent of patients who initially present with skin lesions, but the prevalence of skin lesions in patients who are primarily seen for oral lichen planus is lower and ranges from about 10 to 45 per cent in reported series. Oral lesions may occur before, at the same time as, or after skin lesions.

Oral lichen planus   Key points
- skin lesions may or may not be present
- mucosal lesions are usually bilateral
- non-erosive forms may be symptomless

Clinical features

The characteristic skin lesion is a violaceous, itchy papule which may have distinctive white streaks on the surface (Wickham's striae). The papules may have a variable pattern, discrete, linear, annular, or widespread rashes being described. Almost any area of skin may be involved, but the flexor surface of the wrist is the commonest site. Fingernails are involved in up to 10 per cent of patients, vertical ridges being the usual abnormality. The skin lesions develop slowly and 85 per cent resolve within 18 months, although recurrences are not uncommon. In contrast, oral lichen planus pursues a much more chronic course, in some patients extending over several years.

In patients with oral lichen planus the buccal mucosa is involved in the great majority of cases while the tongue, gingiva, palate, and lips may also be affected. Involvement of the floor of the mouth is very uncommon. Lesions are generally

Management of Dysplastic Lesions
1. Stop assoc. habits
2. treat candidal Infections or Fe deficiency
3. Biopsy to access dysplasia
4. Assess risk of premalignancy on clinical & histological findings
5. Remove Lesion
6. Maintain observation for malignant changes

Management Options For Pre malignant Lesions
1. Observation for early detection of carcinoma
2. Surgical Excision with grafting
3. Cryotherapy
4. Laser excision or vaporization
5. Topical Chemotherapy
6. Retinoids

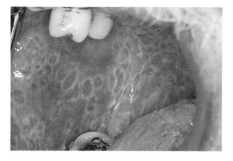

Fig. 9.19 Lichen planus—reticular pattern.

bilateral and a wide spectrum of clinical presentations may occur, alone or in various combinations (Table 9.2). The reticular, plaque-like, and papular patterns (Fig. 9.19) are usually symptom-free, in contrast to the atrophic/erosive types which often occur together (Fig. 9.20). The mucosa in the atrophic/erosive forms has a red and glazed appearance with areas of superficial ulceration of varying extent which may take several weeks to heal. Occasionally, they are preceded by bullae (bullous lichen planus). Erosive lesions are often associated with typical areas of non-erosive lichen planus round the edges of the lesions. Pain and discomfort may be considerable and severe, intractable ulceration is very occasionally seen.

Table 9.2 Clinical types of lichen planus listed in order of frequency of involvement of the oral mucosa

Reticular	—lace-like striae
Atrophic	—diffuse red lesions resembling erythroplakia
Plaque-like	—white plaques resembling leukoplakia
Papular	—small white papules that may coalesce
Erosive	—extensive areas of shallow ulceration
Bullous	—subepithelial bullae

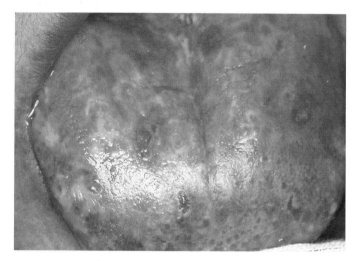

Fig. 9.20 Atrophic/erosive lichen planus.

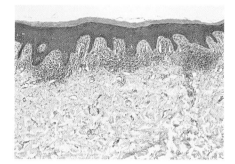

Fig. 9.21 Lichen planus with irregular acanthosis and dense subepithelial lymphocytic infiltration.

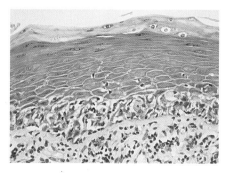

Fig. 9.22 Liquefactive degeneration of basal cells in lichen planus.

Lichen planus involving the gingiva often presents as a desquamative gingivitis (see Chapter 7 and Fig. 7.17). In some patients, more typical non-erosive lesions of lichen planus can usually be found elsewhere on the oral mucosa.

Pathology

In oral lichen planus the epithelium may be ortho- or parakeratinized and it varies considerably in thickness. It may be atrophic or acanthotic, the latter usually resulting in irregular elongation and widening of the rete processes, although a sawtooth pattern, classically described in skin lesions, may be seen (Fig. 9.21). There is a dense, well-defined band of underlying mononuclear inflammatory cell infiltration, consisting mainly of T lymphocytes (Fig. 9.21). Plasma cells are absent or inconspicuous. A characteristic finding is degeneration of basal cells associated with oedema and lymphocytic infiltration of the basal region of the epithelium, described as liquefactive degeneration of basal cells (Fig. 9.22). The degenerating cells appear as hyaline, shrunken/condensed bodies (Civatte bodies) and represent basal cells undergoing apoptosis. In some cases, a lack of cohesion between epithelium and the lamina propria as a result of basal cell degeneration and oedema may result in the formation of subepithelial bullae (blisters). Once ulceration has occurred there is a non-specific inflammatory response which makes histological diagnosis more difficult.

Key points

Lichen planus histopathology
- ortho- or parakeratinized surface
- acanthotic or atrophic epithelium
- subepithelial band of T lymphocytes
- liquefactive degeneration of basal cells

Almost all cases of oral lichen planus run a benign course, but malignant transformation has been described in a very small proportion. It has been suggested that the erosive forms are more likely to undergo such change and if this is so, then epithelial atrophy may be the essential factor. However, there is considerable controversy as to the prevalence of malignant change. This is due, in part, to variation in diagnostic criteria and difficulties in distinguishing, both clinically and histologically, between dysplastic lichen planus and other premalignant lesions such as leukoplakia and erythroplakia. Although the magnitude of the risk is disputed, most studies suggest that the frequency of malignant transformation ranges from about 0.5 to 2.5 per cent of patients over a 5-year-period.

Aetiology

The aetiology of lichen planus is unknown but many factors have been implicated (Table 9.3). Associations with a variety of systemic diseases, such as diabetes mellitus, hypertension, ulcerative colitis, and liver diseases, have been reported, but there is no constant relationship or common mechanism by which such diseases are implicated in lichen planus. However, it is well recognized that lesions which clinically and histologically resemble lichen planus may occur as a reaction to a wide range of drugs, for example, antimalarials and methyl dopa (lichenoid reaction). The mechanisms underlying these reactions are unknown, but in such cases the lesions generally resolve fairly rapidly after withdrawal of the offending drug. Lichenoid lesions have also been reported in some patients to be associated with hypersensitivity to mercuric salts released from corroding amalgam restorations, and in such cases the lesions may be confined to the contact area between the restoration and the mucosa. The majority of these contact lesions regress after replacement of the amalgam, suggesting a type IV hypersensitivity reaction and a contact allergy similar to that occurring in skin in association with other metals such as nickel. Oral and cutaneous lichenoid lesions are also seen as part of a graft-versus-host reaction in patients who have received bone marrow transplants, implicating immunological mechanisms. The dense, band-like inflammatory cell infiltrate of predominantly T lymphocytes and macrophages beneath the epithelium and the beneficial effects of topical steroids in patients with erosive lichen planus also suggest an immunopathogenesis. However, the disease does not have the features of a typical autoimmune disorder as autoantibodies are seldom detected in patients with lichen planus and there is no strong association of the condition with other autoimmune diseases.

Table 9.3 Factors implicated in the aetiology of lichen planus

Genetic predisposition
Infective agents
Systemic diseases
Graft-versus-host disease
Drug reactions
Hypersensitivity to dental materials
Tobacco smoking
Tobacco and/or betel chewing
Vitamin deficiencies
Psychiatric disorders

Pathogenesis

The pathogenesis of lichen planus is not yet understood, but probably involves a cell-mediated immune response to antigenic changes in oral mucosa. It is thought that in response to some external agent, which may be antigenic or may modify the antigenic structure of the epithelial cells, cytokine release is increased from Langerhans cells and keratinocytes. These include factors such as interleukin-1 and interleukin-8, which are chemotactic for leukocytes, and factors which upregulate intercellular adhesion molecules (ICAM-1) to which T lympho-cytes can bind. As a result, there is infiltration of epithelium as well as the lamina propria by both CD4 (helper) and CD8 (cytotoxic/suppressor) lympho-cytes. In addition, the keratinocytes also begin to express class II histocompatibil-ity antigens on their cytoplasmic membranes, particularly HLA-DR. (MHC class II molecules are normally only expressed by immunocompetent cells.) Thus, intraepithelial antigen (either from external sources or from altered ker-atinocytes) can be processed by Langerhans cells, or by keratinocytes expressing class II molecules and then presented to infiltrating CD4 lymphocytes, thereby initiating a cell-mediated immune response. Subsequent activation of cytotoxic CD8 cells is thought to be responsible for the characteristic damage to basal cells (Fig. 9.23).

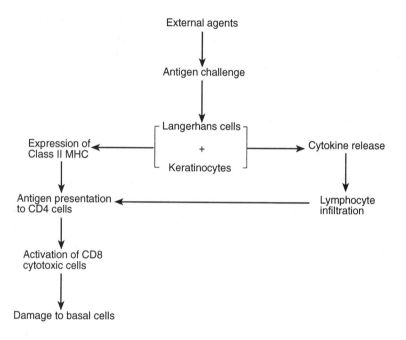

Fig. 9.23 Possible mechanisms involved in the pathogenesis of lichen planus.

Key points	**Pathogenesis of lichen planus**
	• T-cell mediated
	• resembles type-IV hypersensitivity
	• cytotoxic (CD8) lymphocytes damage basal epithelium

Lupus erythematosus

Two main forms of this disease are recognized, chronic discoid lupus erythemato-sus, which is a localized disease, and systemic lupus erythematosus, which is a disseminated disease involving almost every organ of the body. Intermediate forms can also be recognized and some patients with the discoid type may in time develop disseminated disease. Females are affected much more frequently than males.

The lesions in chronic discoid lupus erythematosus are often restricted to the skin and usually occur on the face. They present as scaly red patches which later heal with scar formation. Sometimes the skin lesions in either the discoid or sys-temic types have a symmetrical distribution over the nose and cheek, the so-called butterfly pattern. Oral lesions have been reported in up to 50 per cent of cases of discoid lupus erythematosus, and, although any part of the mucosa may be involved, the cheeks are most frequently affected. When the lips are involved the entire vermilion border may be affected. There is considerable variation in the type of oral lesion seen, but the most usual is a discoid area of erythema or ulceration surrounded by a white keratotic border sometimes with radiating striae (cf. lichen planus) (Fig. 9.24). Histological examination of the oral lesions shows the epithelium to be ortho- or parakeratinized, with areas of hyperplasia and atrophy. Dome-shaped extensions of keratinized cells may extend from the superficial layer down into the hyperplastic rete processes (keratin plugging). Subepithelial and deeply situated perivascular foci of lymphocytes are present in the connective tissue and there may be liquefactive degeneration of basal cells (cf lichen planus) (Fig. 9.25). Immunofluorescent studies show abundant deposits of immunoglobulin (mainly IgG) and complement in the basement membrane zone forming a prominent 'lupus band'.

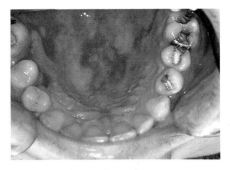

Fig. 9.24 Chronic discoid lupus erythematosus.

The lesions in systemic lupus erythematosus include skin rashes and lymphadenopathy, but the kidneys, liver, lungs, and nervous system are also frequently involved. The skin rashes are maculopapular, photosensitive, and typically occur on the cheeks. Oral lesions are very variable, the most commonly described lesions being superficial erosions and erythematous patches on the buccal mucosa. White, keratotic areas are not so frequently seen as in the discoid type. The histology of oral lesions shows a diffuse infiltration of lymphocytes and the appearances are nonspecific. The systemic disease may end fatally, but the prognosis has improved in recent years due to more effective treatment.

The aetiology of lupus erythematosus is not known, but genetic factors appear to be important, and autoantibodies of several types which are neither species nor organ specific are present in all cases of the systemic form. Antinuclear antibodies are found in most patients, and LE cells (neutrophil leucocytes which have phagocytosed other leucocyte nuclei) can often be demonstrated *in vitro* following incubation of peripheral blood or bone marrow. A few cases of systemic lupus erythematosus are drug induced. The prevailing abnormality in systemic lupus erythematosus appears to be a polyclonal hyperactivity of B lymphocytes.

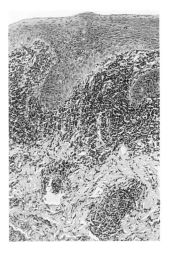

Fig. 9.25 Chronic discoid lupus erythematosus showing perivascular extension of inflammation.

Lupus erythematosus   **Key points**

- females affected more frequently than males
- chronic discoid (localized) form
  —facial skin may be involved
  —cheeks commonest oral site
  —discoid area of erythema with keratotic borders
- systemic form
  —skin rashes and systemic involvement
  —oral lesions variable

FURTHER READING

Axell, T., Pindborg, J. J., Smith, C. J., and van der Waal, I. (1996). Oral white lesions with special reference to precancerous and tobacco-related lesions: conclusions of an international symposium held in Uppsala, Sweden, May 18–21 1994. *Journal of Oral Pathology and Medicine*, **25**, 49–54.

Barnard, N. A., Scully, C., Eveson, J. W., Cunningham, S., and Porter, S. R. (1993). Oral cancer development in patients with oral lichen planus. *Journal of Oral Pathology and Medicine*, **22**, 421–4.

Bratel, J., Hakeberg, M., and Jontell, M. (1996). Effect of replacement of dental amalgam on oral lichenoid reactions. *Journal of Dentistry*, **24**, 41–5.

Brown, R. S., Bottomley, W. K., Puente, E., and Lavigne, G. J. (1993). A retrospective evaluation of 193 patients with oral lichen planus. *Journal of Oral Pathology and Medicine*, **22**, 69–72.

Eversole, L. R. (1989). Oral mucosal disorders of the keratinization process. In *World workshop on oral medicine* (ed. H. D. Millard and D. K. Mason), pp. 95–9. Year Book Medical Publishers, Chicago.

Eveson, J. W. (1983). Oral premalignancy. *Cancer Survey*, **2**, 403–24.

Holmstrup, P. (1991). Reactions of the oral mucosa related to silver amalgam: a review. *Journal of Oral Pathology and Medicine*, **20**, 1–7.

Lumermann, H., Freedman, P., and Kerpel, S. (1995). Oral epithelial dysplasia and the development of invasive squamous cell carcinoma. *Oral Surgery, Oral Medicine, Oral Pathology, Oral Radiology and Endodontics*, **79**, 321–9.

Ostman, P.-O., Anneroth, G., and Skoglund, A. (1994). Oral lichen planus lesions in contact with amalgam fillings: a clinical, histologic, and immunohistochemical study. *Scandinavian Journal of Dental Research*, **102**, 172–9.

Ostman, P.-O., Anneroth, G., and Skoglund, A. (1996). Amalgam—associated oral lichenoid reactions. *Oral Surgery, Oral Medicine, Oral Pathology, Oral Radiology and Endodontics*, **81**, 459–65.

Pindborg, J. J. (1990). Diseases of the skin. In *Oral manifestations of systemic disease* (2nd edn) (ed. J. H. Jones and D. K. Mason), pp. 537–92. W. B. Saunders, London.

Schiodt, M. and Pindborg, J. J. (1984). Oral discoid lupus erythematosus. *Oral Surgery, Oral Medicine, Oral Pathology*, **57**, 46–51, 177–80, and 281–93.

Scully, C. and El-Kom. (1985). Lichen planus: review and update on pathogenesis. *Journal of Oral Pathology*, **14**, 431–58.

Silverman, S., Gorsky, M., and Lozada, F. (1984). Oral leukoplakia and malignant transformation. A follow-up of 2157 patients. *Cancer*, **53**, 563–8.

Wright, J. M. and Wright, B. A. (1988). Premalignancy. In *Oral cancer: clinical and pathological considerations* (ed. B. A. Wright, J. M. Wright, and W. H. Binnie), pp. 33–55. CRC Press, Boca Raton.

Yamamoto, T., Osaki, T., Yoneda, K., and Ueta, E. (1994). Cytokine production by keratinocytes and mononuclear infiltrates in oral lichen planus. *Journal of Oral Pathology and Medicine*, **23**, 309–15.

10 Oral epithelial tumours, melanocytic naevi, and malignant melanoma

10 Oral epithelial tumours, melanocytic naevi, and malignant melanoma

THE main tumours derived from oral epithelium are the squamous cell papilloma and squamous cell carcinoma. The squamous cell papilloma is usually regarded as a benign neoplasm, but a variety of virally induced hyperplasias of oral epithelium may mimic the papilloma clinically and these are included in this chapter. Basal cell carcinoma does not occur in the oral cavity but may arise on the vermilion border of the lip.

The melanocytic naevi and malignant melanomas are hamartomatous and neoplastic lesions, respectively, derived from melanocytes and/or their precursors. Whilst there is an intimate relationship between these cells and the epithelium, melanocytes are derived from the neuroectoderm of the neural crest and are a population of cells distinct from keratinocytes.

SQUAMOUS CELL PAPILLOMA AND OTHER BENIGN LESIONS ASSOCIATED WITH HUMAN PAPILLOMAVIRUS (HPV)

HPV are DNA viruses and more than 70 types are now recognized. They are associated with a number of benign conditions of the skin and oral mucosa characterized by abnormal proliferation of keratinocytes. These include verruca vulgaris, condyloma acuminatum, and focal epithelial hyperplasia. However, certain types of HPV are commonly present in clinically healthy oral mucosa and the identification of HPV in a lesion does not necessarily imply a causal relationship. In particular, the role of HPV in the aetiology of oral squamous cell papilloma is still unclear although HPV DNA, for example to types 6 and 11, has been demonstrated in some cases. The possible role of HPV in the aetiology of squamous cell carcinoma is discussed later in this chapter; their role in leukoplakia is discussed in Chapter 9.

HPV   **Key points**

- infect keratinocytes
- associated with abnormal epithelial proliferation
  —hyperplasia—warts
  —benign neoplasia—papilloma
  —malignant neoplasia—squamous cell carcinoma
- may be present in normal epithelium

Squamous cell papilloma

This common benign tumour is usually a solitary lesion and can occur anywhere on the oral mucosa. Most occur in adults but they may also be seen in children.

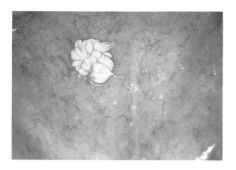

Fig. 10.1 Squamous cell papilloma.

Papillomas vary in size and may be either pedunculated or sessile. They present as warty or cauliflower-like growths with a white or pink surface depending on the amount of keratin present (Fig. 10.1). Histological examination shows finger-like processes of proliferating stratified squamous epithelium supported by thin cores of vascular connective tissue (Fig. 10.2). The epithelium may show hyperkeratosis. Mitotic figures are often seen in the basal layer of the epithelium, but features of epithelial dysplasia are not present.

Malignant change has not been described in a squamous cell papilloma of the oral mucosa and it is not a premalignant lesion.

Verruca vulgaris (common wart)

Clinically, these lesions present as squamous cell papillomas and may be sessile or pedunculated, single or multiple. They appear white because of hyperkeratosis and are seen most often in children when they may be associated with autoinoculation from warts on the fingers and lips.

Histologically, they consist of papillary processes of proliferating, acanthotic, hyperkeratotic squamous epithelium supported by thin cores of vascular connective tissue. The hyperplastic rete ridges around the margins usually slope inwards towards the centre of the lesion (Fig. 10.3). Large vacuolated cells with prominent keratohyalin granules may be present in the stratum granulosum and upper parts of the prickle cell layer (Fig. 10.4).

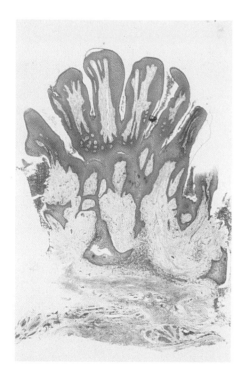

Fig. 10.2 Squamous cell papilloma.

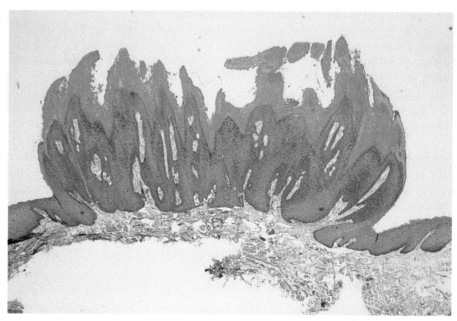

Fig. 10.3 Verruca vulgaris.

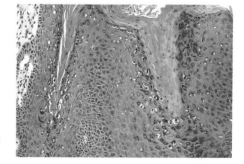

Fig. 10.4 Verruca vulgaris showing vacuolated cells in stratum granulosum.

Common warts on the skin are usually associated with HPV types 2 or 4 infection.

Condyloma acuminatum (venereal wart)

Charactertistically, these warts occur in the anogenital region but they may be seen on the oral mucosa. Clinically, they present as multiple pink nodules which grow and coalesce to form soft, pink, pedunculated or sessile papillary lesions similar in colour to the surrounding mucosa (Fig. 10.5). In some patients they are an oral manifestation of HIV infection (see Chapter 11).

Histologically, the dominant epithelial feature is a prominent acanthosis with marked broadening and elongation of the rete ridges (Fig. 10.6). Vacuolation is often present in the cells of the upper layer of the epithelium. Keratinization is not a feature although there may be a surface layer of parakeratotic cells.

Condyloma acuminatum is associated with HPV types 6, 11, and 16 (Fig. 10.7).

Focal epithelial hyperplasia (Heck's disease)

This rare disease was originally described in native North Americans and Inuit but occurs in other ethnic groups. It is characterized by multiple small elevated epithelial plaques or polypoid lesions most frequently involving the lower lips and buccal mucosa.

Histological examination shows hyperparakeratosis and acanthosis of the oral epithelium with occasional large vacuolated cells.

HPV types 13 and 32 appear to be specific to oral focal epithelial hyperplasia. It is possible that these viruses only produce disease in patients with a genetic predisposition, and this may account for the higher incidence of the disorder in particular populations and ethnic groups.

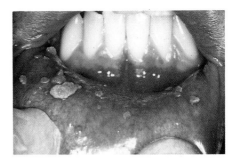

Fig. 10.5 Condyloma acuminatum.

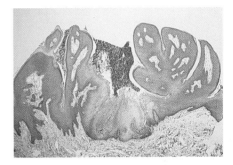

Fig. 10.6 Condyloma acuminatum.

SQUAMOUS CELL CARCINOMA

Epidemiology

Squamous cell carcinoma accounts for 90 per cent or more of all oral malignant neoplasms.

The incidence of oral cancer varies enormously around the world, and data in some cases are difficult to interpret since cancer registration using internationally agreed criteria (based on the WHO International Classification of Diseases (ICD)) is comparatively recent. In the United Kingdom, oral cancer accounts for about 1 per cent of all cancers, in the USA it accounts for about 2–4 per cent, but in parts of India it accounts for 30–40 per cent of all malignant tumours and in some regions a figure approaching 50 per cent has been reported. The incidence rates for large countries, such as India and the USA, conceal regional and ethnic variations. For example, incidence rates tend to be higher in urban as opposed to rural communities, and in the USA are higher for blacks than whites. In the United Kingdom, incidence rates are slightly higher in Scotland than in England and Wales.

In the United Kingdom oral cancer ranks in incidence about 15th of all cancers in men and 20th of all cancers in women, but on a global basis it has been estimated that it is the fourth commonest cancer in men and the sixth commonest in women. When data for both sexes are combined it is the sixth commonest form of malignant disease, and ranks about eighth in incidence for all cancers in developed countries, and third in incidence in developing countries.

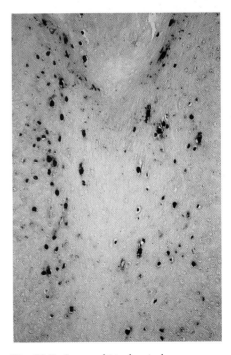

Fig. 10.7 Immunohistochemical demonstration of HPV type 6 (black reaction product) in oral condyloma acuminatum.

In the United Kingdom there are over 2500 new cases and about 1400 deaths per year from oral cancer. The disease is more common in men than in women, although the difference for intraoral cancer is now less marked in England and Wales than previously as incidence rates in men have fallen proportionally more than those for women. The male:female ratio for intraoral cancer in England and Wales is presently about 2:1, and about 3:1 in Scotland. In contrast, lip cancer is some six to eight times more common in men.

Over 90 per cent of oral cancer occurs in patients over the age of 40 years when there is then a sharp and almost linear increase in incidence with age. In England and Wales 85 per cent of cases occur in patients over the age of 50 years.

Although the incidence and mortality rates of oral cancer, particularly in men, have decreased significantly in the United Kingdom and in other developed countries from those of the first half of the twentieth century, there is evidence that the rates are now increasing. In addition, the age of patients with oral cancer, particularly men, has been declining. To what extent this upward trend will continue is unknown but it presumably reflects changes in aetiological factors. In most cases, the reasons for the increasing incidence are unknown but, as discussed later, the increase in cancer of the tongue in the USA has been linked to the increase in use of smokeless tobacco.

Oral carcinoma may occur on any part of the oral mucosa, but there are geographical variations in the sites particularly at risk which partly reflect different aetiological factors. In the United Kingdom the tongue and floor of mouth are the commonest sites. The palate is an unusual location for carcinoma to develop. In contrast, in India the buccal mucosa is the most frequent site, and this can be ascribed to the widespread chewing of betel quid or pan and to smoking habits in that part of the world, as discussed later.

Key points	**Oral cancer**
	• incidence varies around the world
	—1 per cent of all cancers in UK
	—30–40 per cent of all cancers in India
	• globally is one of the 10 commonest cancers
	• incidence in developed countries now on the increase
	• over 2500 new cases/year in UK
	• in the UK is 2–3 times more common in men than women
	• in the UK the death:registration ratio is comparable to that of carcinoma of the uterine cervix

Aetiological factors

No single, clearly recognizable cause has been found for oral carcinoma. It is likely that many factors are involved in the aetiology and that these vary in different ethnic groups. However, epidemiological studies have shown that tobacco and alcohol are the two most important factors for intraoral cancer, and that ultraviolet light is implicated in carcinoma of the lip.

The main factors involved in the aetiology of oral cancer are listed in Table 10.1

Tobacco

A wealth of epidemiological and experimental data implicate tobacco, however used, as an important factor in the aetiology of oral cancer. However, the relative risks associated with different methods of consumption are still unresolved, and the relationship is complicated further by possible synergistic effects when tobacco is combined with other extrinsic factors, such as alcohol and pan chewing (see below).

Polycyclic aromatic hydrocarbons are present in tobacco smoke, but the main carcinogenic agents present in tobacco, regardless of how it is used, are thought to be nitrosamines derived from nicotine, for example N-nitrosonornicotine.

Tobacco smoking

It is now accepted that there is an aetiological relationship between the smoking of tobacco and oral carcinoma regardless of the type of tobacco and method of consumption. Pipe and cigar smoking have been linked with carcinoma of the lip for many years, and the evidence linking cigarette smoking with intraoral carcinoma is now firmly established.

Studies have particularly incriminated heavy cigarette smokers and have shown that those smoking 40 or more cigarettes per day have a significantly increased risk of oral cancer, ranging from about 10 to 20 times that of non-smokers in different series. Other studies have looked at the relative risks at different levels of cigarette consumption and have also compared cigarettes classified as high- or low-tar yield. These have shown a significantly increased risk of oral cancer at all levels of smoking, the level of risk increasing with the amount smoked. The relative risk is decreased for low-tar brands but is still significantly greater, eight times in one study, compared to non-smokers. In subjects who stop smoking the relative risk falls to that of non-smokers after about 10 years.

The type of tobacco, curing methods, and methods of smoking may also influence the relative risk of oral cancer. For example, the high incidence of oral cancer in India is likely to be due, in part, to the widespread smoking of bidis and the habit of reverse smoking (i.e. with the burning end inside the mouth), a habit that is particularly common in women. Reverse smoking is also practised in various other countries, for example Colombia, and is associated particularly with cancer of the palate, one of the rarest sites for oral cancer in other groups. It has been reported that the relative risk of oral cancer for reverse smokers is over 40 times that of non-smokers.

Smokeless tobacco

Snuff is a finely ground or powdered tobacco which may be inhaled dry or used moist in snuff-dipping by placing a pinch of snuff between the gum and the cheek or upper lip. Reports from south-eastern USA, where snuff-dipping is prevalent, and from Sweden indicate that the habit is associated with a significantly increased risk for carcinoma of the gingiva and buccal mucosa. Smokeless tobacco is also available in sachets (resembling tea bags) for oral use, and in the USA it has been suggested that this has led to an increase in oral cancer in young people, but the relative risk is about half that of smoking. The sachets were banned in the United Kingdom in 1990.

Tobacco chewing was relatively common in the United Kingdom in the early part of this century, particularly in occupations such as mining where smoking was environmentally dangerous because of the possibility of explosion. However, in most Western countries the habit has declined, but chewing habits are particularly prevalent in certain parts of the world as discussed below.

Betel quid (pan) and other chewing habits

Pan chewing is one of the most widespread habits in the world and is practised by over 200 million people worldwide. It is particularly common in South-East

Table 10.1 Aetiological factors in oral cancer

| Tobacco smoking |
| pipes |
| cigars |
| cigarettes |
| bidis |
| reverse smoking |
| Smokeless tobacco |
| snuff dipping |
| tobacco sachets |
| tobacco chewing |
| Betel chewing, betel quid, areca nut |
| Alcohol |
| spirits |
| wines and beers quality/quantity |
| alcohol and tobacco synergism |
| Diet and nutrition |
| iron deficiency |
| vitamins A and C |
| nutritional deficiencies and alcoholism |
| Dental factors |
| Ultraviolet light |
| Viruses |
| herpes simplex viruses |
| human papilloma viruses |
| human immunodeficiency virus |
| Immunosuppression |
| Chronic infections |
| candidosis |
| syphilis |
| Occupation |

Asia and India. The composition, type, and quality of the chew vary not only between countries but also between areas within a single country. Basically it consists of betel nut and lime wrapped in a betel leaf, and tobacco, catechu, and other spices are often added according to custom, individual taste, and economic status. Pan is normally chewed after meals, its effects being to satisfy the hunger sensation, to aid digestion, to produce a slight euphoric effect, and to increase salivation. It is frequently kept in the mouth for a long time. Some people take up to 100 pans daily and habitual users may have a pan in their mouth for 24 hours a day. The habit often starts in childhood, even as early as 3 years of age.

This habit induces leukoplakia where the pan is held in the mouth, and malignant transformation is usually evidenced clinically by the development of a papilliferous, ulcerated mass. Unravelling the roles of the constituents of the pan in the aetiology of leukoplakia and squamous cell carcinoma presents major problems which are compounded by possible interactions between components of the pan. For example, slaked lime can hydrolyse one of the alkaloids of betel nut (arecoline) to produce arecoidene which has been shown experimentally to be carcinogenic. The increased incidence of oral cancer in Malaysia and Papua New Guinea where betel nut is chewed with lime, but without tobacco, suggests that such mechanisms could play a role. However, several epidemiological studies have shown that the relative risk of oral cancer is greatly increased when tobacco is present in the pan.

Alcohol

Epidemiological studies from several countries have demonstrated an increased risk of oral cancer in association with alcohol consumption. It is the second major factor, and those who abstain from alcohol have a reduced risk. Although there is evidence to support a dose/time relationship, for example several studies have reported a link between oral cancer and liver cirrhosis, this is less striking than that seen with tobacco smoking. The quality and type of beverage are also factors that have to be considered, and the consumption of unmatured home-stilled spirits containing carcinogenic by-products may be particularly important in certain parts of the world. The relative risk for beer and wine drinkers is as high as, and in some studies greater than, that for spirit drinkers. This is perhaps because the weaker alcohols act as solvents and facilitate penetration of the oral mucosa by other carcinogens that may be present in the mouth, for example tobacco products.

Key points	**Tobacco and alcohol**
	• independent risk factors for oral cancer
	• their effect together is multiplicative
	• relative risks for tobacco vary with method of use and type
	• main carcinogens in tobacco are N-nitrosamines
	• alcohol may enhance transport of carcinogens across mucosal barrier
	• nutritional deficiencies in alcoholics may impair mucosal barrier
	• alcoholic beverages may contain carcinogens

Unravelling the role of alcohol in the aetiology of oral cancer has been complicated because of the close association between drinking and smoking habits. Although alcohol is an important factor independent of smoking, many studies have shown a marked increase in the relative risk when smoking and drinking are practised concurrently, suggesting a synergistic or multiplicative effect.

The mechanisms by which alcohol consumption increases the risk of oral cancer are still unclear. Although pure ethanol is not considered to be carcinogenic, mention has already been made of possible carcinogenic contaminants and congeners that may be present in alcoholic beverages and that such drinks may enhance the penetration of carcinogens across the mucosal barrier. It is also possible that nutritional deficiencies and impaired metabolism which are common in heavy drinkers could damage the ability of the oral mucosa to maintain its barrier function. Histological studies suggest that alcohol and tobacco usage are associated with atrophy of oral epithelium.

Concern has also been expressed regarding the potential risk from mouthwash use. The evidence is inconclusive, but an increased risk of oral cancer has been reported in subjects using high alcohol content (25 per cent or higher) mouthwashes.

Diet and nutrition

The increased risk of oesophageal, pharyngeal, and oral cancer associated with primary sideropenic anaemia (Plummer–Vinson or Patterson–Kelly syndrome) has been recognized for many years. Iron is essential for the maintenance of oral epithelium and it is possible that atrophic changes in iron deficiency anaemia render the mucosa more susceptible to chemical carcinogens. (A similar effect may be associated with other diseases showing epithelial atrophy, such as lichen planus and tertiary syphilis.)

Diet and oral cancer   **Key points**
- deficiencies of vitamins A, C, E and iron are contributory factors to oral cancer
- high fruit consumption decreases the risk of oral cancer

Vitamin A is also important in the maintenance of stratified squamous epithelium, and several epidemiological studies have shown that individuals whose diets are high in the antioxidant vitamins A, C, and E have a decreased risk of oral cancer. The protective effect is related in particular to a diet with a high fruit intake. The possibility of nutritional deficiencies associated with alcoholism has been discussed above.

Dental factors

Poor oral hygiene, faulty restorations, sharp edges of teeth and ill-fitting dentures have all been incriminated in the aetiology of oral cancer, but the evidence for this is meagre. Many patients with oral malignancy have poor dentitions but they also smoke and drink heavily, and the relative importance of the various factors in the aetiology of oral carcinoma is difficult to evaluate. Experimental carcinogenesis has shown that mechanical irritation can act as a promoter, but not as an initiator, and dental factors may have a similar role in oral carcinoma in humans.

Ultraviolet light

High exposure to ultraviolet light is thought to be an important factor in squamous cell carcinoma of the lip. Lip (vermilion border) cancer occurs much more frequently in the lower than the upper lip, is much more common in men than women, and is associated particularly with outdoor occupations. It is rare in dark-skinned races because of the protection conferred against ultraviolet light by melanin pigment. Squamous cell carcinoma of the lip may be preceded by hyper-keratotic and dysplastic changes—solar keratosis.

Viruses

Herpes simplex viruses (HSV)

Laboratory experiments have shown that HSV can be carcinogenic or cocarcino-genic under certain circumstances and so must be considered as possible aetio-logical agents in oral carcinoma. Although viral markers for HSV have been demonstrated in some tumours, this does not necessarily imply a causal relation-ship. If HSV do play a role in the aetiology of oral carcinoma, it remains to be explained why such ubiquitous agents so rarely produce tumours.

Key points	**Viruses and oral cancer**
	• no unequivocal role established
	• evidence for role for HPV in some premalignant lesions and oral carcinomas increasing
	• HSV and EBV are probably incidental passenger viruses

Human papillomaviruses (HPV)

HPV types 16 and 18 are now accepted as important factors in the aetiology of squamous cell carcinoma of the uterine cervix, and several studies have invest-igated the role of these viruses in oral carcinomas and premalignant lesions. The results have been inconsistent, probably because of variation of the sensitiv-ity of the assays used, but in most studies HPV DNA has been found in less than half (generally about 20 per cent) of oral carcinomas compared to 80–90 per cent of cervical lesions. However, detection rates are increasing with more sensitive techniques. HPV 16 is the most common isolate, but interpretation of its role is complicated by reports that the virus may be present in apparently normal mucosa.

HPV contains various genes, but those which are expressed early in viral replication (the E genes) produce proteins which can bind and inactivate the products of two tumour-suppressor genes, p53 and Rb (retinoblastoma gene). The possible significance of mutation or inactivation of p53 in oral leukoplakia has been discussed in Chapter 9 and is discussed later in this chapter in relation to oral cancer. In this respect, HPV was detected in one study in about half of the premalignant lesions examined and in all of those which subsequently developed into invasive squamous cell carcinoma during the long follow-up period.

Although the studies to date do not suggest a major role for HPV in oral cancer, the viruses may act in concert with other factors such as smoking and alcohol. Some evidence suggests that the association between HPV and oral cancer may be more important in patients below the 7th decade. Geographic variations may also exist; a high prevalence of HPV has been reported in a series of oral cancer from India.

Epstein–Barr virus (EBV)

EBV has an aetiological role in the development of some nasopharyngeal carcino-mas (as well as some lymphomas), but a similar role in the development of oral squamous cell carcinoma has not been established. Although the virus has been demonstrated more frequently in carcinoma than in normal epithelium, it is probably present only as a passenger virus.

Human immunodeficiency virus (HIV)

Oral squamous cell carcinoma has been reported as an oral lesion associated with HIV infection, but the evidence is inconclusive (see Chapter 11). However, it is well recognized that patients with immunodeficiencies have an increased incidence of malignant disease in general and of lymphomas in particular.

Immunosuppression

Reports have been published of an increased risk of carcinoma of the lip in patients following renal and other organ transplantation, and it is likely that this is in some way related to the immunosuppressive therapy that such patients receive. Mention has already been made of the possibility of increased risk of oral cancer in patients with AIDS.

Smoking, alcohol, and iron deficiency also reduce the effectiveness of cell-mediated immunity, but the significance of this in their aetiological roles in oral cancer is unknown.

Chronic infections

Chronic candidal infection

This is often associated with speckled leukoplakias, and such lesions are particularly prone to undergo malignant transformation (see Chapter 9). It has been suggested that the fungus is in some way responsible for the transformation. Chronic hyperplastic candidosis (see Chapter 11) also presents as a leukoplakic lesion and may have premalignant potential. However, chronic oral candidal infections, such as those seen in patients with chronic mucocutaneous candidosis, do not undergo malignant transformation, even though there may be an associated immune deficiency or abnormality. The role of candidal infection in malignant transformation must, therefore, be regarded as uncertain.

Syphilis

Historically, tertiary syphilis has been linked with oral cancer, particularly on the dorsum of the anterior two-thirds of the tongue. Development of carcinoma may be preceded by syphilitic leukoplakia. It is possible that epithelial atrophy in the late stages of the disease renders the mucosa more susceptible to other carcinogens. However, it is also likely that the high incidence of oral cancer reported in the past resulted, in part, from medicaments (for example arsenicals) used to treat the infection. Late-stage syphilis is now rare and with modern treatment plays an almost insignificant role in the aetiology of oral cancer today.

Occupation

A high incidence of oral carcinoma has been reported in textile workers, particularly in those exposed to dust from raw cotton and wool. It has also been suggested that there is an increased risk among workers in the printing trades, but the evidence is inconclusive.

Oncogenes and tumour-suppressor genes

Oral cancer has a multifactorial aetiology and is the result of genetic damage allowing uncontrolled proliferation of cells. It is a multistep process involving multiple sequential mutations particularly to the genes which regulate cell growth and proliferation. These genes are the growth-promoting proto-oncogenes found in normal cells, and the tumour-suppressor genes that encode for growth inhibitory proteins. Under normal circumstances cellular proliferation is controlled by the balance between these growth-promoting and growth-inhibiting genes. During carcinogenesis a proto-oncogene may undergo mutation and become an activated oncogene, resulting in enhanced activity, and/or tumour-suppressor genes may be mutated or their products inactivated. The result in both cases leads to deregulation of cell proliferation and tumour formation.

Oncogenes

The main oncogenes that have been studied in oral cancer are members of the c-myc and ras families and erb B-1. Over-expression of these genes has been reported in oral squamous cell carcinoma, but the underlying mechanisms are not fully understood and results from different studies are sometimes at variance. For example, alterations of the ras genes (mutation or amplification) which could account for over-expression of the oncoprotein occur in about a third of oral cancers in India but only in about 5 per cent in western Europe and the USA. This may be associated with specific tobacco smoking and chewing habits in India. Although the sequence of genetic events in the development of oral cancer is far from being defined, over-expression of ras oncogenes may be an early event, whereas over-expression of c-myc genes occurs later in the progression of the disease and may be associated with a poor prognosis. The erb B-1 gene encodes for the epidermal growth factor receptor (EGFR) which is a transmembrane glycoprotein that stimulates cell proliferation on contact with its ligand, epidermal growth factor. Over-expression of erb B-1 has been reported in about 50 per cent of squamous cell carcinomas and may also be important in the transition from a premalignant lesion to invasive carcinoma.

Tumour-suppressor genes

Abnormality of the p53 gene which gives rise to altered p53 protein is one of the most common genetic changes seen in a wide variety of human cancers, including oral squamous cell carcinoma. The p53 gene is essential for normal cell growth and plays a key role in the control of cell division by blocking the cycle in the G_1 phase, the phase before DNA synthesis (S phase), if there is damage to the DNA. This G_1 checkpoint control allows time for repair of the damaged DNA thus preserving the integrity of the genome and preventing transmission of mutations to daughter cells. If DNA repair fails p53 may also trigger apoptosis. Mutations of the p53 gene can therefore result in loss of regulation of the normal cell cycle and allow cells with damaged DNA to undergo replication. As discussed in Chapter 9, abnormalities of the p53 gene are thought to be an early event in the development of oral cancer. In this respect, it has been shown that p53 mutations and over-expression of mutant p53 protein correlate with heavy drinking and tobacco consumption.

Key points	**Oncogenes**
	• derived from mutated proto-oncogenes of normal cells
	• mutation results in enhanced or inappropriate gene expression
	• code for growth-promoting factors
	• excess or abnormal oncogene product may lead to uncontrolled cell growth
	• over-expression of certain oncogenes is involved in the aetiology of oral cancer

Clinical presentation

The clinical presentation of oral squamous cell carcinoma can take many forms. Early diagnosis is the most important factor influencing prognosis, and clinicians must be suspicious of any lesion for which no cause can be found or which does not respond as expected when putative causes have been eliminated. Oral cancer is also a relatively uncommon disease and lesions may present in areas of the mouth that are difficult to examine. Clinicians must therefore be vigilant in their examination of the mucosa. Vigilance and suspicion are key words in the diagnosis of early carcinoma.

Early lesions are usually asymptomatic. Common modes of presentation are a white patch, a small exophytic growth which in the early stages may show no ulceration or erythema, a small indolent ulcer, or an area of erythroplakia (Figs 10.8–10.11). Pain is seldom present. Clinical features which should arouse suspicion of an early carcinoma are persistent ulceration, induration, and fixation of affected tissue to underlying structures, and underlying bone destruction in the case of alveolar lesions. Lymph node involvement may occur early in oral carcinomas, but enlarged regional nodes do not necessarily indicate metastatic spread as they may show only non-specific changes of reactive hyperplasia. Carcinoma developing on the vermilion border of the lip is clearly visible and so may be noticed at an early stage as a slightly raised swelling or a crusty, inconspicuous lesion resembling delayed healing of herpes labialis (Fig. 10.12).

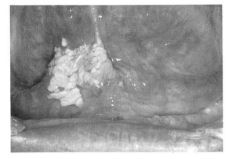
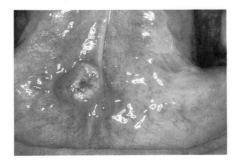
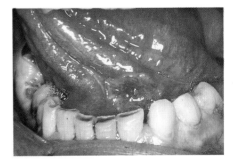

Fig. 10.8 **Fig. 10.9** **Fig. 10.10**

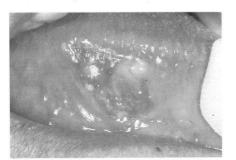
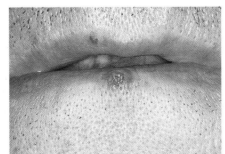

Figs 10.8, 10.9, 10.10, and 10.11 Clinical appearances of early oral squamous cell carcinomas presenting as a white patch, exophytic growth, indolent ulcer, and red patch, respectively.

Fig. 10.12 Early squamous cell carcinoma of lip.

Fig. 10.11 **Fig. 10.12**

An advanced or late lesion may present as a broad-based, exophytic mass with a rough, nodular, warty, haemorrhagic, or necrotic surface, or as a deeply destructive and crater-like ulcer with raised, rolled everted edges. Infiltration of the oral musculature may result in functional disturbances, particularly if the tumour involves the tongue or floor of mouth. Because of reduced mobility of the tongue patients may complain of impaired speech or of difficulty in swallowing. Pain may be a feature of an advanced lesion. Bone invasion may be detected on radiographs and may be suggested clinically by mobility of teeth, and in the mandible, by altered sensation over the distribution of the mental nerve, or pathological fracture.

It is important to note that the size of the surface lesion does not indicate the extent of underlying invasion.

Key points	Clinical features of oral squamous cell carcinoma

	• variable appearances
	   —vigilance
	   —suspicion
	• local invasion
	   —destruction and
	   —distortion of tissues leading to
	   —dysfunction
	• metastatic spread to regional nodes

Pathology

There is considerable variation in the histological appearances of oral squamous cell carcinoma. However, all show invasion and destruction of local tissues, and it is this that accounts for the induration and tethering or fixation that may be detected clinically (Fig. 10.13).

In well-differentiated tumours, the neoplastic epithelium is obviously squamous in type and consists of masses of prickle cells with a limiting layer of basal cells around the periphery. Intercellular bridges are readily recognizable. Keratin pearls are often found within the masses of infiltrating cells, each pearl consisting of a central area of keratin surrounded by whorls of prickle cells (Fig. 10.14). In less well-differentiated tumours the keratin pearls are sparse or absent, and the prickle cells and their nuclei are much more pleomorphic. Mitotic figures are usually abundant and many may be atypical (Fig. 10.15). In poorly differentiated or anaplastic tumours the malignant cells are even more irregular and may hardly be recognizable as epithelial cells (Fig. 10.16). In such cases, immuno-histochemistry to demonstrate cytokeratins (intermediate filament proteins that characterize epithelia) is particularly valuable (Fig. 10.17).

There is variable lymphocytic and plasma cell infiltration in the stroma supporting the invasive malignant epithelium, which probably represents a reaction by the host's immune system to tumour antigens as well as a response to tumour necrosis and ulceration.

Most oral squamous cell carcinomas are extremely locally destructive. The pattern of infiltration of the adjacent tissues by the neoplastic epithelium is variable. In some tumours the appearances suggest a broad front of invasion, but in others apparently separate islands of carcinoma or even individual malignant cells may be seen well in advance of the main growth. Lymphatic permeation, vascular invasion, sarcolemmal, and perineural spread may occur. Slender cords of malignant epithelium may infiltrate for considerable distances within muscle fibres and along nerve bundles necessitating excision of a wide margin of surrounding tissue in the surgical management of such a tumour. Invasion of bone

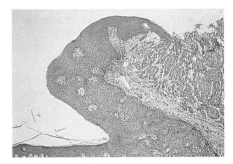

Fig. 10.13

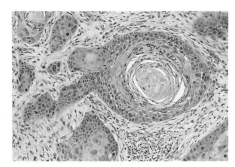

Fig. 10.14

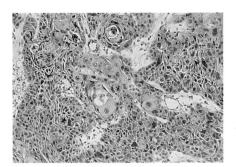

Fig. 10.15

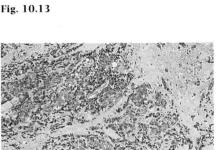

Fig. 10.16

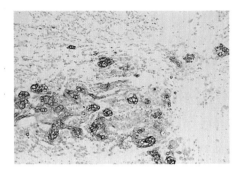

Fig. 10.17

Fig. 10.13 The edge of a malignant ulcer showing invasive squamous cell carcinoma.

Fig. 10.14 Well-differentiated squamous cell carcinoma showing keratin pearls.

Fig. 10.15 Moderate/poorly-differentiated squamous cell carcinoma.

Fig. 10.16 Anaplastic squamous cell carcinoma.

Fig. 10.17 Immunohistochemical demonstration of cytokeratin (brown reaction product) in anaplastic malignant cells of tumour shown in Fig. 10.16.

occurs as a result of local spread. In the edentulous jaws (Fig. 10.18) the main route of entry appears to be through the crest of the ridge, following the path of vessels communicating between the marrow and periosteum rather than through the cortical plates. In the dentate patient, tumour may also invade via the periodontal ligament. Within the jaws the tumour spreads through the marrow spaces (Fig. 10.19) between the cancellous trabeculae and, particularly in the mandible, along neurovascular bundles. The extent of bone involvement may, therefore, be greater than that suggested on routine radiographs.

Lymphatic spread to the regional lymph nodes is a variable feature, but the frequency of cervical metastasis tends to increase with increasing size of the primary tumour. As the metastatic carcinoma destroys and replaces the nodal lymphoid tissue it may also invade through the capsule of the node into the surrounding tissues, resulting in fixation of the node on clinical examination. Extracapsular spread is an important feature which has an adverse affect on prognosis. Blood-borne metastases occur late in the clinical course of the disease but many patients die before distant metastases become apparent.

Pathology of oral squamous cell carcinoma   **Key points**
- cytologically malignant squamous epithelium
- keratinization varies with degree of differentiation
- local invasion
  —lymphatic permeation
  —sarcolemmal spread   related to
  —perineural spread   clinical features
  —bone, edentulous/dentate   and management
- metastatic spread to nodes
  —intracapsular/extracapsular

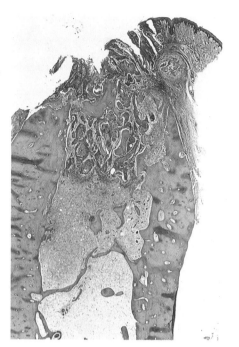

Fig. 10.18 Invasion of the mandible by squamous cell carcinoma spreading from the alveolar crest.

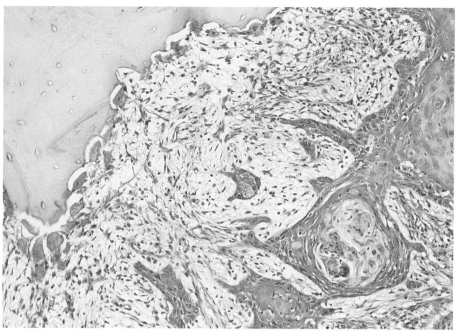

Fig. 10.19 Destruction of bone associated with infiltration of marrow spaces by squamous cell carcinoma.

Prognosis

The survival rate of patients with oral carcinoma depends on a number of factors, but early diagnosis is by far the most important. It is influenced by the site of the lesion, and generally the further back in the mouth the tumour, then the worse the prognosis. This is probably because tumours at the back of the mouth tend not to be diagnosed at an early stage, but the rich lymphatic drainage around the base of the tongue may also favour early metastatic spread. Carcinomas in females have a better prognosis than carcinomas in males, possibly because they tend to be diagnosed and treated at an earlier stage. This probably reflects the fact that more females are regular dental attenders than males. Age affects prognosis, partly because with increasing age the patient becomes less well able to withstand extensive surgery or radiotherapy. Reduction in the effectiveness of cell-mediated immune responses may also be involved.

Attempts have been made to grade carcinomas numerically depending on their degree of histological differentiation and several schemes have been devised, the best known of which is Broders' classification which graded carcinomas on a scale of 1–4 ranging from well-differentiated to undifferentiated tumours. However, the relationship between such grading and prognosis is controversial and it is also unrealistic to grade small biopsies as many carcinomas are not microscopically homogeneous.

The major factors thought to influence prognosis have been incorporated into clinical staging systems which assess the extent of disease in the patient. The most widely used is the TNM system (Table 10.2) which is based on three parameters—T, the size of the primary lesion; N, the extent and distribution of metastases in the regional lymph nodes; M, the presence or not of distant metastases. Other more complicated systems have been proposed, such as the STNMP system which takes account of the site (S), the extent or size of the tumour (T), the condition of the regional lymph nodes (N), the absence or presence of distant metastases (M), and the pathology (P).

Table 10.2 Clinical staging of malignant neoplasms of the oral cavity (IDC9, 140, 141, 143–145) based on the TNM system

Tumour
T1 Greatest diameter of primary tumour 2 cm or less
T2 Greatest diameter of primary tumour > 2 cm but not > 4 cm
T3 Greatest diameter of primary tumour > 4 cm
T4 Massive tumour > 4 cm with gross local invasion

Nodes
N0 No clinically positive nodes
N1 Single ipsilateral node not greater than 3 cm diameter
N2 (a) Single ipsilateral node > 3 cm but not > 6 cm diameter
    (b) Multiple ipsilateral nodes not > 6 cm diameter
    (c) Bilateral or contralateral nodes not > 6 cm diameter
N3 Any node > 6 cm diameter

Metastasis
M0 No distant metastases
M1 Distant metastases

Clinical staging

Stage 1	T1	N0	M0	
Stage 2	T2	N0	M0	
Stage 3	T3	N0	M0	or
	T1, T2, or T3	N1	M0	
Stage 4	T4	N0 or N1	M0	or
	any T	N2 or N3	M0	or
	any T	any N	M1	

Prognosis   **Key points**

- early diagnosis is the major factor determining the prognosis of oral cancer

---

The reduction in survival rates related to metastatic spread is well established. For example, in one study the 5-year survival rate for patients without lymph node metastasis was 86 per cent compared to 44 per cent for those with metastasis. This illustrates the importance of early diagnosis as the major factor influencing prognosis.

Verrucous carcinoma

This is considered to be a distinctive pathological variety of low-grade squamous cell carcinoma occurring on the oral mucosa and also on the skin and other squamous mucosal surfaces. In the mouth it is found most commonly in the mandibular buccal sulcus and adjacent buccal mucosa. It is a disease of the elderly and is seen particularly in tobacco chewers and snuff takers.

Verrucous carcinoma presents clinically as a thick white plaque of heaped-up folds of tissue with deep cleft-like spaces between the folds. It grows slowly and erodes rather than invades the adjacent soft tissues and bone relatively late in its growth. Metastases are said not to occur. The diagnosis can only be made by histological examination, which shows large, heavily keratinized fronds of neoplastic epithelium with bulbous rete processes invading the connective tissue to a similar depth, and so not giving the pattern of invasion usually associated with squamous cell carcinoma. The epithelium is well differentiated, there is little or no cytological atypia, and the basement membrane is intact. Mitoses are rare. The adjacent connective tissue is characteristically heavily infiltrated by chronic

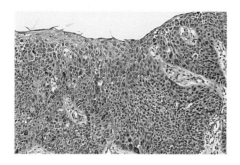

Fig. 10.20 Carcinoma-*in-situ* of the oral mucosa.

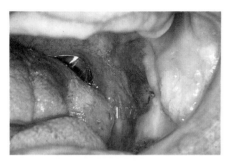

Fig. 10.21 Carcinoma-*in-situ* presenting as erythroplakia.

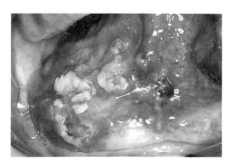

Fig. 10.22 Multifocal invasive carcinoma arising in an extensive field change of carcinoma-*in-situ* presenting as erythroplakia.

inflammatory cells. Reports have been published of anaplastic transformation of verrucous carcinoma treated by radiotherapy, and so surgical excision is usually advised.

The diagnosis of verrucous carcinoma is difficult and strict criteria must be adopted. The tumour must be differentiated from a well-differentiated papillary squamous cell carcinoma or from leukoplakic lesions with warty surfaces, variously called verrucous hyperplasia or verrucous leukoplakia.

Carcinoma-*in-situ*

This term is used to describe severe epithelial dysplasia in which the whole, or almost the whole, thickness of the epithelium is involved but the basement membrane is intact and there is no invasion of the lamina propria (Fig 10.20). Although in the uterine cervix nearly all cases of invasive carcinoma develop from such lesions, this is not so for invasive carcinoma of the oral mucosa. The majority of oral carcinomas are not preceded by a recognizable premalignant lesion (see below).

Oral carcinoma-*in-situ* usually presents clinically as leukoplakia or erythroplakia (Fig. 10.21). The natural history of oral carcinoma-*in-situ* is not well understood. Although in some patients the lesion may progress with time to invasive carcinoma, this is not inevitable and in some cases it remains static and may even regress. It is not uncommon to find histological changes of carcinoma-*in-situ* in the epithelium surrounding an invasive carcinoma, which might suggest a field change in a wide area of mucosa. It is probable that some carcinomas thought to be recurrent tumours represent new primary lesions arising in such a field change (Fig. 10.22).

PREMALIGNANT (OR PRECANCEROUS) LESIONS AND CONDITIONS

A premalignant (or precancerous) lesion is defined as a morphologically altered tissue in which cancer is more likely to occur than in its normal counterpart, for example leukoplakia. That is, the lesion itself undergoes malignant transformation. In contrast, a premalignant (or precancerous) condition is a generalized disorder associated with a significantly increased risk of cancer developing somewhere in the mouth, for example oral submucous fibrosis. However, it must be remembered that relatively few oral carcinomas are preceded by a recognizable premalignant lesion or condition.

The following may be described as premalignant lesions or conditions of the oral mucosa and most are discussed elsewhere:

(1) leukoplakia and erythroplakia;
(2) oral epithelial atrophy occurring in syphilis, oral submucous fibrosis, sideropenic dysphagia, and possibly some vitamin deficiencies;
(3) chronic hyperplastic candidosis;
(4) lichen planus.

EXFOLIATIVE CYTOLOGY

Cells are continually desquamating from the surface of the oral mucosa and from the surface of mucosal lesions. Their collection and microscopic examination can help in diagnosis and this is the basis of exfoliative cytology.

Several epithelial cell types may be seen in a smear from normal oral mucosa (Table 10.3) depending on the site from which it is obtained and the force used in its collection (Fig. 10.23).

Various changes have been described in cells from squamous cell carcinomas and premalignant lesions of the oral mucosa, including enlarged hyperchromatic nuclei, an increased nuclear to cytoplasmic ratio, and coarse clumping of the nuclear chromatin (Fig. 10.24). The size and form of the nuclei and cells may be irregular and several nucleoli may be present. Although the use of exfoliative cytology is well established in screening for carcinoma of the cervix, the technique has not proved reliable in the mouth. It is of little value in assessing keratotic lesions since only surface cells are likely to be sampled, and in lesions where the surface is eroded, ulcerated, or relatively atrophic, secondary inflammatory and degenerative changes may so distort the appearance of the cells as to render interpretation impossible.

BASAL CELL CARCINOMA (RODENT ULCER)

This is a common neoplasm of the skin of the face, particularly in elderly patients with a history of long exposure to ultraviolet radiation (Fig. 10.25). Occasionally, basal cell carcinomas present on the lips, particularly the upper lip, but many are probably skin tumours that have spread to involve the vermilion. Multiple naevoid basal cell carcinomas arising at a younger age and on non-sun-exposed sites are a characteristic feature of the multiple basal cell naevus syndrome (see Chapter 6).

Table 10.3 Cytological appearances and types of exfoliated squamous cells

Cornified squames	anuclear, fully keratinized
Superficial cells	pyknotic nuclei, quadrilateral-shaped cells
Intermediate cells	larger nuclei with fine chromatin pattern; ovoid cells
Parabasal cells	nuclei with fine chromatin pattern; ovoid cells about half the size of above
Basal cells	round nucleus, finely dispersed chromatin, small ovoid cells

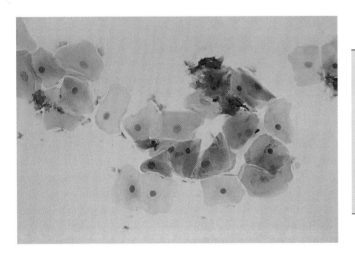

Fig. 10.23

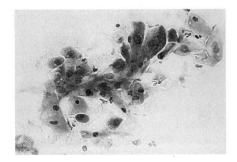

Fig. 10.24

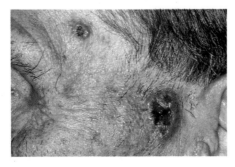

Fig. 10.25

Fig. 10.23 Normal superficial parakeratinized squames.

Fig. 10.24 Exfoliated cytologically malignant squames.

Fig. 10.25 Basal cell carcinoma (rodent ulcer).

The typical basal cell carcinoma presents as a slow-growing nodule that eventually ulcerates centrally. Histologically, it consists of cytologically malignant basaloid cells, arranged in a variety of patterns, invading adjacent tissues.

Melanocytes are dendritic cells located mainly in the basal layer of the epidermis and in some mucous membranes. They are widely distributed and present in large numbers in the oral mucosa of clinically pigmented and non-pigmented races, the difference being one of activity rather than of number. Their function is to produce melanin which they then pass to the adjacent keratinocytes. Melanocytes are of neuroectodermal origin and do not contain intermediate filaments of the cytokeratin family.

A variety of lesions are associated with abnormality of melanocytes. Those presenting as tumours or tumour-like conditions (i.e. the naevi and neoplastic proliferations) are considered in this chapter. Other types of hypermelanosis of the oral mucosa, some of which are associated with systemic disease, are discussed in Chapter 13.

Melanocytic naevi

A naevus is any developmental blemish on skin or mucosa (Latin *naevus*, birthmark). Melanocytic naevi (often referred to as moles) are exceedingly common, particularly in the skin of the head and neck. Most present in childhood and adolescence and every person develops between 20 and 30 naevi. Despite their abundance in skin, they are rare in the oral mucosa. Most of those reported have presented in adult life as slightly elevated, pigmented lesions on the hard palate or buccal mucosa. Melanocytic naevi are hamartomatous lesions formed by proliferation of melanocytes or their precursors. The amount of melanin pigment they contain is highly variable.

Junctional, compound, and intramucosal (intradermal) naevi

These lesions represent different stages in the natural history of melanocytic naevi and are separated histologically depending on the location of the melanocytes (Figs 10.26–10.28). In a junctional naevus nests of melanocytic cells are seen along the epithelial-connective tissue junction. A lesion with junctional and connective tissue components is a compound naevus. As the lesion matures, junctional activity disappears and the lesion is located entirely within the lamina propria (dermis) giving rise to an intramucosal (intradermal) naevus. Most oral melanocytic naevi are of this type.

Although malignant change can occur in naevi this is exceedingly rare bearing in mind how common naevi are. However, the presence of junctional activity in a lesion from an adult must be viewed with caution.

Blue naevus

This is the second most frequent type of intraoral naevus. It is located deeper in the connective tissues than the intramucosal naevus, and is characterized by an ill-defined proliferation of elongated spindle-shaped, usually heavily pigmented melanocytes derived from melanocytic cells that have failed in their fetal migration to reach the basal layer of the epithelium. Blue naevi are not part of the natural history of the other naevi described above; junctional activity is not a

Fig. 10.26 Junctional naevus.

Fig. 10.27 Compound naevus.

Fig. 10.28 Intradermal naevus.

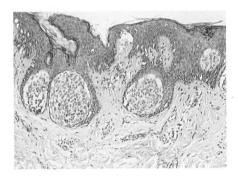

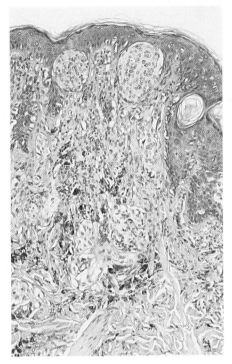

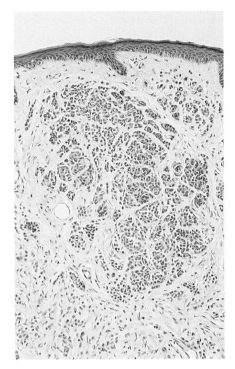

Fig. 10.26

Fig. 10.27

Fig. 10.28

feature. Although they usually contain abundant melanin pigment they appear clinically as bluish rather than brown lesions because of their deeper location.

Malignant melanoma *in situ* and malignant melanoma

Since excessive exposure to ultraviolet light is the most important predisposing factor for malignant melanoma of the skin, many tumours arise in the head and neck region.

Skin tumours may present as pigmented plaques or nodular lesions and may be preceded by malignant melanoma *in situ*. This is characterized by horizontal spread within the epithelium. Vertical spread into the dermis characterizes invasive malignant melanoma and the prognosis depends mainly on the depth of invasion at the time of diagnosis.

Malignant melanoma of the oral mucosa is rare. It is slightly more common in men than women, and over 70 per cent of cases involve the posterior maxillary alveolar ridge and hard palate (Fig. 10.29). Most are advanced and extensively invasive lesions at presentation, but in about a third of cases there is a history of previous pigmentation in the area.

Most oral malignant melanomas present as dark-brown or bluish-black slightly raised lesions with an uneven nodular or papillary surface (amelanotic lesions tend to appear reddish in colour). Growth may be rapid and there may be extensive destruction of bone with loosening of the teeth. Both regional lymph node and blood-borne metastases are common, and the prognosis for most patients is very poor.

Histologically, malignant melanomas are highly pleomorphic neoplasms. The amount of melanin pigment is variable and in some may be absent (Fig. 10.30). Immunohistochemical studies using specific markers for malignant melanocytes are useful in such cases. Ultrastructural examination to identify immature melanosomes can also be used.

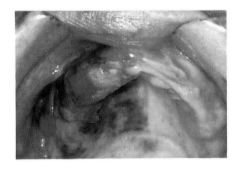

Fig. 10.29 Malignant melanoma.

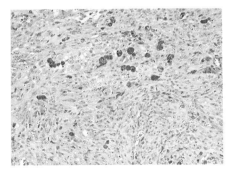

Fig. 10.30 Malignant melanoma (pigmented).

Key points

Oral malignant melanoma

- rare
- most frequent in posterior maxillary region
- may be preceded by melanosis
  —vigilance, suspicion
- nodular or plaque-like with irregular surface

FURTHER READING

Abbey, L. M., Page, D. G., and Sawyer, D. R. (1980). The clinical and histopathologic features of a series of 464 oral squamous papillomas. *Oral Surgery, Oral Medicine, Oral Pathology*, **49**, 419–42.

Binnie, W. H. and Rankin, K. V. (1984). Epidemiological and diagnostic aspects of oral squamous cell carcinoma. *Journal of Oral Pathology*, **13**, 333–41.

Binnie, W. H. Rankin, K. V., and Mackenzie, I. C. (1983). Etiology of oral squamous cell carcinoma. *Journal of Oral Pathology*, **12**, 11–29.

Boyle, P., Macfarlane, G. J., Maisonneuve, P., Zheng, T., Scully, C., and Tedesco, B. (1990). Epidemiology of mouth cancer in 1989: a review. *Journal of the Royal Society of Medicine*, **83**, 724–30.

Buchner, A., Leider, A. S., Merrell, P. W., and Carpenter, W. M. (1990). Melanocytic naevi of the oral mucosa: a clinicopathologic study of 130 cases from northern California. *Journal of Oral Pathology and Medicine*, **19**, 197–201.

Field, J. K. (1992). Oncogenes and tumour-suppressor genes in squamous cell carcinoma of the head and neck. *Oral Oncology, European Journal of Cancer*, **28B**, 67–76.

Field, J. K., Pavelic, Z. P., Spandidos, D. A., Stambrook, P. J., Jones, A. S., and Gluckman, J. L. (1993). The role of the p53 tumour suppressor gene in squamous cell carcinoma of the head and neck. *Archives of Otolaryngology Head and Neck Surgery*, **119**, 1118–22.

Jacobsen, S. and Shear, M. (1972). Verrucous carcinoma of the mouth. *Journal of Oral Pathology*, **1**, 66–75.

Miller, C. S. and White, D. K. (1996). Human papillomavirus expression in oral mucosa, premalignant conditions, and squamous cell carcinoma. *Oral Surgery, Oral Medicine, Oral Pathology, Oral Radiology and Endodontics*, **82**, 57–68.

Rapini, R. P., Golitz, L. E., Greer, R. O., Krekorian, E. A., and Poulson, T. (1985). Primary malignant melanoma of the oral cavity: a review of 177 cases. *Cancer*, **55**, 1543–51.

Raybaud-Diogène, H., Tétu, B., Morency, R., Fortin, A., and Monteil, R. A. (1996). P53 overexpression in head and neck squamous cell carcinoma: review of the literature. *Oral Oncology, European Journal of Cancer*, **32B**, 143–9.

Scully, C. (1982). The immunology of cancer of the head and neck with particular reference to oral cancer. *Oral Surgery, Oral Medicine, Oral Pathology*, **53**, 157–69.

Scully, C. (1992). Oncogenes, onco-suppressors, carcinogenesis and oral cancer. *British Dental Journal*, **173**, 53–9.

Scully, C. (1992). Viruses and oral squamous cell carcinoma. *Oral Oncology, European Journal of Cancer*, **28B**, 57–9.

Scully, C. (1993). Oncogenes, tumour suppressors and viruses in oral squamous carcinoma. *Journal of Oral Pathology and Medicine*, **22**, 337–47.

Scully, C. (1995). Oral precancer: preventive and medical approaches to management. *Oral Oncology, European Journal of Cancer*, **31B**, 16–26.

Shafer, W. G. (1975). Oral carcinoma *in situ*. *Oral Surgery, Oral Medicine, Oral Pathology*, **39**, 227–38.

Shafer, W. G. and Waldron, C. A. (1975). Erythroplakia of the oral cavity. *Cancer*, **36**, 1021–8.

Shear, M. and Pindborg, J. J. (1980). Verrucous hyperplasia of the oral mucosa. *Cancer*, **46**, 1855–62.

Smith, C., Pindborg, J. J., and Binnie, W. H. (1990). *Oral cancer: epidemiology, etiology and pathology*. The Cancer Series. Hemisphere Publishing Corporation, New York.

van der Waal, R. I., Snow, G. B., Karim, A. B., and van der Waal, I. (1994). Primary malignant melanoma of the oral cavity: a review of eight cases. *British Dental Journal*, **176**, 185–8.

Winn, D. (1995). Diet and nutrition in the etiology of oral cancer. *American Journal of Clinical Nutrition*, **61** (suppl), 437S–45S.

Woods, K. V., Shillitoe, E. J., Spitz, M. R., Schantz, S. P., and Adler-Storthz, K. (1993). Analysis of human papillomavirus DNA in oral squamous cell carcinomas. *Journal of Oral Pathology and Medicine*, **22**, 101–8.

Woolgar, J. A., Scott, J., Vaughan, E. D., Brown, J. S., West, C. R., and Rogers, S. (1995). Survival, metastasis and recurrence of oral cancer in relation to pathological features. *Annals of the Royal College of Surgeons of England*, **77**, 325–31.

Wright, B. A., Wright, J. M., and Binnie, W. H. (1988). *Oral cancer: clinical and pathological considerations*. CRC Press, Boca Raton.

11 Infections of the oral mucosa

11 Infections of the oral mucosa

The common oral mucosal infections are caused by viruses, bacteria, and fungi. Helminthic and protozoal infections may involve oral tissues, but discussion of these is outside the scope of this book.

VIRAL INFECTIONS

The laboratory confirmation of the diagnosis of many viral diseases is slow and difficult and, therefore, the diagnosis of most viral infections of the oral mucosa is based mainly on clinical features. However, there are three main laboratory methods of diagnosis available:

1. Virus may be isolated from the lesions and identified after cultivation in tissue culture, fertilized eggs, or laboratory animals.
2. Virus particles or characteristic histological changes may be found in affected tissue using either light or electron microscopy. Viral antigens may be demonstrated in infected cells by immunofluorescent, immunocytochemical or *in-situ* hybridization techniques.
3. Serological studies can be used to demonstrate a significant rise in antibody titre (at least fourfold) against a particular virus between the acute and convalescent sera. Alternatively, the identification of specific IgM (the first class of antibody produced in acute infection) to a particular virus in the acute serum is helpful in diagnosis.

The main viral infections of the oral mucosa are listed in Table 11.1; some of the diseases are discussed elsewhere in this book. Human immunodeficiency virus (HIV), mumps, and influenza are included in the table since there may be associated mucosal lesions. HIV is discussed later in this chapter. Mumps primarily affects salivary glands (see Chapter 14), but may be associated with a non-specific stomatitis because of the reduced salivary flow. An acute non-specific stomatitis may also be seen as an early feature in patients with influenza.

Herpetic stomatitis

The herpes simplex viruses (HSV) are DNA viruses and are the most frequent cause of a viral infection of the mouth. There are two types of HSV with serological, biological, and clinical differences. Type 1 is traditionally associated with infections of the skin and oral mucous membranes, and type 2 virus with infections of the genitalia. However, it now appears that this distinction is much less clear-cut; type 2 virus is being increasingly found in herpetic stomatitis and vice versa. HSV have also been implicated in recurrent erythema multiforme (see Chapter 12).

Table 11.1 Viral infections causing, or associated with, diseases of the oral mucosa

Disease	Virus
Herpetic stomatitis, primary/recurrent	Herpes simplex viruses, types 1 and 2
Chickenpox and shingles (herpes zoster)	Varicella-zoster virus
Herpangina	Coxsackie A virus
Hand, foot, and mouth disease	Coxsackie A virus
Infectious mononucleosis	Epstein–Barr virus
Measles	Paramyxovirus
Hairy leukoplakia	Epstein–Barr virus
Viral warts/epithelial hyperplasias	Human papillomaviruses
Oral manifestations of:	
HIV infection	Human immunodeficiency virus
Mumps	Paramyxovirus
Influenza	Influenza virus
Cytomegalovirus infection	Cytomegalovirus

Primary infection with HSV type 1 is frequently subclinical or causes a mild pharyngitis, but in some patients presents as primary herpetic gingivostomatitis. The infection is transmitted by droplet spread or contact with the lesions. Two main age-groups are affected, young children and young adults. Following an incubation period of about 5 days the patient complains of prodromal symptoms of malaise and fever, and within a day or two the mouth becomes uncomfortable with the development of numerous small vesicles on any part of the oral mucosa and lips. The vesicles soon ulcerate (Fig. 11.1) and become secondarily infected and this is accompanied by regional lymphadenitis. There is usually a widespread inflammation of the gingiva which is erythematous and oedematous (Fig. 11.2). Fresh crops of vesicles develop over the next few days, but the symptoms begin to subside about the sixth day of fever with the oral lesions taking 10–14 days to resolve. Circumoral crusting lesions on the lips may be seen, the crusting being due to coagulation of serum which exudes from ruptured vesicles. Extraoral lesions may also be present, particularly in children. For example, vesicles may occur on the skin of the chin as a result of drooling of saliva and on the fingers as a result of sucking. Infections involving the nail-bed, herpetic whitlow, may be quite painful and infection may be transmitted to the eyes by rubbing.

Key points	**Primary infection with HSV**
	• mainly young children/young adults
	• mainly transmitted by saliva
	• frequently subclinical or
	• acute stomatitis with vesicles, ulcers, and malaise

Histological examination of an intact herpetic vesicle shows an intraepithelial blister (Fig. 11.3). The vesicle results from distension and rupture of the virally infected epithelial cells by intracellular oedema and the coalescence of disrupted cells. The infected cells are swollen and have eosinophilic cytoplasm and large, pale vesicular nuclei. These changes are described as ballooning degeneration. Giant cells containing many such nuclei (up to 20 or more) also form as a result of fusion of the cytoplasm of infected cells (Fig. 11.4). The balloon cells and mult-inucleate giant cells can often be identified in smears taken from an intact vesicle

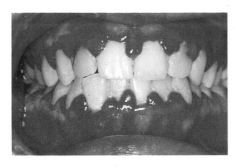

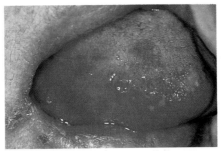

Figs 11.1 and 11.2 Acute herpetic stomatitis showing acute gingivitis and lingual ulceration.

Fig. 11.3 Intraepithelial vesicle in herpes labialis.

Fig. 11.4 Cytopathic changes and multinucleate cells in smear from a herpetic vesicle.

Fig. 11.1

Fig. 11.2

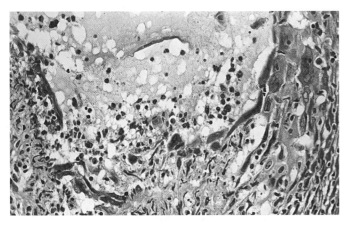

Fig. 11.3

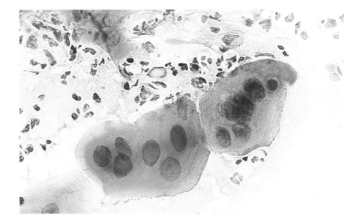

Fig. 11.4

or from one which has recently ruptured. The lamina propria shows a variable inflammatory infiltrate, the density of which depends on the stage and severity of the disease, and inflammatory cells also extend into the epithelium.

Pathology of HSV infection   **Key points**

- infection of epithelial cells
- cytopathic changes
- degeneration and rupture of infected cells
- intraepithelial vesicles

About one in three of those who have had a primary infection, either clinical or subclinical, later develop recurrent infections which are characterized by marked local symptoms unaccompanied by systemic illness. Herpes labialis is the most frequent type of recurrent infection (Fig. 11.5), and appears as clusters of vesicles on the lips and adjacent skin appearing a few hours after prodromal symptoms of itching or tingling. The vesicles rupture within a short time and become crusted. They usually heal within a week. Recurrences may be brought on by a number of different stimuli including mild febrile infections, such as the common cold, ultraviolet light, mechanical trauma, menstruation, stress, and immunosuppression. Recurrent intraoral lesions occur occasionally, almost always on the hard palate or gingiva. Genetic factors may partly determine which people develop recurrent HSV infection as an association with certain HLA types has been suggested.

Recurrent HSV infections are caused by reactivation of virus which following the primary infection has remained latent in the sensory ganglion of the trigeminal

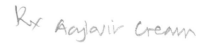

Rx Acylavir Cream

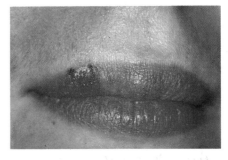

Fig. 11.5 Recurrent herpes labialis.

nerve. Transcription of HSV DNA is blocked in the latency state and so the virus is not affected by antiviral drugs. The sensory ganglion also appears to be an immunoprivileged site so the virus is effectively sequestered from the immune system. There is probably a decrease in latent viral DNA with time. Various stimuli may alter the latency state, permitting the block in HSV transcription to be overcome. The virus then migrates down the sensory nerve axons to the nerve endings where it may be eliminated by immune mechanisms. However, if cell-mediated immunity is impaired the virus can replicate in epithelial cells adjacent to the nerve endings on the lips and adjacent skin or oral mucosa resulting in recurrent herpes. Alternatively, there may just be asymptomatic shedding of HSV into the oral cavity and saliva. Recurrent infections appear to be associated with transient immunosuppression, but patients with a generalized impairment of cell-mediated immunity (for example those receiving immunosuppressive or cytotoxic therapy, or those infected with HIV) are particularly prone to recurrent herpes and may develop intractable infections.

Key points	**Recurrent HSV**
	• reactivation of latent virus in trigeminal sensory ganglion
	• triggered by a variety of factors
	• usually a minor problem, mainly lips
	• severe recurrences in immunocompromised patients

Chickenpox and herpes zoster (shingles)

Both chickenpox and herpes zoster are caused by the same DNA virus (the varicella-zoster virus) which is morphologically similar to the herpes simplex virus.

The lesions of chickenpox may be found on the oral mucosa, especially the soft palate and fauces, and may precede the characteristic skin rash. The oral lesions usually present as small ulcers. Intact vesicles are seldom seen but when examined histologically show cytopathic effects indistinguishable from those of herpes simplex. Zoster is the manifestation of recurrent infection following a primary attack of chickenpox, and in this respect, is similar to recurrent herpes simplex infection except that repeated attacks of zoster are unusual.

Following infection by chickenpox, the virus remains latent in the sensory ganglia probably for the remainder of the life of the host. Reactivation of the virus to cause zoster is uncommon but may occur apparently spontaneously or when the host defences are depressed. Severe infection may be seen in immuno-compromised patients. The lesions are localized to the distribution of one or more sensory nerves. The characteristic unilateral vesicular eruption is frequently preceded by prodromal symptoms of pain and paraesthesia for up to two weeks. When the trigeminal nerve is involved the first division (ophthalmic) is most frequently affected. Involvement of the second or third division causes facial pain and the patient may complain of toothache, followed by the development of vesicles in the distribution of one or more branches of the trigeminal nerve (Figs 11.6, 11.7). The vesicles may be entirely intraoral where they rapidly ulcerate and become secondarily infected. The disease usually runs a course of about 14 days. The most distressing complication of zoster is post-herpetic neuralgia, probably caused by fibrosis in and around the sensory nerves and ganglia. Although zoster involves sensory nerves it occasionally presents with lower motor neurone-type facial paralysis as the Ramsay-Hunt syndrome. The syndrome is due to extension of primary involvement of the geniculate ganglion to affect the facial nerve.

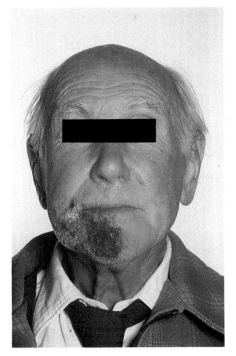

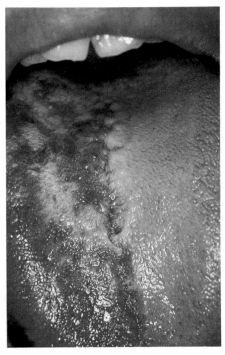

Fig. 11.6

Fig. 11.7

Figs 11.6 and 11.7 Herpes zoster involving the mandibular division of the trigeminal nerve. The skin shows recently ruptured, crusted vesicles. The tongue shows a later stage with healing ulcers.

Herpangina

This infection is caused by various types of coxsackievirus A. Coxsackieviruses are RNA viruses.

The infection is seen most commonly in children and is characterized, clinically, by the sudden onset of a mild illness with fever, anorexia, dysphagia, and sore throat. Vesicles, which rapidly break down into ulcers 1–2 mm in diameter, are seen on the tonsils, soft palate, and uvula (Fig. 11.8). The symptoms persist for 2–3 days only. Clinically, it may be difficult to distinguish from acute primary herpes. However, the latter is a gingivostomatitis, whereas herpangina is an oropharyngitis. No specific histopathological changes have been described.

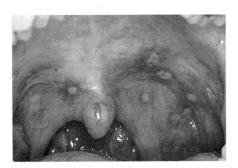

Fig. 11.8 Herpangina.

Hand, foot, and mouth disease

This infection is also caused by various types of coxsackievirus A, especially type 16. It occurs predominantly in children and is transmitted in conditions of close association such as within households. The disease is characterized by the development of shallow ulcers 2–8 mm in diameter situated on the gingiva, tongue, cheeks, and palate, together with vesicles and ulcers on the palms of the hands and the soles of the feet (Figs 11.9–11.11). The lesions may persist for up to 2 weeks. No specific histopathological changes have been described.

In those cases of herpangina or hand, foot, and mouth disease where the diagnosis may be in doubt, estimation of specific IgM in acute sera is helpful.

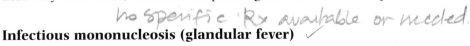

no specific Rx available or needed.

Infectious mononucleosis (glandular fever)

This infection is caused by the Epstein–Barr virus (EBV), a member of the herpes group. It occurs predominantly in teenagers and young adults and is transmitted by kissing either from an infected patient or a healthy carrier.

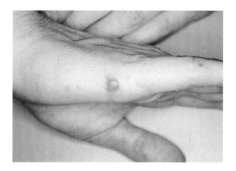

Fig. 11.9

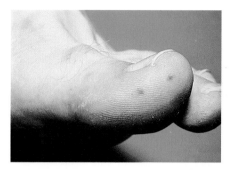

Fig. 11.10

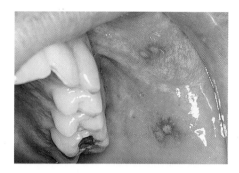

Fig. 11.11

Figs 11.9, 11.10, and 11.11   Hand, foot, and mouth disease.

The disease is characterized by lymph node enlargement, fever, and inflammation of the pharynx, and may be associated with prolonged periods of malaise lasting months or more. Petechial haemorrhages at the junction of the soft and hard palate and inflammation and ulceration of the oral mucosa may be seen, but the oral changes are non-specific. Cases have also been reported presenting as pericoronitis in association with bilateral submandibular lymphadenitis, even if the pericoronitis is unilateral.

Diagnosis may be confirmed by testing acute serum for IgM antibodies to EBV capsid antigen or by a specific monospot slide test. Such investigations have largely replaced the classical Paul–Bunnell test.

As discussed in previous chapters, EBV is associated with Burkitt's lymphoma and has also been detected in oral squamous cell carcinoma. It is also the cause of hairy leukoplakia which is discussed later in this chapter.

Measles ✗

This infection occurs predominantly in children, and in developed countries is usually a mild disease with low mortality. In other countries the mortality is high. Prodromal symptoms may resemble a common cold and are accompanied by the appearance of Koplik's spots on the oral mucosa, especially the buccal mucosa opposite the molar teeth. They present as pin-point bluish white spots against an erythematous background, and range from few in number to several hundred. They are likely to be overlooked particularly as they start to disappear as the characteristic skin rash develops some three to four days later.

In parts of West Africa, gangrenous stomatitis (cancrum oris, noma) may occur as a complication of measles in malnourished patients.

Cytomegalovirus (CMV) ✗

Cytomegalovirus (CMV) is a herpes group virus that rarely causes disease in immunocompetent individuals but which is an important pathogen in immuno-compromised hosts, for example AIDS patients and organ transplant patients. However, subclinical infection is common, affecting 40–80 per cent of adults. Previously uninfected transplant patients may acquire the virus from the transplanted organ or transfused blood.

The most common oral manifestation is non-specific oral ulceration. CMV infection of salivary glands is also common but usually asymptomatic (see Chapter 14). However, it has been reported that the virus is strongly associated with the xerostomia seen in AIDS patients. It has also been suggested that it may play a role in cyclosporin-associated gingival overgrowth in transplant patients, following CMV infection of gingival fibroblasts and endothelial cells.

BACTERIAL INFECTIONS

It is surprising how few specific bacterial infections of the oral mucosa occur in view of the enormous number of bacteria and the wide range of species (including pathogens) normally present in the oral cavity. This is presumably at least partly related to the normal host defences against infection. An intact oral mucosa acts as a barrier against infection, but it is possible for bacteria to cross a damaged epithelial barrier (for example an ulcer) and undamaged oral epithelium is permeable to numerous molecules including some bacterial toxins. Saliva has a mechanical, cleansing action on the oral mucosa, and also contains non-specific and specific antibacterial substances, such as lysozyme and immunoglobulins. Secretory IgA in saliva is derived from the salivary gland secretions, while IgG, IgM, and serum IgA are derived from the gingival crevice fluid. The immunoglobulins in saliva may prevent the attachment of bacteria and viruses to the oral mucosa and teeth, and may possibly opsonize bacteria for phagocytosis by neutrophil leucocytes and macrophages. Phagocytosis may also be enhanced in the oral cavity by complement activation. Large numbers of phagocytic cells (predominantly neutrophil leucocytes) are continually released into the oral cavity, mostly from the gingival crevice, and many of these cells are capable of phagocytosis.

Acute ulcerative gingivitis (AUG) (acute necrotizing ulcerative gingivitis (ANUG))

This condition is now relatively uncommon in industrialized countries, although there has been a global increase associated with HIV infection. In industrialized countries the disease occurs mostly in young adults, and is more common in males than females, but in developing countries it is seen almost exclusively in children, related to poverty and malnutrition.

The infection presents with necrosis and crater-like, punched-out ulceration of the interdental papillae of sudden onset which may also involve the gingival margins (Fig. 11.12). The ulcers are covered with a greyish-green pseudomembrane demarcated from the surrounding mucosa by a linear erythema. Other signs and symptoms include gingival bleeding, either spontaneously or on minor trauma, pain or soreness of the gums, marked halitosis, a bad taste often described as metallic, and increased salivation. Malaise, cervical lymphadenopathy, and fever may be present in advanced cases. There is a high recurrence rate of infection unless underlying predisposing factors are adequately treated.

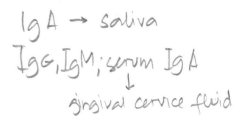

Fig. 11.12 Acute ulcerative gingivitis.

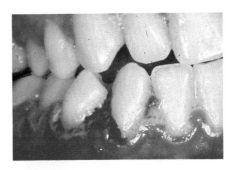

Fig. 11.13 Fusospirochaetal complex in acute ulcerative gingivitis.

AUG **Key points**

- polymicrobial, endogenous infection
- disturbance of host–parasite relationship
- overgrowth of fusospirochaetal complex
- gingival necrosis

Histological examination shows that the surface epithelium of the papillary and marginal gingiva is destroyed and replaced by a pseudomembrane variably composed of fibrin, necrotic epithelial cells, red and white blood cells, bacteria, and cellular debris. The underlying connective tissue shows marked acute inflammatory changes. Gram-stained smears of the pseudomembrane show a multiplicity of organisms (Fig. 11.13) with a great preponderance of spirochetes, pleomorphic rods, and fusiform organisms (the fusospirochaetal complex) (Table 11.2). Superficial bacterial invasion of the tissues has also been demonstrated by

Table 11.2 Microorganisms implicated in acute ulcerative gingivitis

Treponema species for example	*T. vincentii*
Prevotella species for example	*P. intermedia*
Porphyromonas species for example	*P. gingivalis*
Selenomonas species for example	*S. sputigena*
Fusobacterium species for example	*F. fusiformis*
Leptotrichia species for example	*L. buccalis*

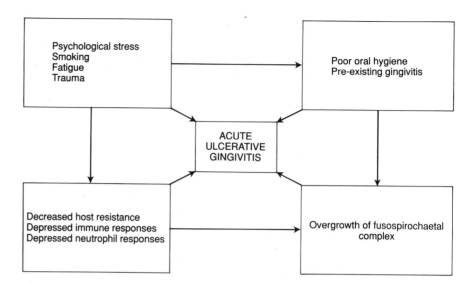

Fig. 11.14 Factors involved in the aetiology of acute ulcerative gingivitis.

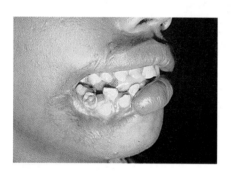

Fig. 11.15 Noma (cancrum oris).

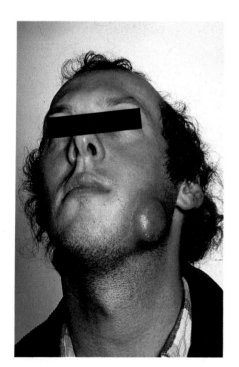

Fig. 11.16 Actinomycosis.

electron microscopy. The precise role of the various types of bacteria is unclear, but the disease is usually regarded as an endogenous, opportunistic polymicrobial infection.

It is likely that a variety of factors may disturb the normal symbiotic host-parasite relationship facilitating overgrowth of the organisms of the fuso-spirochaetal complex. These include reduced host resistance, at a local or general level, and pre-existing gingival tissue damage such as its present in chronic gingivitis (Fig. 11.14).

A persistent form of necrotizing gingivitis is associated with HIV infection (see later) and AUG is an important factor in the development of noma (see below).

Noma (cancrum oris)

Noma is a severe, rapidly developing gangrene of the orofacial tissues and jaws that occurs almost exclusively in developing countries, especially sub-Saharan Africa. The majority of cases are preceded by AUG followed by rapid spread of necrosis from the original gingival lesions into the cheek and development of an area of demarcated gangrene of the orofacial tissues (Fig. 11.15). The histological and bacteriological features are similar to AUG. Almost all cases of noma appear to develop in malnourished children whose resistance has been lowered still further by intercurrent infection such as measles or malaria.

Actinomycosis

Actinomyces are bacteria which are normal inhabitants of the oral cavity. Originally, *Actinomyces israelii* was considered to be the principal cause of human actinomycosis, but it is now realized that other species such as *A. viscosus* and *A. naeslundi* may also be associated with the disease, which is always a mixed infection.

The soft tissues of the submandibular area and neck are most commonly involved in cervicofacial actinomycosis. The infection is characterized by multiple foci of chronic suppuration. It presents with the development of firm swellings which eventually soften and are accompanied by the formation of pus which discharges through multiple sinuses (Fig. 11.16). Pain is variable and the swellings are often painless. The multiple abscesses which eventually form tend to point on

polymorphonuclear leucocytes
surrounded by pus (w/ actinomyces)

Rx Penicillin ⎤
   Erythromycin ⎥ 4-6 wks
   Doxycillin ⎥
   Tetracyclin ⎦

to the skin rather than the mucosal surface and are accompanied by marked fibrosis of the surrounding tissues. Infection is endogenous, and either a tooth socket, most commonly a lower third molar, or an infected root canal are thought to be the portals of entry. It is almost always confined to the soft tissues, but actinomycotic osteomyelitis may occur.

Actinomycotic lesions develop as areas of granulomatous inflammation surrounded by abundant granulation tissue and fibrous tissue. Fresh foci of infection develop adjacent to the primary site following transport of some of the organisms by phagocytic cells, and a central area of suppurative necrosis eventually develops in most of these foci. Granules consisting of tangled meshes of Gram-positive filaments of actinomyces with radiating filaments projecting on the surface are present in the pus (Fig. 11.17). The peripheral filaments are often Gram-negative and may show terminal clubbing. The organisms may be seen clinically as 'sulphur granules' in pus from actinomycotic lesions. Although actinomyces predominate in the lesions, other organisms are present and hence the clinical disease is a mixed infection. The other organisms may provide improved conditions for anaerobic growth of actinomyces and can lower host or local tissue resistance.

Actinomyces may also be isolated from some dental abscesses, but the organisms are most likely opportunistic colonizers. Such abscesses do not behave as actinomycotic lesions.

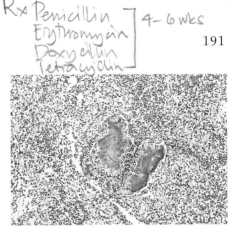

Fig. 11.17 Colony of actinomyces in pus.

- spreads into lung, thorax, pleura by aspiration or direct from pharynx or neck (THORACIC ACTINOMYCOSIS)
- spread into retroperitoneal tissue, multiple sinuses in abd wall. Liver also involved (ABD. ACTINOMYCOSIS)

Syphilis (primary, secondary, tertiary, congenital) ✓PAINLESS

Syphilis is an infection caused by the spirochaete *Treponema pallidum*. The incidence in Western countries has declined significantly over the past decade. The primary lesion (chancre) usually occurs on the genitalia, but in a minority of patients may present on the oral mucosa, usually the lips. It is typically described as a clean-based, painless, shallow ulcer with considerable induration of the subjacent connective tissue. The regional lymph nodes are also enlarged. Histologically, the chancre consists of ulcerated granulation tissue with a dense mononuclear inflammatory cell infiltrate chiefly composed of plasma cells.

The chancre heals spontaneously over a period of a few weeks and secondary lesions develop about 6 weeks later, some 2–3 months after the initial exposure. A generalized skin rash is the predominant feature and may be accompanied by oral lesions. In the mouth, a diffuse erythema or the characteristic mucous patch which is a necrotic slough covering an area of chronic inflammation, may be seen. Mucous patches may coalesce to produce lesions of irregular outline called snail-track ulcers. Histological examination shows no distinguishing features except that numerous spirochaetes may be demonstrated by silver staining.

In tertiary syphilis, a gumma may occur in the tongue (Fig. 11.18) or palate, initially presenting as an indurated swelling which subsequently may become necrotic and ulcerated to form a deep painless ulcer. Histologically, a gumma consists of a central mass of coagulative necrosis surrounded by granulation tissue infiltrated by lymphocytes, plasma cells, and macrophages with occasional giant cells. Spirochaetes are very scanty or absent.

Endarteritis obliterans is thought to be the cause of the atrophic glossitis which is also a feature of tertiary syphilis, the smooth surface of the tongue being broken up by fissures resulting from atrophy and fibrosis of the tongue musculature. Hyperkeratosis (syphilitic leukoplakia) (Fig. 11.19) frequently follows, and carcinoma of the tongue develops with far greater frequency than coincidence would permit. However, tertiary syphilis is now a rare factor in the aetiology of oral cancer (see Chapter 10).

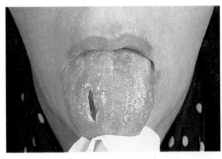

Fig. 11.18 Syphilitic gumma. coag necrosis surrounded by granulation tissue. full of lymphocytes, plasma cells, giant cells macrophages

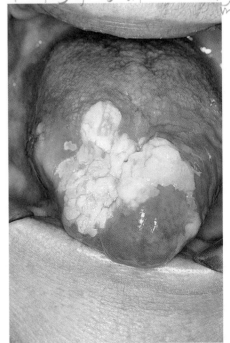

Fig. 11.19 Syphilitic leukoplakia.

Rx Penicillin
   tetracycline
   erythromycin

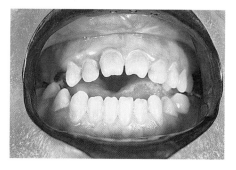

Fig. 11.20 Hutchinson's incisors.

Congenital syphilitic infection is associated with infection of the developing tooth germs of the permanent incisors (Hutchinson's incisors) (Fig. 11.20) and first molars (Moon's molars or mulberry molars). The maxillary central incisors are most frequently involved and are characterized by central notching of the incisal edge and a tapering 'screw-driver' appearance. Mulberry molars, usually the first permanent molars, are characterized by hypoplastic defects of the occlusal surface and defective cusp development with rounded, globular masses of hard tissue producing their mulberry appearance.

Collapse of the bridge of the nose, due to infection and destruction of the developing nasal bones, produces the characteristic saddle deformity of the bridge and the 'dished' appearance of the face.

Tuberculosis

Tuberculosis is an infection caused by mycobacteria, usually *Mycobacterium tuberculosis*, but *M. bovis* and other atypical mycobacteria may also cause disease in man.

Globally, about 8 million people develop tuberculosis each year. Although in Western countries the disease is still relatively uncommon there has been a steady increase in incidence over the past decade associated, in part, with socio-economic factors such as poverty and homelessness, HIV infection, and the emergence of organisms resistant to antituberculous drugs. Primary lesions of the oral mucosa may occur, but secondary infections associated with the coughing-up of infected sputum from pulmonary tuberculosis are more likely. A chronic, painless undermined ulcer covered with a greyish-yellow slough occurring most commonly on the tongue is the classical description of oral tuberculosis, but other types of ulcer and granulating gingival lesions have also been described. Patients may also present with tuberculous lymphadenitis, most frequently affecting the cervical nodes, but the intra- and extraparotid groups are occasionally involved.

Key points	Granulomatous infections
	• Actinomycosis
	—endogenous polymicrobial infection
	—submandibular swellings
	—chronic suppuration; multiple sinuses
	—'sulphur' granules in pus
	• Syphilis
	—primary: chancre
	—secondary: snail-track ulcers, mucous patches
	—tertiary: gumma, lingual leukoplakia
	—congenital: dental anomalies, 'dished' face
	• Tuberculosis
	—oral usually secondary to pulmonary
	—painless, chronic lingual ulcer
	• Leprospy
	—oral lesions in lepromatous type
	—secondary to nasal involvement
	—nodular masses palate/anterior maxilla

Diagnosis usually follows a biopsy, and the finding of typical tuberculoid granulomas, but tubercle bacilli must be demonstrated either in stained sections or by culture of the tissue before the diagnosis can be established. Other chronic granulomatous diseases, such as sarcoidosis and cat-scratch disease, may show a similar histological appearance, but tubercle bacilli cannot be demonstrated in these lesions.

Leprosy

Leprosy is another infection caused by a mycobacterium, *Mycobacterium leprae*. It is rare in Northern Europe and America but endemic to certain tropical areas. Two forms of infection exist depending on the immune response of the host to the organism. In the lepromatous type there is no cell-mediated response to *M. leprae*, although the humoral response is high, and there is widespread infection throughout the body. In the tuberculoid type the converse is true: cell-mediated responses are high, humoral responses low, and the infection remains localized.

Oral lesions occur almost exclusively in the lepromatous type and have been reported in about 50 per cent of patients. They present as nodular inflammatory masses which tend to ulcerate and heal with fibrosis. The hard and soft palates, anterior gingivae in the maxilla, and the tongue are most often affected. Oral lesions are usually secondary to nasal involvement.

Patients with lepromatous leprosy may show varying degrees of facial deformity associated with bone lesions, particularly of the nasomaxillary complex.

Gonorrhoea

Gonorrhoea is a venereal disease caused by *Neisseria gonorrhoea*. Although the oral mucosa is considered to be highly resistant to gonococcal infection, tonsillar and oropharyngeal lesions have been reported in sexually active adults, particularly homosexuals. The oral manifestations vary from a generalized painful erythematous stomatitis to vesiculation and ulceration associated with burning and pain on speaking and swallowing. Lesions have been reported from all areas of the mucosa.

Reiter syndrome

Reiter syndrome is considered here for convenience since, although its aetiology is still unknown, gonorrhoea has been suggested as an aetiological factor as have mycoplasmal infection, genetic predisposition, and autoimmune mechanisms. HLA-B27 correlates highly with Reiter syndrome.

The syndrome usually occurs in males between the ages of 20 and 35 years, and the classical triad consists of arthritis, conjunctivitis, and urethritis, but a variety of other features, for example oral lesions, are now included. Oral manifestations are variable, but include slightly elevated areas of erythema on the buccal mucosa, lips and gingivae, and purpuric spots on the palate.

Acute streptococcal stomatitis

There is doubt as to whether a specific streptococcal infection of the oral mucosa exists as a clinical entity. Generalized erythema of the oral mucosa together with a marked acute gingivitis, submandibular lymphadenitis, and a mild degree of malaise and fever are the features usually described. However, viral infections of the mouth with streptococci acting as secondary colonizing opportunists could produce the same clinical features.

FUNGAL INFECTIONS

Candida species and opportunistic infection

The fungal infections of the oral mucosa most frequently encountered are those due to species of the genus *Candida*. *Candida albicans* is the principal species associated with infection, but other species such as *C. glabrata, C. tropicalis, C. krusei*, and *C. parapsilosis* are also pathogenic for man. Most *Candida* species are dimorphic and exist as ovoid yeast forms or hyphae. They multiply primarily by the production of buds from ovoid yeast cells.

Candida species, principally *C. albicans*, are commensal organisms in the mouth, but the reported rates of carriage vary greatly depending on the population studied and the sensitivity and timing of sampling. In healthy adults the average carriage rate is about 20 per cent, but in the presence of any medical condition this is increased to about 40 per cent. Carriage rates are also increased in pregnancy and in tobacco smokers and denture wearers. In children the peak carriage, about 45 per cent, occurs during the first 18 months of life. *Candida* is also found as a commensal organism in the throat, large bowel, and vagina. The primary oral reservoir for the organism in carriers is the dorsum of the tongue. There is an overlap in the candidal counts in saliva from carriers and from individuals showing infection, and so isolation of *Candida* from the mouth of an adult is not confirmatory evidence of infection and must be considered together with the clinical findings. It is often presumed that *Candida* has a direct aetiological relationship with a lesion if hyphae are present in smears or in histological sections of the lesion, the presence of yeasts alone not being regarded as confirmatory evidence.

Key points	*Candida* species
	• commensal organisms
	• carriage rates very variable
	• opportunistic pathogens
	• *C. albicans* the most common pathogenic species

Table 11.3 Factors predisposing to oral candidal infection

Local factors
  Mucosal trauma
  Denture (appliance) wearing
  Denture (appliance) hygiene
  Tobacco smoking
  Carbohydrate-rich diet

Age
  Extremes of age:
    neonates/infants; old age

Drugs
  Broad-spectrum antibiotics
  Steroids, local/systemic
  Immunosuppressant/cytotoxic agents

Xerostomia
  Drugs, radiotherapy
  Sjögren syndrome

Systemic disease
  Iron deficiency; iron deficiency
    anaemia
  Megaloblastic anaemias
  Acute leukaemia
  Diabetes mellitus
  HIV infection and AIDS
  Other immunodeficiency states

Candida species are notorious opportunistic pathogens, and both general and local predisposing factors are important in the pathogenesis of oral candidal infections (Table 11.3). For example, debilitated patients, such as those receiving antibiotic, steroid, or cytotoxic therapy, are particularly susceptible to candida infections, with local factors, such as tobacco smoking and trauma from an unclean or ill-fitting denture, also being important.

Non-specific and specific factors are involved in protection of the oral mucosa from candidal infection. Non-specific factors include shedding of epithelial cells, salivary flow, antimicrobial factors in saliva, commensal bacteria, and the phagocytic activity of neutrophils and macrophages.

Specific antibodies to *Candida* are present in the sera of most individuals, and increased titres of humoral antibodies against *Candida* species are found in patients with candidal infections when compared with control subjects. However, poor resistance to candidal infection can be found in patients despite high titres of candidal antibodies, suggesting that the systemic humoral immune response may not confer protection from infection. Secretory immunity may be more important than systemic immunity in protection of the oral mucosa. For example, secretory IgA levels in saliva are raised in patients with oral candidosis and may inhibit adherence of the organisms to oral epithelium.

There is considerable evidence to suggest that cell-mediated immune responses are impaired in patients with chronic mucocutaneous candidosis—a syndrome associated with a range of distinct immune abnormalities. Cellular immune defects have also been found in patients with other types of chronic oral candidal infection but no consistent pattern has been demonstrated.

The mechanisms by which *Candida* species exert a pathological effect on the tissues are not known. Secreted hydrolytic enzymes such as proteinases, lipases, and a number of toxins are produced and the toxins are probably antigenic.

stimulating an immune response in the affected tissues. The tissue changes may, therefore, be due to a direct effect of the toxin on the tissues, a delayed hypersensitivity reaction, or enzymatic breakdown of the infected epithelium. Adherence of the organism to epithelial cells is also required for colonization, carriage, and the development of infection. A number of mechanisms involving surface proteins have been identified.

Classification of oral and perioral candidosis

A variety of candidal infections involve the oral mucosa and perioral tissues and a number of classifications have been proposed. However, most share similar features in that they distinguish between acute and chronic infections and between infections confined to the oral and perioral tissues, and those where oral infection is a manifestation of a generalized systemic candidosis. Most of the latter are associated with various types of immunodeficiency.

In addition, *Candida* may be found in association with other mucosal lesions, for example, speckled leukoplakia, hairy leukoplakia, median rhomboid glossitis, and black hairy and other coatings on the tongue, where a causal relationship has not been fully established. These disorders are discussed elsewhere in this book.

The classification of candidal infections used in this chapter is given in Table 11.4.

Oral candidal infection is an almost universal finding in patients with severe cell mediated (T cell) immunodeficiencies, particularly in patients suffering from HIV infection. The types of infection seen in these patients do not fall easily into this classification. For example, as discussed later in this chapter, chronic pseudomembranous and chronic erythematous candidoses are seen in patients with HIV infection.

Acute pseudomembranous candidosis

The development of acute pseudomembranous candidosis (commonly referred to as thrush) is generally associated with some prior local disturbance or systemic illness (see Table 11.3). Antibiotic, corticosteroid (including inhaled corticosteroids used to control asthma) and immunosuppressive drug therapy, diabetes mellitus, anaemia, blood dyscrasias such as leukaemia, advanced malignancy, and immunodeficiency states are common predisposing factors. Thrush occurs in up to 5 per cent of newborn infants, when it is probably associated

Table 11.4 Classification of oral candidosis

Group 1: Candidoses confined to the oral mucosa
Acute
    Acute pseudomembranous candidosis (thrush)
    Acute atrophic (erythematous) candidosis

Chronic
    Chronic atrophic candidosis
      (denture stomatitis)
    Candida-associated angular cheilitis
    Chronic hyperplastic candidosis
      (candidal leukoplakia)

Group 2: Oral manifestations of generalized candidoses
Chronic mucocutaneous candidoses

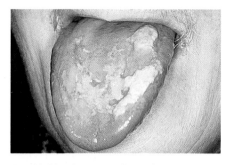

Fig. 11.21 Acute pseudomembranous candidosis in debilitated elderly patient.

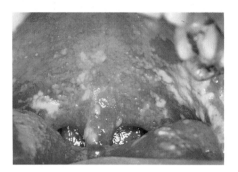

Fig. 11.22 Acute pseudomembranous candidosis associated with use of steroid inhaler in an asthmatic patient.

with immature antimicrobial defences, *Candida* being picked up from the birth canal. The infection is also seen in about 10 per cent of elderly debilitated patients.

The disease presents clinically as a thick white coating (the pseudomembrane) on the affected mucosa, said to resemble milk curds (Figs 11.21, 11.22) which can be wiped away (albeit with difficulty in some cases) to leave a red, raw, and often bleeding base. Lesions may occur on any mucosal surface of the mouth and vary in size from small drop-like areas to confluent plaques covering a wide area.

Histological examination shows the involved epithelium to be hyperplastic with the superficial necrotic and desquamating parakeratotic layers infiltrated both by candidal hyphae and yeasts, and by inflammatory cells which are predominantly neutrophil leucocytes. The neutrophils may accumulate to form microabscesses. It is along the junction between the superficial infected layer (the pseudomembrane) and the deeper epithelium that the pseudomembrane separates when the lesion is firmly wiped. In addition, there is infiltration of the lamina propria by acute and chronic inflammatory cells. The candidal hyphae appear as weakly basophilic, thread-like structures with haematoxylin and eosin staining, but are seen much more clearly after special staining such as in periodic acid–Schiff (PAS) preparations. Examination of a smear made of the pseudomembrane shows necrotic material and leucocytes with epithelial cells partly matted together by candidal hyphae and yeasts (Fig. 11.23).

Acute atrophic (erythematous) candidosis *(Antibiotic Sore tongue)*

This condition is seen most commonly on the dorsum of the tongue in patients undergoing prolonged corticosteroid or antibiotic therapy, but it may develop after only a few days of topical application of an antibiotic. Antibiotic therapy alters the oral bacterial flora allowing resistant organisms, such as *Candida*, to flourish, and the condition is commonly referred to as antibiotic sore tongue. It presents as a red and often painful area of oral mucosa (most commonly the tongue) which resembles thrush without the overlying pseudomembrane. Indeed, small patches of thrush may be found elsewhere in the mouth, particularly in areas protected from masticatory or similar trauma, and it is likely that, in some patients, the acute atrophic form develops when the pseudomembrane is shed.

Rx:
· Stop causative antibodies if possible
· Use a narrower spectrum drug
· Topical antifungal therapy
   ↓
   – nystatin suspension
   – miconazole gel

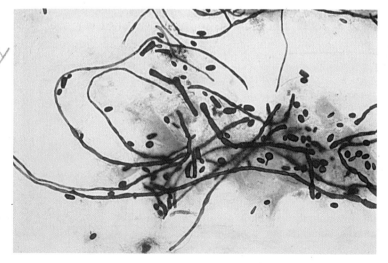

Fig. 11.23 Candidal hyphae and yeasts in smear from a patient with oral candidosis.

Histological examination of such lesions is rarely carried out, but shows a thin, atrophic, non-keratinized epithelium with occasional candidal hyphae penetrating the superficial layers. There is an associated inflammatory infiltrate, both in the epithelium and the underlying connective tissue. The appearances are essentially the same as for acute pseudomembraneous candidosis without the pseudomembrane.

-atrophic
-non-keratinized
-candidal hyphae present.

Chronic atrophic candidosis (denture stomatitis)

50%, ♀ > ♂, more in max denture

This common and usually symptomless condition has been found in about 50 per cent of randomly selected denture wearers, and is seen more frequently in women than in men. It is regarded as being a secondary candidal infection of tissues modified by the continual wearing of often ill-fitting dentures and is associated with poor denture hygiene. The condition is characterized clinically by chronic erythema and oedema of the mucosa directly covered by the denture, the affected mucosa being clearly delineated by the outline of the denture. The palate is almost invariably affected but it is very unusual to see lesions related to lower dentures, probably because they fit much less closely than upper dentures and so an environment favouring the overgrowth of *Candida* is not present. The condition may also occur under orthodontic appliances.

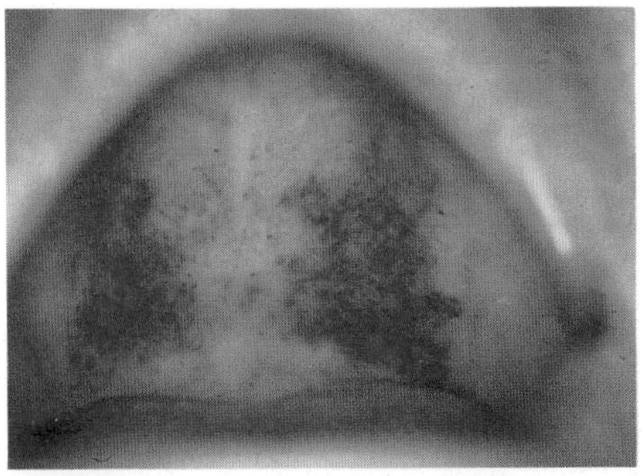

Fig. 11.24 Pin-point pattern of inflammation in chronic atrophic candidosis (denture stomatitis).

Clinically, three patterns of inflammation can be identified:

(1) pin-point areas of erythema—localized inflammation (Fig. 11.24);

(2) diffuse areas of erythema—generalized inflammation;

(3) erythema associated with a granular or multinodular mucosal surface (Fig. 11.25)—chronic inflammatory papillary hyperplasia (see Chapter 8).

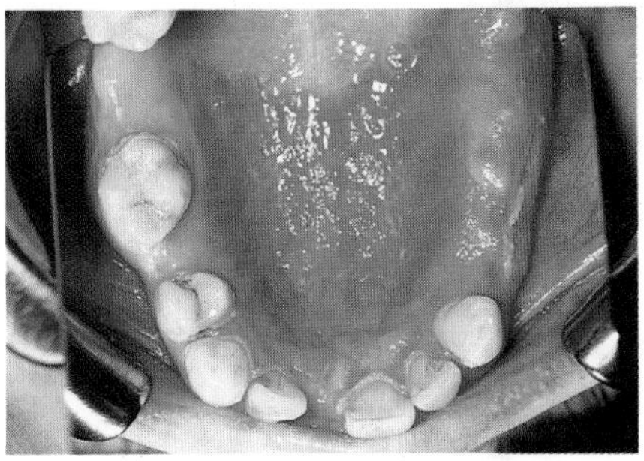

Fig 11.25 Chronic atrophic candidosis associated with papillary hyperplasia.

The confined space between the mucosa and the upper denture, inadequate cleaning of the fitting surface, and wearing the denture throughout the night, all appear to favour the overgrowth of *Candida* resulting in a local imbalance of the host-parasite relationship. The disease has also been initiated experimentally in humans and in animal models by inoculation of *C. albicans* beneath dentures or other appliances covering the palatal mucosa. Sucrose rinses favour the initiation of experimentally induced infections by enhancing the multiplication of yeasts, and clinical studies have also shown that a high-carbohydrate diet predisposes to infection. *Candida* can be recovered more readily from the fitting surface of the denture than from the surface of the mucosa, and evidence suggests that microscopic pores and irregularities on the fitting surface of a denture provide a suitable environment for growth and retention of the organisms. It is thought that a delayed hypersensitivity response to candidal antigens contributes to the inflammation.

Histologically, the epithelium may show hyperplasia and/or atrophy, with the surface being either parakeratinized or non-keratinized. Leucocytes infiltrate the epithelium, sometimes forming microabscesses in the superficial layers, and there is a chronic subepithelial inflammatory cell infiltrate of varying intensity. Invasion of the epithelium by candidal hyphae is not a feature of the condition.

TREATMENT
1. Topical Amphotericin (Tab)
2 Topical Nystatin (Tab)
3 Soak denture overnight in 0.1% hypochlorite
4 Apply miconazole gel on denture - then wear it.
Reapply 3x day for 2 wks.

Candida-associated and other forms of angular cheilitis

Angular cheilitis is a multifactorial disease of infectious origin. It occurs predominantly in denture wearers and is seen in about 30 per cent of patients with denture stomatitis and less frequently with other types of oral candidosis. In patients with no evidence of candidal infection *Staphylococcus aureus* or, less frequently, beta-haemolytic streptococci may be involved. In some cases, combinations of these organisms are implicated.

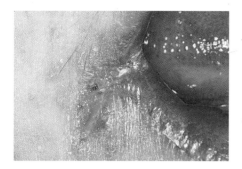

Fig. 11.26   Angular cheilitis.

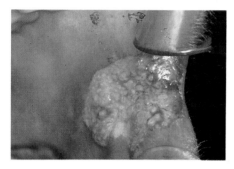

Fig. 11.27   Chronic hyperplastic candidosis.

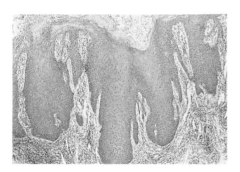

Fig. 11.28   Prominent acanthosis in chronic hyperplastic candidosis.

Clinically, angular cheilitis is characterized by soreness, erythema, and fissuring at the corners of the mouth (Fig. 11.26). Deep folds of skin at the angles of the mouth, which may be associated with loss of occlusal height in old age or result from incorrectly designed or old dentures, may be contributory factors. The folds predispose to infection because of local maceration of the keratinized layers of the skin as a result of continual wetting by saliva. Nutritional deficiencies, in particular iron deficiency and deficiencies of riboflavin, folic acid, and of vitamin B_{12}, are predisposing factors in some cases.

Chronic hyperplastic candidosis   X

This form of candidosis (commonly referred to as candidal leukoplakia) presents clinically as a persistent white patch on the oral mucosa which is indistinguishable from leukoplakia. Characteristically, the lesions present as dense, opaque white patches of irregular thickness and density with a rough or nodular surface. They cannot be removed by scraping, but fragments may be detached and identification of hyphae in smears of such material assists in the diagnosis. In some cases, areas of erythematous mucosa are present within the plaque producing a speckled leukoplakia (Fig. 11.27). Lesions are seen most frequently on the buccal mucosa adjacent to the commissure of the lips and present as roughly triangular, often bilateral white plaques tapering posteriorly. They are often associated with angular cheilitis. Less frequently, the palate or tongue may be involved and when multiple sites are affected the term chronic multifocal oral candidosis is sometimes applied. In many patients there is a strong association with tobacco smoking. Other local factors, such as denture wearing and occlusal friction, may also be involved.

Histologically, the epithelium is parakeratinized and is generally markedly hyperplastic and acanthotic (Fig. 11.28). Many of the cells in the parakeratinized surface of the epithelium are separated by oedema and numerous neutrophil leucocytes, the neutrophils often collecting together as microabscesses (Fig. 11.29). Candidal hyphae invade the parakeratin more or less at right angles to the surface, but never penetrate deeper into the prickle cell layers (Fig. 11.30). A variable number of acute and chronic inflammatory cells are present throughout the prickle cell layer and there is a mixed chronic inflammatory cell infiltrate, in which plasma cells are often prominent, in the lamina propria. Areas of atrophic epithelium may be present within the lesion and in these areas the superficial layers of candida-infected parakeratin may be missing. Focal absence of the infected parakeratin layer may be responsible for the speckled erythematous appearances seen clinically. The histological distinction from acute pseudomembranous candidosis may be difficult.

Chronic hyperplastic candidosis is considered to be a premalignant lesion and epithelial dysplasia is seen in about 50 per cent of cases. *Candida* species can gen-

Fig. 11.29   Superficial microabscess formation in chronic hyperplastic candidosis.

Fig. 11.30 .   Invasion of parakeratin by candidal hyphae in chronic hyperplastic candidosis.

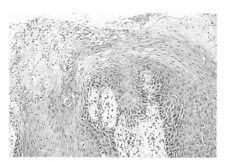

Fig. 11.29

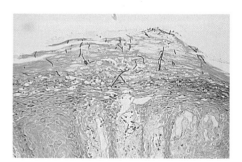

Fig. 11.30

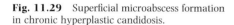

erate carcinogens such as nitrosamines. As with idiopathic leukoplakia (see Chapter 9) the severity of dysplasia and the risk of malignant transformation are increased in speckled, non-homogeneous lesions.

It has not been conclusively shown whether chronic hyperplastic candidosis is primarily leukoplakia with a secondary candidal infection, or whether it is primarily a chronic candidal infection which in time leads to epithelial hyperplasia and acanthosis. About a third of all leukoplakias are infected by candidal species but only the minority show the characteristic histological features described above, which are common to other candidal infections. The raised antibody titre to *C. albicans* in patients with lesions showing such features is further evidence supporting an aetiological role for the fungus, and some lesions do respond to prolonged antifungal therapy.

Candidal infections: clinical aspects   **Key points**
- acute pseudomembranous and chronic hyperplastic present as white lesions
- pseudomembrane can be wiped away
- acute atrophic and chronic atrophic present as red patches
- chronic atrophic virtually confined to palate
- chronic types mainly associated with angular cheilitis
- local and/or systemic factors must be sought in all cases

Candidal infections: pathological aspects   **Key points**
- mycelial invasion of parakeratin except in chronic atrophic
- neutrophil infiltration of epithelium with superficial microabscesses
- no mycelial invasion in chronic atrophic, organism colonizes denture base
- prominent acanthosis in chronic hyperplastic
- epithelial dysplasia in chronic hyperplastic

Chronic mucocutaneous candidoses

This is a rare group of disorders characterized by persistent superficial candidal infections of mucosae, nails, and skin, the oral mucosa being involved in almost all cases (Fig. 11.31). Oral lesions resemble those seen in chronic hyperplastic candidosis and may involve any part of the mucosa.

The disorders in this group can be classified in a variety of ways, but four main subgroups are identified based on clinical features and age of onset, a fifth group can be added where chronic candidosis is associated with primary immunodeficiencies and HIV infection (Table 11.5).

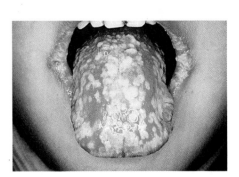

Fig. 11.31 Chronic mucocutaneous candidosis.

Familial chronic mucocutaneous candidosis

This presents within the first year of life and is associated with an autosomal recessive pattern of inheritance. Most patients are only mildly affected.

Diffuse chronic mucocutaneous candidosis

This presents within the first five years of life as a sporadic disease or with an autosomal recessive pattern of inheritance. It is a severe disorder with extensive oral candidosis and severe skin involvement associated with multiple, disfiguring skin lesions (candida granulomas).

Table 11.5   Classification of chronic mucocutaneous candidoses (CMC)

Subgroup	Onset	Inheritance	Features
Familial CMC	early	autosomal recessive	mainly oral; skin mild
Diffuse CMC	early	sporadic/autosomal recessive	severe skin and oral lesions candida granulomas
Candidosis endocrinopathy syndrome	early	autosomal recessive/sporadic	mild/moderate oral and skin lesions hypoparathyroidism Addison's disease
Late-onset CMC	late	sporadic	mild skin and oral lesions thymoma
CMC associated with primary immunodeficiencies	early	sporadic and hereditary types	oral and skin, variable involvement

Candidosis endocrinopathy syndrome (autoimmune polyendocrinopathy syndrome)

This rare disorder appears to be transmitted as an autosomal recessive pattern of inheritance but sporadic cases occur. It usually manifests by the second decade and chronic oral candidosis is a common presenting feature.

The chronic candidosis may precede the manifestations of endocrine abnormalities by several years. Hypoparathyroidism is seen most frequently, but hypoadrencorticism (Addison's disease), hypothyroidism, and diabetes mellitus, alone or in combinations, may also develop. The hypoparathyroidism may be associated with enamel hypoplasia affecting the permanent teeth.

Late-onset chronic mucocutaneous candidosis

Mild chronic candidosis mainly affecting the oral mucosa may occur in middle-aged or elderly patients who develop thymoma.

Chronic mucocutaneous candidosis associated with primary immunodeficiencies and HIV infection

Chronic candidosis may be a feature in patients with primary immunodeficiency syndromes and in those with defective polymorphonuclear leucocyte function.

Unusual forms of chronic candidosis are also prevalent in HIV-infected patients as discussed later in this chapter.

Oral manifestations of the deep visceral mycoses

The systemic or deep-seated visceral mycoses are rare diseases outside endemic areas and are found mainly in South America and in parts of the USA (Table 11.6). In non-endemic areas they are increasing in frequency in immunocompromised patients. Oral lesions are relatively uncommon presenting most frequently as non-specific ulceration or as nodular granulomatous lesions. They are usually associated with lesions elsewhere, especially the respiratory tract.

Table 11.6   Deep-seated mycotic infections

Disease	Organism	Geographical distribution
Blastomycosis (North American blastomycosis)	*Blastomyces dermitidis*	mainly North-Central and South-Eastern USA
Coccidioidomycosis	*Coccidioides immitis*	arid zones of South-Western USA, Central, and South America
Cryptococcosis	*Cryptococcus neoformans*	widespread; most prevalent in USA and Australia
Histoplasmosis	*Histoplasma capsulatum*	worldwide, especially Central USA, Central and South America, Far East
Paracoccidioidomycosis (South American blastomycosis)	*Paracoccidioides brasiliersis*	Central and South America

HUMAN IMMUNODEFICIENCY VIRUS (HIV) INFECTION AND AIDS

HIV is transmitted by the exchange of blood or body fluids principally through sexual contact (both homosexual and heterosexual), the injection of blood or blood products (for example intravenous drug abusers and haemophiliacs), or from mother to child (perinatal infection). Transmission of the virus may be followed by infection which is detected by the appearance of HIV antibodies in the blood (seroconversion). This generally occurs within three months of exposure. A few patients have an acute HIV infection at this time, the clinical features of which include pyrexia, skin rash, headache, diarrhoea, sore throat, and erythema of the buccal and palatal mucosa. The clinical responses to HIV infection are shown in Fig. 11.32.

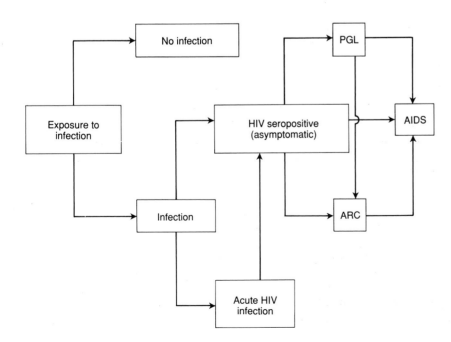

Fig. 11.32   Clinical responses to HIV.

Following seroconversion most patients remain symptom-free for many years (HIV seropositive), but in time may develop persistent generalized lymphadenopathy (PGL). In both PGL and asymptomatic HIV-seropositive patients there may then be progression to the AIDS-related complex (ARC) which is characterized by lymphadenopathy, persistent pyrexia, diarrhoea, weight loss, fatigue, and malaise. The final stage of infection is fully developed AIDS (acquired immune deficiency syndrome), characterized by opportunistic infections, Kaposi's sarcoma and non-Hodgkin's lymphoma, but patients may also develop thrombocytopenia and neurological disease. AIDS always has a fatal outcome.

Infection by HIV involves the binding of the virus to many target cells, but binding to the CD4 receptor of T-helper lymphocytes plays a major role in the pathogenesis of HIV disease. In due course, infected T-helper cells die with a consequent reduction in the number of T-helper cells and a decrease in CD4 helper/CD8 suppressor cell ratios. The ability to mount a normal immune response is, therefore, impaired, particularly in response to T-cell dependent antigens such as viruses, fungi, and encapsulated bacteria, and this accounts for most of the clinical manifestations of the disease. Other cells to which HIV may bind include bone marrow stem cells, macrophages, endothelial cells, lymph node dendritic cells, and possibly Langerhans cells, but these cells are generally not killed by the virus. HIV infection is also characterized by a polyclonal B-cell stimulation leading to hyperglobulinaemia with antibodies directed against HIV-infected cells.

The oral manifestations of HIV infection are numerous and have been divided into three groups based on the strength of their association with HIV infection. The main lesions in each group are listed in Table 11.7. Some of these conditions are described elsewhere in this book.

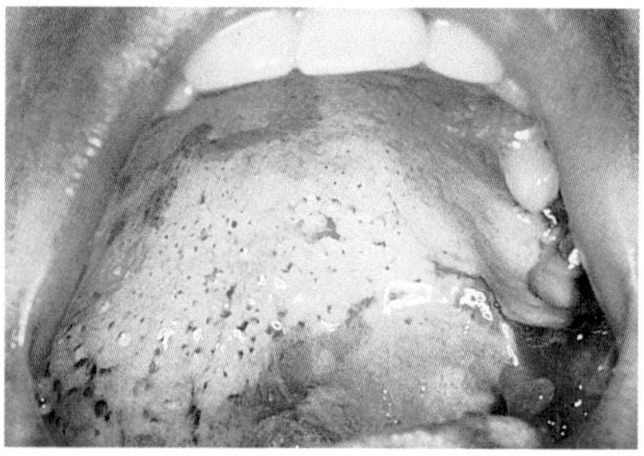

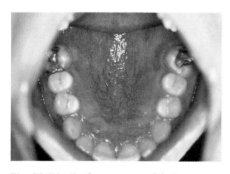

Fig. 11.33 Severe pseudomembranous candidosis associated with HIV.

Oral candidosis

This is the most frequent oral manifestation of HIV infection and has been reported in over 90 per cent of patients with AIDS and in about 25 per cent of HIV-positive patients who have not developed AIDS. The more severe the immune impairment the more likely the patient is to have oral candidosis. Xerostomia is another important predisposing factor. The pseudomembranous and erythematous varieties are seen most frequently but, unlike their counterparts in non-HIV infected patients, they may persist for months. Pseudomembranous candidosis (Fig. 11.33) may involve any part of the oral mucosa but the palate, cheeks, lips, and dorsum of the tongue are most frequently affected. Erythematous candidosis (Fig. 11.34) presents as a red lesion, and most commonly affects the palate and dorsum of the tongue where it is also associated with loss of the filiform papillae and resembles median rhomboid glossitis. Hyperplastic candidosis is most frequently seen on the cheeks but the commisures are rarely involved, as is usually the case in HIV-seronegative patients.

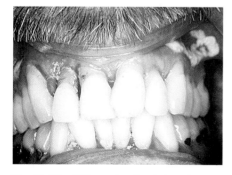

Fig. 11.34 Erythematous candidosis associated with HIV.

HIV-associated periodontal diseases

It is well established that HIV infection is associated with severe periodontal disease in some patients (Fig. 11.35), but the prevalence of periodontal disease within the population of HIV-seropositive patients remains controversial and unresolved. Recent studies suggest that the general periodontal health in this group of patients is better than previously thought. The pathogenesis of HIV-associated periodontal disease is also unresolved. Although it has been suggested that the immune deficiency allows a shift in the gingival crevicular flora towards a more pathogenic plaque, other studies have shown that the complex mixed flora in periodontal disease is similar in HIV-positive and HIV-negative patients.

Fig. 11.35 HIV-associated periodontal disease together with an area of pesudomembranous candidosis.

Table 11.7 Classification of oral lesions associated with HIV infection

Group I: Lesions strongly associated with HIV infection

Candidosis
  Erythematous
  Hyperplastic
  Pseudomembranous

Hairy leukoplakia (EBV)

HIV associated periodontal disease
  HIV-gingivitis
  Necrotizing ulcerative gingivitis
  HIV-periodontitis
  Necrotizing stomatitis

Kaposi's sarcoma

Non-Hodgkin's lymphoma

Group II: Lesions less commonly associated with HIV infection

Atypical ulceration (oropharyngeal)

Idiopathic thrombocytopenic purpura

Salivary gland disorders
  Dry mouth, decreased salivary flow rate
  Uni- or bilateral swelling of major glands

Viral infections (other than EBV)
  Cytomegalovirus
  Herpes simplex virus
  Human papillomavirus
  Varicella-zoster virus

Group III: Lesions possibly associated with HIV infection

Bacterial infections other than gingivitis/periodontitis

Fungal infection other than candidosis

Melanotic hyperpigmentation

Neurologic disturbances
  Facial palsy
  Trigeminal neuralgia

Increase in attachment loss has been reported in HIV-positive patients when CD4 cell counts in peripheral blood were below 200/mm^3.

Gingivitis is seen as a distinctive red line at the free gingival margin with bleeding either spontaneously or associated with tooth brushing. It may also be referred to as linear gingival erythema. Severe and progressive loss of periodontal bone associated with necrosis of interdental and marginal tissues, exposure of bone, and severe pain is seen in periodontitis. Persistent acute necrotizing ulcerative gingivitis which does not respond to conventional treatment is characteristic of HIV infection. A necrotizing stomatitis associated with extensive soft-tissue necrosis, exposure of bone, and sequestration of dead bone fragments may also occur, and may develop from HIV-associated periodontitis.

Viral infections

Infections with herpes simplex and varicella-zoster viruses in association with HIV infection are more severe and extensive than when occurring in an HIV-seronegative patient, and frequently recur. Viral warts are often seen in the mouths of patients infected with HIV, and unusual types of HPV have been identified in some of these lesions. Disseminated CMV infection may be seen in AIDS, and EBV is the cause of hairy leukoplakia and may be associated with some lymphomas. Kaposi's sarcoma is associated with a herpesvirus.

Hairy leukoplakia

Lesions of hairy leukoplakia (HL) are usually asymptomatic and most commonly occur bilaterally on the lateral borders of the tongue, with lesions being described occasionally elsewhere on the oral mucosa. Clinically, the lesions are non-removable white patches with wide variation in size, severity, and surface characteristics. The most characteristic lesions present as vertical white folds on the lateral border of the tongue with a raised, corrugated or hairy surface (Fig. 11.36). However, the lesions may also have a smooth flat surface. Histological examination of HL typically shows acanthotic, parakeratinized epithelium (Fig. 11.37) often with long, finger-like surface projections of parakeratin producing the hairy or corrugated appearance seen clinically. Candidal hyphae may be present in the parakeratin in about half the cases, but the candidosis is a secondary rather than a causal infection. There is an absence of associated inflammatory cells both in the epithelium and in the lamina propria. Swollen or balloon cells with prominent cell boundaries are present as a band in the prickle cell layer beneath the parakeratin (Fig. 11.38). Some have small, darkly staining nuclei and perinuclear vacuoles. The swollen cells contain Epstein–Barr virus and have been described as koilocytes or koilocyte-like cells (Fig. 11.39). (Strictly, the term koilocyte should be confined to cells infected with HPV.) Demonstration of EBV is essential to confirm the diagnosis.

HL is seen in HIV-seropositive patients from all risk groups and it has been suggested that, at any one time, between 20 and 30 per cent of HIV-seropositive

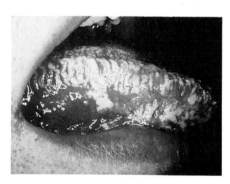

Fig. 11.36

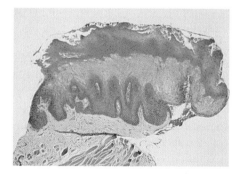

Fig. 11.37

Fig. 11.36 HIV-associated hairy leukoplakia.

Fig. 11.37 Hairy leukoplakia showing hyperkeratosis and underlying balloon cells.

Fig. 11.38 Ballooned cells with perinuclear vacuoles in hairy leukoplakia.

Fig. 11.39 *In situ* DNA hybridization for Epstein–Barr virus showing positive signals (black) over nuclei in ballooned cells.

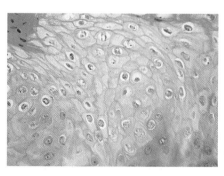

Fig. 11.38

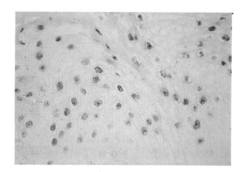

Fig. 11.39

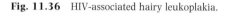

patients may have HL. Cases of HL have also been described in HIV-seronegative patients receiving immunosuppressive therapy (for example for renal or heart transplants), and a small number of extremely rare cases have been reported in apparently healthy persons.

It appears highly probable that HL is due to opportunistic infection of the oral epithelium by EBV in association with HIV infection or in other immuno-compromised patients. A long-term carrier state for EBV generally follows natural infection with EBV, which in most people occurs either subclinically during childhood or as acute infectious mononucleosis (glandular fever) in teenage years (as discussed earlier in this chapter). The main reservoir for the carrier state is thought to be the circulating B lymphocytes, but epithelial cells in the oropharynx and possibly the salivary glands are other reservoirs. Repeated direct infection of epithelial cells with EBV from saliva is required to maintain HL, and the need for continuous EBV shedding may explain why the disease is almost restricted to immunocompromised patients. EBV can be found in the saliva of most HIV-seropositive individuals. A marked depletion of Langerhans cells has also been described in HL, and the impaired antigen handling that results, in association with the impaired systemic immune response, may allow EBV to enter the oral epithelium and viral replication to occur. The characteristic site distribution on the lateral border of the tongue might result from it being an area particularly liable to trauma which could allow access of EBV from the saliva to viral receptors on the prickle cells.

HL is a common finding among patients with AIDS or late-stage HIV infection, and it is an indication of declining immunocompetence. There is no evidence to suggest that HL is a premalignant condition.

Kaposi's sarcoma (KS)

As first described by Kaposi in 1872, this tumour was a sarcoma of multifocal origin, found mostly in Jews, and occurring mainly on the skin of the extremities. However, in the 1960s it became apparent that the tumour was endemic in Southern Africa (up to 10% of all tumours in some areas). In endemic areas it presents in one of two forms. In one, individuals up to 40 years of age are affected with involvement of the skin of the arms and legs—the tumour has a good prognosis. The other occurs in children with spread to lymph nodes and visceral organs, and has a poor prognosis.

KS is the commonest tumour associated with HIV infection, occurring in up to 1 in 4 AIDS patients with a male to female ratio of 20:1. There is a higher frequency in whites and homosexuals than in blacks and intravenous drug abusers. Recently, it has been demonstrated that KS in both HIV-positive patients and other populations is associated with infection by a herpesvirus known as KS-associated herpesvirus (KSHV) or human herpesvirus 8 (HHV-8). The evidence suggests that the virus has a causal role.

KS in AIDS presents on the skin or mucosal surfaces with single or multiple lesions which may be macules, papules, or nodules that have a pink, red, or violet colour. Skin lesions become darker and larger with time; the tip of the nose is the most frequent facial site. Oral lesions are seen most frequently on the palate (Fig. 11.40), with the gingiva and tongue being less frequent sites. They present as blue, black, or red macules which later become darker, raised, and ulcerated. The lesions are painless unless ulcerated.

Early lesions of KS consist of proliferating endothelial cells and atypical, often cleft-like, vascular channels together with extravasated erythrocytes, haemosiderin, and inflammatory cells. A few atypical spindle-shaped cells may be seen in the interstitial tissues. Distinction from granulation tissue and other vascular lesions

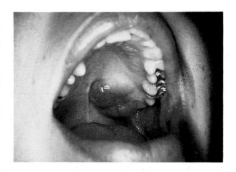

Fig. 11.40 Oral Kaposi's sarcoma associated with HIV.

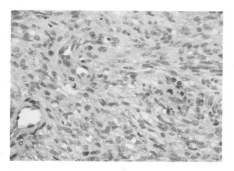

Fig. 11.41 Kaposi's sarcoma showing atypical spindle cells and vascular channels.

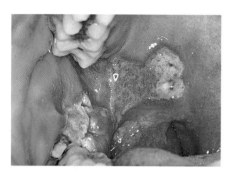

Fig. 11.42 Atypical oral ulceration associated with HIV.

such as haemangiomas and pyogenic granulomas may be difficult. However, in the later stages the vascular component decreases and the atypical spindle cells predominate (Fig. 11.41). There is no curative treatment, but the lesions may respond to radiotherapy or chemotherapy.

Non-Hodgkin's lymphoma (NHL)

An increased incidence of NHL is seen in AIDS patients (as in other groups of immunocompromised patients), and oral mucosal involvement has been described. Some of these lymphomas are associated with EBV.

Neurological disturbances

HIV is neurotropic and may directly involve the central nervous system leading, for example, to peripheral neuropathy or dementia. Facial nerve palsy may follow involvement of neurones in the central nervous system.

Atypical ulceration

Atypical ulceration (Fig. 11.42), particularly of the oropharynx, has been described in AIDS risk groups and may resemble aphthous stomatitis. Some may be associated with viral infection such as CMV.

Idiopathic thrombocytopenic purpura

Small purpuric lesions or larger areas of bruising may be seen on the oral mucosa, associated with thrombocytopenia resulting from an autoimmune response.

HIV-associated salivary gland disease

Xerostoma and salivary gland enlargement associated with lymphocytic infiltrates may occur in up to 10 per cent of adult patients with AIDS (see Chapter 14). Lymphoepithelial cysts may also arise.

Oral pigmentation

Melanin pigmentation of the oral mucosa has been described in patients with HIV, but whether this is directly related to the infection, or associated with drug therapy, or adrenal gland insufficiency has not been determined.

Key points	**HIV infection**
	• oral signs and symptoms may be the initial manifestation
	• a wide variety of oral manifestations described
	• opportunistic infections are a major feature
	• oral candidosis is a frequent early manifestation
	• HL often indicates progression to AIDS
	• severe, specifically related periodontal diseases occur in some patients

FURTHER READING

Barr, C. E. (1995). Periodontal problems related to HIV-1 infection. *Advances in Dental Research*, **9**, 147–51.

Cannon, R.D. Holmes, A. R., Mason, A. B., and Monk, B. C. (1995). Oral candida: clearance, colonization or candidiasis. *Journal of Dental Research*, **74**, 1152–61.

Challacombe, S. J. (1994). Immunologic aspects of oral candidiasis. *Oral Surgery, Oral Medicine, Oral Pathology*, **78**, 202–10.

Chang, F., Syrjanen, S., Kellokoski, J., and Syrjanen, K. (1991). Human papillomavirus (HPV) infections and their association with oral disease. *Journal of Oral Pathology*, **20**, 305–17.

EEC Clearinghouse on Oral Problems Related to HIV Infection (1991). An update of the classification and diagnostic criteria of oral lesions in HIV infection. *Journal of Oral Pathology and Medicine*, **20**, 97–100.

Eng, H.-L., Lu, S.-Y., Yang, C.-H., and Chen, W.-J. (1996). Oral tuberculosis. *Oral Surgery, Oral Medicine, Oral Pathology, Oral Radiology, Endodontics*, **81**, 415–20.

Epstein, J. and Scully, C. (1993). Cytomegalovirus: a virus of increasing relevance to oral medicine and pathology. *Journal of Oral Pathology and Medicine*, **22**, 348–53.

Epstein, J. B., Sherlock, C. H., and Wolber, R. A. (1993). Oral manifestations of cytomegalovirus infection. *Oral Surgery, Oral Medicine, Oral Pathology*, **75**, 443–51.

Eversole, L. R. (1992). Viral infections of the head and neck among HIV-seropositive patients. *Oral Surgery, Oral Medicine, Oral Pathology*, **73**, 155–63.

Greenberg, M. S. (1996). Herpesvirus infections. *Dental Clinics of North America*, **40**, 359–68.

Greenspan, D. and Greenspan, J. S. (1992). Significance of oral hairy leukoplakia. *Oral Surgery, Oral Medicine, Oral Pathology*, **73**, 151–4.

Greenspan, D. and Greenspan, J. S. (1996). HIV-related oral disease. *Lancet*, **348**, 729–33.

Holmstrup, P. and Westergaard, J. (1994). Periodontal diseases in HIV-infected patients. *Journal of Clinical Periodontology*, **21**, 270–80.

Johnson, B. D. and Engel, D. (1986). Acute necrotizing ulcerative gingivitis. A review of diagnosis, etiology and treatment. *Journal of Periodontology*, **57**, 141–50.

Lynch, D. P. (1994). Oral candidiasis. History, classification, and clinical presentation. *Oral Surgery, Oral Medicine, Oral Pathology*, **78**, 189–93.

MacFarlane, T. W. and Samaranayake, L. P. (1990). Systemic infections. In *Oral manifestations of systemic disease* (2nd edn) (ed. J. H. Jones and D. K. Mason), pp. 339–86. W. B. Saunders, London.

Samaranayake, L. (1992). Oral mycoses in HIV infection. *Oral Surgery, Oral Medicine, Oral Pathology*, **73**, 171–80.

Samaranayake, L. P. and MacFarlane, T. W. (1990) (ed). *Oral candidosis*. Wright, Bristol.

Scully, C. (1992). Oral infections in the immunocompromised patient. *British Dental Journal*, **172**, 401–7.

Scully, C., el-Kabir, M., and Samaranayake, L. P. (1994). Candida and oral candidosis: a review. *Critical reviews in Oral Biology and Medicine*, **5**, 125–57.

12 Oral ulceration and vesiculobullous diseases

12 Oral ulceration and vesiculobullous diseases

CLASSIFICATION OF ORAL ULCERATION

Injury to the oral mucosa, from whatever cause, may result in a localized defect of the surface in which the covering epithelium is destroyed leaving an inflamed area of exposed connective tissue. Such defects are called ulcers or erosions, the latter term sometimes being used to describe a superficial ulcer. Ulceration is the most common lesion of the oral mucosa and is a manifestation of many local and general disorders. Oral ulceration may be classified on an aetiological basis and the main causes are listed in Table 12.1. Several of these conditions are dealt with elsewhere in this book. This chapter is primarily concerned with traumatic ulceration, recurrent aphthous stomatitis, and ulceration associated with systemic diseases and the vesiculobullous diseases.

TRAUMATIC ULCERATION

Mechanical trauma from biting, sharp cusps, outstanding teeth, or ill-fitting intraoral appliances is a common cause of oral ulceration (Fig. 12.1). Such ulcers do not usually present a problem in clinical diagnosis, but three criteria should be fulfilled:

1. A cause of trauma must be identified.
2. The cause must fit the site, size, and shape of the ulcer.
3. On removal of the cause the ulcer must show signs of healing within 10 days.

Problems in diagnosis may arise with chronic traumatic ulcers, for example related to overextended flanges of a denture. Such ulcers may have been present for several weeks and may be deep crater-like lesions with rolled edges which are indurated on palpation because of surrounding fibrosis. Differentiation from a neoplastic ulcer may, therefore, be difficult. Biopsy is indicated when a presumed traumatic ulcer does not shown signs of healing within 10 days. A traumatic ulcer shows the histological features of chronic non-specific inflammation.

A wide variety of chemicals may cause oral ulceration. These include irritant or caustic agents used in dental practice that may be accidentally applied to the oral mucosa, and preparations used by patients in self-treatment of oral complaints. The latter include various antiseptic mouthwashes, particularly if inadequately diluted, and aspirin misused by some patients as a local obtundant for the relief of toothache. The caustic action of aspirin is dose- and time-related and reactions vary in severity from oedema through to necrosis of the epithelium. The oedematous epithelium resembles leukoedema; the necrotic epithelium presents as soggy white plaques which slough off to leave areas of ulceration (see Fig. 9.8).

Table 12.1 Causes of oral ulceration

1. *Infective*
    Bacterial
    Viral
    Fungal

2. *Traumatic*
    Mechanical
    Chemical
    Thermal
    Factitious injury
    Radiation
    Eosinophilic ulcer (traumatic granuloma)

3. *Idiopathic*
    Recurrent aphthous stomatitis
        minor aphthous ulcers
        major aphthous ulcers
        herpetiform ulcers

4. *Associated with systemic disease*
    Haematological diseases
    Gastrointestinal tract diseases
    Behçet syndrome
    HIV infection
    Other diseases

5. *Associated with dermatological diseases*
    Lichen planus
    Chronic discoid lupus erythematosus
    Vesiculobullous diseases

6. *Neoplastic*
    Squamous cell carcinoma
    Other malignant neoplasms

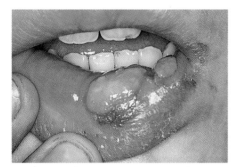

Fig. 12.1   Traumatic ulcer due to lip biting.

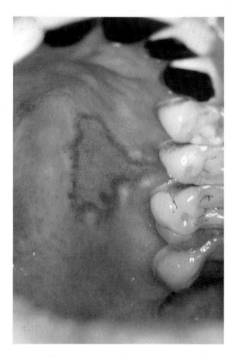

Fig. 12.2   Traumatic ulcer due to thermal burn.

Fig. 12.3, 12.4   Factitious ulcer caused by finger-nail. Notice also bite marks on thumb.

Fig. 12.5   Eosinophilic ulcer (traumatic granuloma).

Ulceration due to acute thermal trauma, for example from taking very hot food or drink, can occur on any part of the oral mucosa but is most commonly seen in the palate (Fig. 12.2).

Factitious ulcers are self-inflicted and may be a manifestation of stress, anxiety, or more severe emotional disturbance. Their appearances and distribution vary considerably depending on how they are induced. Common causes are biting or chewing of lips, cheeks or tongue, and damage, for example to the gingivae, from sharp finger-nails (Figs 12.3, 12.4).

In patients undergoing radiotherapy for head and neck cancer the oral mucosa may suffer immediate damage due to the direct effects of radiation on the cells, or delayed effects due to epithelial atrophy and damage to the underlying vascular bed. The immediate effects include erythema, radiation mucositis, and ulceration. These changes usually appear within 2–3 weeks and heal within a similar period, after completion of the therapy. Oedema due to obstruction of the regional lymphatics may also occur. The later effects of vascular damage and epithelial atrophy render the mucosa susceptible to trauma and even minimal trauma can cause ulceration which may take months to heal. Ulcers occurring at the site of the original neoplasm may be difficult to differentiate from recurrent tumour, but radiation ulcers are generally painful whereas this is not a common symptom of early malignant disease.

An unsual type of ulceration, sometimes referred to as eosinophilic ulcer, traumatic granuloma, or eosinophilic granuloma of soft tissues, appears to be associated particularly with trauma and crush injury to muscle, although the pathogenesis of the lesion is unclear. It occurs most commonly on the tongue and presents clinically as a chronic, well-demarcated ulcer which may mimic a squamous cell carcinoma (Fig. 12.5). Histological examination shows an ulcer covered by a thick layer of fibrinous exudate with a dense, chronic inflammatory cell infiltrate in its base involving underlying damaged muscle. The deeper parts of the lesion are characterized by an infiltrate rich in histiocytes and eosinophils, as reflected in the various names applied to this lesion. However, true granulomas are not present and the condition has no relationship to eosinophilic granuloma of bone.

RECURRENT APHTHOUS STOMATITIS (RAS)

Although a variety of oral ulcers may recur, for example those associated with mechanical trauma and dermatological diseases, there is a group of idiopathic ulcers whose natural history is characterized by frequent recurrences over a number of years. It is to this group that the collective term recurrent aphthous stomatitis (RAS) is applied.

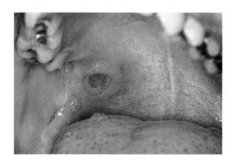

Fig. 12.3

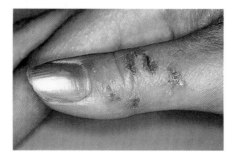

Fig. 12.4

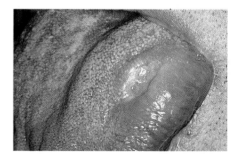

Fig. 12.5

The prevalence varies with the population studied, but a reasonable estimate would be that between 11 per cent and 20 per cent of the population may be affected. Generally, the condition is more common in females than males and in the majority of patients the onset of RAS is in the first three decades of life. Three types of ulcers are recognized, based primarily on their clinical features:

(1) minor aphthous ulcers;

(2) major aphthous ulcers;

(3) herpetiform ulcers.

In addition, any of the three types may be associated with Behçet syndrome (see later).

Clinical features of RAS

Prodromal symptoms described as soreness, burning, or prickling sensations are recognized by many patients 1–2 days before the onset of ulceration. The mucosa may appear normal at this stage or there may be erythematous macules at the sites of future ulcers. The salient clinical features of the three types of RAS are listed in Table 12.2.

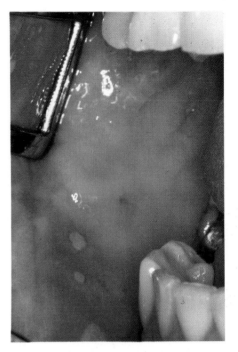

Fig. 12.6 Minor aphthous ulceration.

Minor aphthous ulceration

Minor aphthous ulceration accounts for 80 per cent or more cases of RAS. The condition is characterized by the occurrence of from one to five, shallow, round or oval ulcers which affect the non-keratinized areas of the oral mucosa (Figs 12.6, 12.7). The ulcers are less than 10 mm in diameter (generally they are about 4–5 mm across), and have a grey/yellow base with an erythematous margin. They heal without scarring, usually within 7–10 days, and they tend to recur at 1–4 month intervals, although this is very variable.

Major aphthous ulceration

Major aphthous ulcers are larger than minor aphthae and are usually greater than 10 mm in diameter (Fig. 12.8). They may occur at any of the sites of minor aphthae but may also involve the keratinized oral mucosa and commonly the soft palate, tonsillar areas, and oropharynx. The number of ulcers varies from one to ten and they may take 4–6 weeks to heal, and may heal with scarring. They tend to recur at less than monthly intervals, so that in severe cases ulceration of the oral cavity is virtually continuous and may be associated with severe

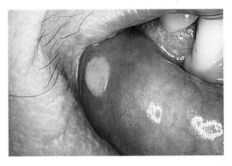

Fig. 12.7 Minor aphthous ulceration.

Table 12.2 Clinical features of recurrent aphthous stomatitis

	Minor	Major	Herpetiform
Age of onset (years)	10–19	10–19	20–29
Number of ulcers	1–5	1–10	10–100
Size of ulcers (mm)	< 10	> 10	1–2 but often coalesce
Duration (days)	7–14	> 30	10–30
Principal sites	Lips, cheeks, tongue	As for minor plus palate, pharynx	As for minor plus floor of mouth, palate, pharynx, and gingiva

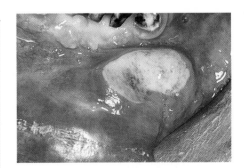

Fig. 12.8 Major aphthous ulceration.

discomfort and with difficulty in eating and speaking. Unlike the shallow ulceration of minor aphthae, major aphthae extend deeper and may present as crater-like ulcers with rolled margins which are indurated on palpation because of underlying fibrosis. Differentiation of an isolated lesion from a malignant ulcer may be difficult. It should be appreciated that major and minor aphthae represent a spectrum of the same disease process and intermediate forms may be seen.

Key point	**Recurrent aphthous stomatitis**
	• differential diagnosis of the three subtypes is based entirely on clinical features.

Herpetiform ulceration

Herpetiform ulceration is characterized by multiple, small, pin-head sized ulcers (about 1–2 mm across) that can occur on any part of the oral mucosa (Fig. 12.9). As many as a hundred ulcers may be present. When several ulcers are clustered together, confluence can result in larger areas of ulceration of irregular outline. The ulcers usually heal within 2–3 weeks. Large confluent ulcers may take longer and may heal with scarring, but this is not otherwise prominent. The ulcers tend to recur at less than monthly intervals and, as for major aphthae, may be associated with severe discomfort.

Aetiology of RAS

The aetiology of RAS is far from clear, but there is increasing evidence that damaging immune responses are involved. In addition, a number of local and general factors have also been incriminated (Table 12.3) and one or more of these may play a contributory role in a proportion of cases. These factors include the following.

Hereditary predisposition

A family history is found in up to 45 per cent of patients, but the mode and pattern of inheritance has not been established. Although some studies have suggested an increased prevalence associated with certain of the genetically determined histocompatibility antigens, no consistent patterns have been established.

Table 12.3 Aetiological factors in recurrent aphthous stomatitis

Hereditary predisposition
Trauma
Emotional stress and other psychological factors
Bacterial and viral infection
Allergic disorders
Haematological and deficiency disorders
Gastrointestinal diseases
Hormonal disturbance

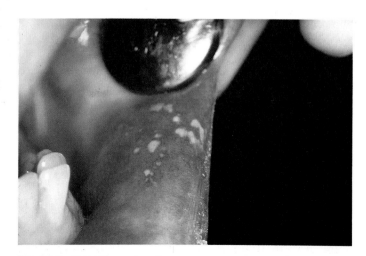

Fig. 12.9 Herpetiform ulceration.

However, HLA-B51, which is strongly associated with Behçet syndrome, appears to have a negative association with RAS and this may help to differentiate the conditions. Although the genetic basis predisposing to RAS is far from understood, immune responses play a role in the pathogenesis of many of the diseases known to be associated with HLA antigens in man.

Trauma

Trauma may precipitate and influence the site of some ulcers but does not play an essential role in the aetiology of RAS.

Emotional stress

Epidemiological studies have suggested that emotional stress may be a precipitating factor but it is unlikely to be the direct cause of ulceration. Stress may also be associated with pernicious habits, such as cheek biting, which may precipitate and influence the pattern of ulceration. Cigarette smoking has been reported to protect against RAS, and the onset of RAS in some patients has been associated with cessation of tobacco smoking. Whether the protective effect is related to increased keratinization of the mucosa or to a systemic mechanism is unknown.

Infective agents

Various microorganisms have been isolated from recurrent oral ulcers but attempts to incriminate them as causal factors have been largely unsuccessful. Hypersensitivity to *Streptococcus sanguis* antigens has been implicated in the pathogenesis of RAS, but studies of hypersensitivity to the organism in patients and control subjects have produced conflicting results. Nevertheless, there is some evidence of cross-reacting antigens between *Streptococcus sanguis* and oral mucosa and there is a possibility that these could be involved in the immuno-pathogenesis of RAS.

A viral aetiology for herpetiform ulceration has been suggested but there is little evidence to support such a hypothesis. Although clinically the ulceration is similar to that produced by infection with herpes simplex virus (hence herpetiform), herpes simplex virus is not associated with the ulcers.

Adenoviruses have been isolated occasionally from RAS but there is no evidence that they are causal. They are ubiquitous organisms and their presence may be purely incidental, as so-called passenger viruses. A rise in IgM antibody titres to varicella-zoster virus and to cytomegalovirus has also been reported during recurrences, but the significance of this is unknown.

Allergic disorders

Some patients with RAS associate the onset of ulceration with certain foods and this, together with the raised level of IgE found in some patients, has led to the claim that food allergies play a role in the aetiology of RAS. However, the evidence is often anecdotal, and results from controlled studies in which patients were challenged with specific foods are inconclusive.

Haematological disorders

Haematological abnormalities associated with deficiencies of haematinics may be found in up to 20 per cent of patients with RAS. Iron (ferritin) deficiency, which may or may not be associated with anaemia, occurs most frequently, but in the majority of patients no underlying cause can be identified. Deficiencies of folate and/or vitamin B_{12} are also associated with RAS, but much less frequently than iron.

The role of haematological deficiency states in the aetiology of RAS is unclear, although it is known that deficiencies of iron, folate, vitamin B_{12} can produce atrophic changes in the oral mucosa. However, the ulceration in some patients improves when the deficiency is corrected, suggesting a causal role.

In some patients haematological deficiency states are secondary to gastrointestinal disease.

Gastrointestinal diseases

RAS has been reported in patients with a variety of gastrointestinal diseases, some of which are associated with secondary haematological abnormalities as a result of malabsorption or chronic blood loss. An association with coeliac disease (idiopathic steatorrhoea or gluten-sensitive enteropathy) is well recognized, but the incidence of coeliac disease in patients with RAS is low, probably only about 2–4 per cent. In contrast RAS, usually of the minor aphthous type, is a common symptom amongst patients with coeliac disease. RAS may also be seen in patients with ulcerative colitis and Crohn's disease.

Key points	Aetiology of RAS
	• cause remains unknown
	• haematinic deficiency and/or underlying systemic disease associated in a minority of patients
	• a variety of factors may operate in an individual patient

Hormonal disturbance

In a small number of female patients a relationship between RAS and the menstrual cycle has been reported. It has been suggested that the degree of cornification of the mucosa is reduced in the low oestrogen, premenstrual phase and that this may render the mucosa more susceptible to trauma which could trigger the ulcers. Further evidence of a hormonal association in some patients is suggested by observations that the onset of ulceration may coincide with puberty and that remissions may occur in pregnancy. However, a recent extensive retrospective review of the literature concluded that no associations between RAS and the premenstrual period, pregnancy, or the menopause has been established.

Immunological and histopathological features of RAS

Although the aetiology of RAS is unknown there is considerable evidence that immune mechanisms are associated with the pathogenesis of the lesions.

Circulating antibodies to oral mucosal antigens have been demonstrated in 70–80 per cent of patients with minor or major aphthae and in patients with Behçet syndrome as compared with 10 per cent of controls, but their role in the pathogenesis of the lesions is uncertain. They maintain a relatively constant level and do not fluctuate with periods of activity and remission of ulceration, therefore, they may be simply a reflection of epithelial damage due to some other cause. However, patients with RAS have enhanced antibody-dependent cellular cytotoxicity activity (ADCC) early in the disease, suggesting a role for such a mechanism in the pathogenesis of the ulcers. Circulating immune complexes have also been demonstrated in some patients with RAS and in patients with

Behçet syndrome, the amount of immune complex being closely associated with disease activity. Immune complexes may cause tissue damage by activating complement. Despite these observations it appears unlikely that humoral immune mechanisms play a significant role in the pathogenesis of RAS.

In contrast, there is strong evidence that T-cell reactions are implicated in RAS from both histopathological and immunological studies. Microscopic examination of preulcerative lesions (premonitory stage) shows focal vacuolation and degeneration of suprabasal epithelial cells accompanied by a mononuclear, mainly lymphocytic, infiltrate in the lamina propria. In the deeper parts of the lesion the infiltrate has a mainly perivascular distribution and a similar pattern is seen in some other type IV delayed hypersensitivity reactions. Small numbers of lymphoid cells also infiltrate the epithelium. As the ulcerative stage approaches there is increased infiltration of the tissues, particularly the epithelium, by mononuclear cells accompanied by more extensive oedema and degeneration of the epithelium progressing to frank ulceration. Ultrastructural studies have demonstrated that the degeneration of prickle cells is associated with apoptosis and that the apoptotic debris is phagocytosed by macrophages in the mononuclear infiltrate. As the epithelium breaks down the cellular exudate becomes more mixed and includes large numbers of neutrophil leucocytes. These features resemble those seen in lichen planus except that in RAS the epithelial damage is not confined to the basal strata.

Immunohistochemical studies have shown changes in the T-cell subpopulations as the ulcers develop. The preulcerative lesion is characterized by mainly CD4 positive (inducer/helper) lymphocytes with smaller numbers of CD8 (suppressor/cytotoxic) cells in a ratio of about 2:1 (CD4:CD8). In contrast, the ulcerative stage is characterized by a marked increase in CD8 cells (CD4:CD8 approximately 1:10). As the ulcerative phase ends and the healing lesions becomes established there is a striking reversal of this ratio and CD4 cells predominate (CD4:CD8 approximately 10:1). These cyclical changes support a role for lymphocytotoxicity in the pathogenesis of the ulcers. It has been shown that peripheral blood lymphocytes from patients with RAS are cytotoxic to oral epithelial cells. The cytokine tumour necrosis factor (TNF) is also elevated in such lymphocytes suggesting that it may be involved in cell lysis.

Pathogenesis of RAS   **Key points**

- T cell reactions are involved
- mechanisms resemble those implicated in lichen planus
- immune response against keratinocyte-associated antigen
- keratinocyte death mediated by cytotoxic T cells

Changes in the expression of histocompatibility antigens by epithelial cells in RAS lesions accompany the changes in T-cell subpopulations, similar to those described for lichen planus in Chapter 9. In particular, the epithelial cells express the class II major histocompatibility antigens which are normally only expressed by immunocompetent cells. In the preulcerative stage these class II MHC antigens are found on the plasma membranes of the basal cells, but as the ulcerative phase develops they are expressed throughout the thickness of the epithelium. Expression declines to zero as the ulcers heal. Whether or not these changes play an active role in the pathogenesis of RAS has yet to be determined. They may merely reflect changes in lymphocyte populations and cytokine production.

In conclusion, the pathogenesis of RAS is similar to that of lichen planus. There is infiltration of the epithelium by T lymphocytes (epidermotropism) in response to some, as yet, unidentified keratinocyte-associated antigen. This results in the differentiation of cytotoxic T cells and T cell mediated cell death throughout all strata of the epithelium, probably involving TNF. However, why epithelial cell death is so focal in RAS, producing the discrete and varying patterns of ulceration seen clinically, is unknown.

Behçet syndrome

Behçet syndrome is a rare disease originally characterized by the classical triad of RAS of any of the types listed above, genital ulceration, and eye lesions, especially uveitis. However, not all patients show the classical triad (although 90 per cent or more have RAS), and a variety of other manifestations, which include cutaneous, joint, neurological, vascular, and intestinal disorders, are now recognized as components of the syndrome. The disease is more common in males than in females and occurs especially in Japan.

On clinical and prognostic grounds Behçet syndrome can be divided into various subgroups, although these should not be regarded as distinct entities but as representing a spectrum of activity. The main clinical types are:

1. *Mucocutaneous type*: the mouth, genitals, skin, and conjuctiva may be involved.
2. *Arthritic type*: involvement of one or more large joints in addition to one or more of the manifestations of the mucocutaneous type.
3. *Neurological type*: involvement of the central nervous system in addition to some or all of the manifestations of types 1 and 2.
4. *Ocular type*: uveitis in addition to some or all of the manifestations of types 1, 2, and 3.

The aetiology of Behçet syndrome is unknown but there is a strong association with the histocompatibility antigen HLA-B51. Many of the systemic manifestations are probably related to the deposition of immune complexes.

VESICULOBULLOUS DISEASES

The vesiculobullous diseases are included in this chapter because they usually present as oral ulceration following rupture of the vesicles or bullae. The latter are collections of clear fluid within or just below the epithelium, which patients may refer to as blisters. The distinction between a vesicle and a bulla is simply one of size, the distinction being somewhat arbitary, but the term bulla is generally applied to a lesion greater than 5 mm in diameter.

Classification

The vesiculobullous diseases are divided into two major groups depending on the histological location of the lesions. In the first, the lesions form within the epithelium—intraepithelial vesicles; in the second, they form between the epithelium and the lamina propria (or dermis of the skin)—subepithelial vesicles.

The intraepithelial vesiculobullous diseases can be subdivided into two groups depending on the mechanisms of formation of the lesion.

1. Acantholytic vesicles and bullae, for example pemphigus. The lesions are produced by breakdown of the specialized intercellular attachments (desmosomes) between epithelial cells.
2. Non-acantholytic vesicles and bullae, for example viral infections of oral mucosa. The lesions are produced by death and rupture of groups of epithelial cells.

The main vesiculobullous diseases which may affect the oral mucosa are listed in Table 12.4.

Erythema multiforme is listed in the subepithelial group for convenience although, as its name implies, the manifestations are very variable and may include intraepithelial vesicles. Some forms of epidermolysis bullosa are also associated with intraepithelial vesicles but the majority are subepithelial in type.

The viral infections have been dealt with in Chapter 11. Darier's disease and bullous lichen planus are discussed in Chapter 9 since they usually present in the mouth as white lesions. The remaining conditions are all uncommon and are essentially skin diseases with oral manifestations.

Pemphigus

Pemphigus is an uncommon autoimmune disease which exists in several clinical forms, the most common and most severe being pemphigus vulgaris. This usually presents in middle-age, predominantly in women, and occurs more commonly in Ashkenazi Jews than in other ethnic groups. It is characterized by widespread bullous eruptions involving the skin (Fig. 12.10) and mucous membranes. The oral mucosa is ultimately involved in nearly all patients and in about 50 per cent of cases is the site of the initial lesions. In some patients the disease remains confined to the oral cavity. The bullae are fragile and readily rupture forming crusted or weeping areas of denudation on the skin and irregular, ragged mucosal ulcers (Fig. 12.11). Any part of the oral mucosa may be involved but

Table 12.4   Vesiculobullous diseases affecting the oral mucosa

I.   *Intraepithelial vesiculobullous diseases*

    Acantholytic lesions

        Pemphigus
            pemphigus vulgaris *(most severe)*
            pemphigus foliaceous
            pemphigus vegetans

        Familial benign chronic pemphigus
            (Hailey–Hailey disease)
            Darier's disease

    Non-acantholytic lesions

        Viral infections
            herpes simplex infections
            herpes zoster
            coxsackie infections

II.   *Subepithelial vesiculobullous diseases*

    Erythema multiforme

    Pemphigoid group
        bullous pemphigoid
        benign mucous membrane (cicatricial) pemphigoid

    Dermatitis herpetiformis

    Linear IgA disease

    Epidermolysis bullosa group
        inherited forms
        epidermolysis bullosa acquisita (acquired type)

    Oral blood blisters (angina bullosa haemorrhagica)

    Bullous lichen planus

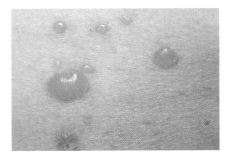

Fig. 12.10   Skin bullae in pemphigus vulgaris.

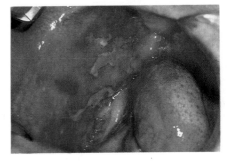

Fig. 12.11   Ragged oral ulcers in pemphigus vulgaris.

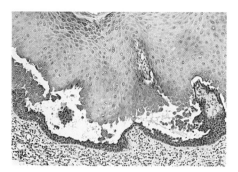

Fig. 12.12 Intraepithelial vesicle in pemphigus vulgaris.

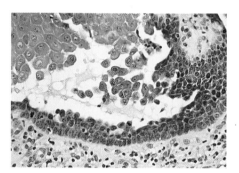

Fig. 12.13 Pemphigus vulgaris vesicle and acantholytic cells.

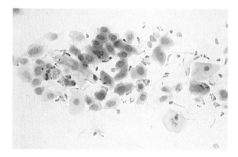

Fig. 12.14 Acantholytic (Tzanck) cells in smear from pemphigus vesicle.

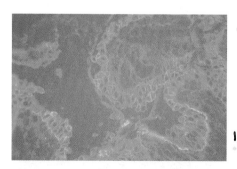

Fig. 12.15 Immunofluorescent demonstration of epithelial-bound autoantibody in pemphigus bulla.

the soft palate, buccal mucosa, and gingiva are most frequently affected. The bullae are produced as a result of acantholysis and this process extends laterally into the surrounding epithelium, often for a considerable distance. As a result of this lateral extension the superficial layers of the epithelium can be slid over and detached from the deeper layers by gentle lateral pressure (Nikolsky's sign). The lateral extension also allows pressure exerted by the accumulation of fluid within the blister to dissipate so the bullae tend to be flaccid rather than tense.

Before the introduction of corticosteroid therapy the prognosis was very poor and many patients survived less than two years following the onset of lesions. Treatment with high doses of corticosteroids and other immunosuppressants has significantly reduced the mortality and in many patients the disease can now be controlled, with prolonged remissions being reported.

Histological examination shows characteristic intraepithelial vesicles or bullae and cleft-like spaces produced by acantholysis. Typically, these changes occur between stratum spinosum cells just above the basal cell layer (Fig. 12.12). The basal cells forming the base of the lesion remain attached to the lamina propria and project into the bulla like a row of tombstones. There is remarkably little inflammatory cell infiltration until the lesion ruptures, but occasional eosinophils may be seen in the epithelium in early lesions. Acantholytic stratum spinosum cells occurring singly or in small clumps are found lying free within the blister fluid (Fig. 12.13). Unlike normal polyhedral stratum spinosum cells they are small and rounded and contain enlarged hyperchromatic nuclei (Tzanck cells). Their identification in cytological smears taken from a blister is helpful in establishing a diagnosis (Fig. 12.14).

Immunological studies are important in establishing and confirming the diagnosis. Pemphigus is an autoimmune disease, and circulating autoantibodies to the intercellular substance of stratified squamous epithelium can be demonstrated in the serum of patients. The antibodies are predominantly of the IgG class, but IgM and occasionally IgA classes may be represented. The autoantibody titre is correlated with the severity of the disease, and repeated tests on patients' sera to detect changes in titre may be helpful in assessing the clinical course of the disease and response to treatment. However, circulating pemphigus-like antibodies occasionally appear in association with other conditions, for example following severe burns. Direct binding of autoantibodies to the intercellular substance of stratum spinosum cells can also be demonstrated by immunofluorescent techniques applied to biopsy specimens from involved epithelial (Fig. 12.15). The autoantibodies are thought to be responsible for the acantholysis as discussed below.

Oral lesions have also been reported in pemphigus foliaceous, where acantholysis occurs at a higher level in the epithelium, and in pemphigus vegetans. The latter is considered to be a milder form of pemphigus vulgaris and is characterized by the formation of vegetative masses of exuberant granulation tissue which develop following rupture of the bullae. Although any part of the oral mucosa may be involved, in most of the reported cases the lesions have involved the angles of the mouth.

There is considerable experimental evidence that the autoantibodies in pemphigus are involved in acantholysis and that the acantholytic activity resides in the IgG fraction. Three main mechanisms have been proposed:

1. *Complement activation via the classical pathway resulting in generation of lytic activity*

Experimental studies suggest this is probably not an important mechanism. Acantholysis can be induced in explants of skin in organ culture by complement-free pemphigus serum.

Pemphigus

- intraepithelial, acantholytic vesicles and bullae
- ragged oral ulcers
- oral lesions often the presenting feature
- autoantibodies to desmosomal protein

2 *Protease production*

Binding of the autoantibody to antigen on the surface of epithelial cells results in the release of proteolytic activity which causes acantholysis. There is evidence that this is associated with activation of tissue plasminogen within the epithelium and generation of the proteolytic enzyme plasmin, which is then thought to be responsible for degradation of cell adhesion molecules. However, increased production of plasminogen activator by keratinocytes is seen in other diseases of skin not associated with acantholysis.

3. *Direct binding of autoantibody to intercellular adhesion molecules*

Recent studies have shown that the pemphigus antigen is a protein component of the desmosome belonging to the cadherin family. These transmembrane proteins are involved in cell–cell adhesion, and it is proposed that binding of the antibody to the proteins in the desmosomes prevents cell–cell adhesion directly by steric interference. Once acantholysis is initiated, plasminogen release and complement-mediated lysis may amplify the process.

Familial benign chronic pemphigus (Hailey-Hailey disease)

This rare and relatively benign disorder has an autosomal dominant pattern of inheritance and is characterized by recurrent acantholytic vesicular eruptions on the skin. Oral involvement has been reported. Despite the acantholysis the immunological findings are negative and this, together with the family history, helps differentiate it from pemphigus vulgaris.

Erythema multiforme

Erythema multiforme is a disease of abrupt onset involving skin and mucous membranes and has a wide range of clinical presentations, hence 'multiforme'. The pathogenesis of the disease is unknown, although many precipitating factors have been implicated including drugs (particularly sulphonamides) and preceding infection (especially herpes simplex infection). However, many cases appear to arise spontaneously. It has been suggested that the disease represents a hypersensitivity reaction and that the manifestations may be related to deposition of immune complexes in which the antigen may be of drug, bacterial, or viral origin.

Erythema multiforme occurs mainly in young adults and is more common in males than in females. There may be a prodromal phase with upper respiratory infection, headache, malaise, nausea, and sometimes arthralgia. The severity of the disease varies considerably. In its most severe form, the Stevens–Johnson syndrome, there is widespread involvement of the skin and oral, genital, and ocular mucosae. Ocular involvement (Fig. 12.16) can lead to conjunctival scarring and visual impairment. Milder forms usually involve the oral mucosa, with or without skin lesions, or the skin alone may be involved. Generally, the disease tends to subside after 10–14 days but recurrences may occur. Recurrent erythema multiforme is associated in particular with recurrent attacks of herpes simplex virus infection.

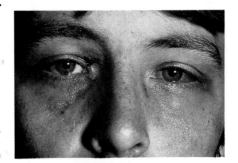

Fig. 12.16 Ocular lesions in erythema multiforme.

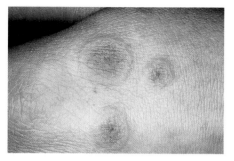

Fig. 12.17 Target skin lesions in erythema multiforme.

The skin lesions have a variety of forms, including erythematous maculopapular rashes and vesiculobullous eruptions in addition to the characteristic and virtually diagnostic target or iris lesions (Fig. 12.17) These consist of concentric rings of varying erythema and oedema in the centre of which may be an intact or ruptured and crusted bulla. The hands and feet are most commonly involved.

Oral lesions may involve any part of the mucosa, although the lips and anterior parts of the mouth are most commonly affected (Figs 12.18, 12.19). The appearance of the lesions varies with time. Erythematous patches are quickly followed by vesiculobullous eruptions which rapidly break down into erosions as the bullae disintegrate. The erosions on the lips are accompanied by bleeding and crusting. Circumoral crusting, haemorrhagic lesions are an important sign in arriving at a clinical diagnosis: somewhat similar lesions may be seen in acute herpetic gingivostomatitis.

Key points	**Erythema multiforme**
	• mucosal vesicles and bullae variable
	• oral ulceration/circumoral crusting, haemorrhagic lesions
	• target/iris skin lesions
	• precipitated by drugs/herpesvirus antigens
	• immune complex vasculitis

The diagnosis of erythema multiforme is based primarily on the clinical findings. The histopathological features are non-specific (although biopsy may be useful to exclude other diseases) and a wide spectrum of histological changes has been described. Epithelial changes include inter- and intracellular oedema, and varying degrees of necrosis of keratinocytes leading to intraepithelial vesiculation. Alternatively, bullae may form subepithelially following degeneration of basal cells and detachment of the full thickness of the epithelium from the lamina propria (Fig. 12.20). The epithelium forming the lid of the bulla is often necrotic. The lamina propria is oedematous and there is a variable, mononuclear inflammatory cell infiltration which extends perivascularly into the deeper tissues.

Immunological findings in erythema multiforme are either negative or non-specific but deposits of IgM and C3 may be found in the superficial vessels, suggesting that the disease is mediated in part by deposition of immune complexes and a type III hypersensitivity reaction. Deposition of immune complexes leads to complement activation, chemotaxis of neutrophils, and vasculitis, resulting eventually in ischaemic necrosis of epithelium. Neutrophils may also release lysosomal enzymes which could cause direct damage to keratinocytes. Circulating immune complexes have been detected in patients with erythema multiforme and in some cases they have been associated with herpes simplex viral antigens.

Figs 12.18, 12.19 Oral lesions in erythema multiforme.

Fig. 12.20 Vesicle in erythema multiforme.

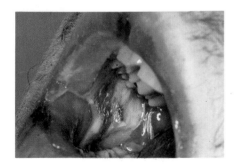

Fig. 12.18

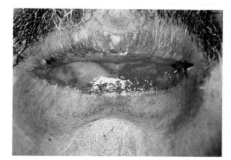

Fig. 12.19

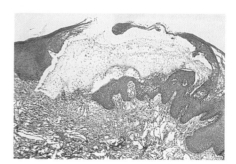

Fig. 12.20

Pemphigoid

The general heading of pemphigoid includes bullous pemphigoid and benign mucous membrane pemphigoid. The term benign is often omitted and the latter may also be referred to as cicatricial pemphigoid. It is probable that the conditions are related and represent manifestations of a spectrum of disease, although it may be possible to separate them on clinical and, to some extent, immunological grounds. Both are autoimmune disorders characterized by the formation of subepithelial bullae. Pemphigoid is about twice as common in women as men and the mean age of onset is about 60 years. The disease is not life-threatening but may run a chronic course over many years.

Bullous pemphigoid primarily involves the skin, presenting as large tense bullae typically involving the limbs and lower abdomen. Oral lesions occur in a minority of patients but it is very rare for these to precede the skin eruptions. When present, the oral manifestations are indistinguishable from those of benign mucous membrane pemphigoid.

In contrast, the oral mucosa is almost always affected in benign mucous membrane pemphigoid (Fig. 12.21), whereas the skin is only minimally involved. In most cases oral lesions precede those in other locations and may be the only manifestations of the disease.

Bullae, which are occasionally haemorrhagic, occur anywhere on the oral mucosa. Unlike those seen in pemphigus vulgaris they tend to be tense and, because the lid consists of a full thickness epithelium, are relatively tough and may remain intact for a few days. When they rupture they give rise to erosions which heal slowly, sometimes with scarring, hence the alternative name for this disease—cicatricial pemphigoid (Fig. 12.22). Although bullae can occur on any part of the mucosa, the most consistent oral lesions in dentate patients, occurring in over 90 per cent of cases, involve the gingiva where the condition presents as desquamative gingivitis (Fig. 12.23). In some patients this is the only manifestation of the disease.

In addition to the oral mucosa the conjunctiva and mucosae of the nose, larynx, pharynx, oesophagus, and genitalia may be involved. Ocular involvement is the most serious complication with scarring leading to adhesions between the bulbar and palpebral conjunctiva, opacity of the cornea, and blindness (Fig. 12.24).

Histopathological examination of established pemphigoid lesions shows separation of the full thickness of the epithelium from the lamina propria producing a subepithelial bulla, with a thick roof (Fig. 12.25). Developing bullae are characterized by foci of oedema in the basement membrane zone which enlarge to form vesicles. Initially, there is no evidence of an inflammatory reaction in the lamina propria but as the vesicle develops there is infiltration by variable numbers of neutrophils and eosinophils around and within the developing bulla. These changes

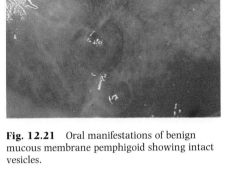

Fig. 12.21 Oral manifestations of benign mucous membrane pemphigoid showing intact vesicles.

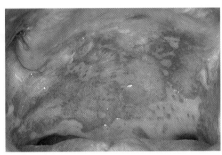

Fig. 12.22 Extensive oral ulceration associated with benign mucous membrane pemphigoid.

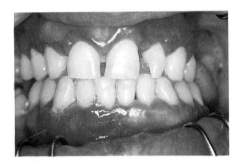

Fig. 12.23 Benign mucous membrane pemphigoid presenting as desquamative gingivitis.

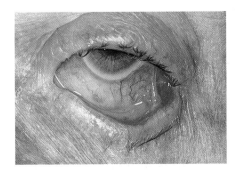

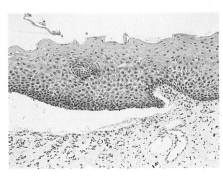

Fig. 12.24 Ocular lesions in benign mucous membrane pemphigoid.

Fig. 12.25 Subepithelial bulla in benign mucous membrane pemphigoid.

Fig. 12.24   **Fig. 12.25**

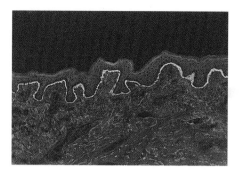

Fig. 12.26 Linear binding of IgG in the basement membrane zone in benign mucous membrane pemphigoid.

are accompanied by a perivascular mononuclear, mainly lymphocytic, infiltrate in the lamina propria, the intensity of which increases as the lesion develops.

Electron microscopic studies have shown that separation occurs through the lamina lucida of the basement membrane, between the cell membranes of the basal cells and the lamina densa. Loss of hemidesmosomes and disorganization of tonofilaments within basal cells have also been described.

Immunopathological investigations involving direct immunofluorescence studies of fresh, unfixed biopsy material to detect tissue-bound immune products and indirect immunofluorescence techniques to detect circulating autoantibodies in the patient's serum are essential to establish the diagnosis (Table 12.5). In both bullous and benign mucous membrane pemphigoid, direct immunofluorescence shows linear binding of immunoglobulin, predominantly IgG but occasionally other classes, in the basement membrane zone (Fig. 12.26). Linear deposits of complement products, principally C3, are also bound to the basement membrane zone.

By indirect immunofluorescence techniques circulating autoantibodies of IgG type against basement membrane antigens of skin and mucosa can be demonstrated in about 75 per cent of patients with bullous pemphigoid. In contrast, the serum of patients with benign mucous membrane pemphigoid rarely contains circulating anti-basement membrane antibodies.

The immunopathological findings suggest that bulla formation involves binding of autoantibody, activation of complement, generation of chemotactic factors, and leucocyte-mediated damage associated with the accumulation and release of proteolytic enzymes from neutrophils. It is highly likely that the leucocyte-mediated damage also involves the activity of eosinophils.

Patients with bullous pemphigoid have antibodies to two hemidesmosome-associated antigens. One is located intracellularly, whilst the other is a transmembrane protein with intra- and extracellular components. The autoantigen in mucous membrane pemphigoid has not been precisely characterized but is thought to be similar or identical to the transmembrane protein identified in bullous pemphigoid.

Key points

Mucous membrane pemphigoid
- subepithelial vesicles and bullae
- occasionally intact oral vesicles and bullae
- extensive oral ulceration
- desquamative gingivitis (dentate pts. esp.)
- autoantibodies to hemidesmosomal proteins

Dermatitis herpetiformis

Dermatitis herpetiformis is a chronic, intensely pruritic subepidermal autoimmune blistering disease of skin. Oral manifestations are variable and range from small symptomless erythematous areas to extensive erosions. Their incidence is difficult to establish but in some series they have been reported in up to 75 per cent of patients.

Histologically, the lesions are characterized by the formation of microabscesses at the tips of the connective tissue (dermal) papillae beneath the epithelium. Neutrophils predominate, but as the lesions develop increasing numbers of eosinophils are seen. Immunofluorescence studies show granular deposits of IgA in the tips of the connective tissue papillae together with complement components (Table 12.5). Activation of the alternative complement pathway by IgA

Table 12.5 Major immunological findings in subepithelial bullous disorders

Disease	Direct IF	Indirect IF (circulating antibodies)
1 Bullous pemphigoid	Linear, IgG, C3; BM zone	Positive (75 %) IgG
2 Benign mucous membrane pemphigoid	Linear, IgG, C3; BM zone	Negative
3 Dermatitis herpetiformis	Granular IgA, C3; tips of dermal papillae	Negative
4 Linear IgA disease	Linear, IgA, C3; BM zone	Negative
5 Epidermolysis bullosa acquisita	Linear IgG, C3; BM zone	Positive (30–40 %) IgG

and the subsequent generation of chemotactic factors are thought to be important in the pathogenesis of the lesions, but T-lymphocyte reactions and cytokine release may also be involved.

Many patients with dermatitis herpetiformis also have abnormalities of their jejunal mucosa associated with gluten hypersensitivity, but the precise relationship between the intestinal, oral, and skin lesions is uncertain.

Linear IgA disease

This is a rare subepidermal blistering disease of skin which clinically overlaps with dermatitis herpetiformis and bullous pemphigoid. Oral lesions have been reported. Patients may have gluten hypersensitivity, but this is much less common than in dermatitis herpetiformis. There is a strong association with internal malignancy, especially lymphoma.

Immunopathological studies show linear binding of IgA along the basement membrane zone similar to the pattern seen in pemphigoid, but different from the clumped granular deposits of dermatitis herpetiformis (Table 12.5).

Epidermolysis bullosa

The inherited forms of epidermolysis bullosa form a diverse and complex group of syndromes of which over 30 types have been reported.

In general, they are characterized by the formation of skin bullae which may be manifest at birth or appear shortly afterwards. There is extreme fragility of the skin and the bullae usually develop in response to minimal trauma or pressure, but they may arise spontaneously. Hands, feet, knees, elbows, buttocks, and occiput are common sites. Oral and other mucosae may be involved. The bullae tend to heal slowly with scarring which can result in claw-like deformity of the hands (Fig. 12.27) and other complications, such as difficulties in eating, speaking, and swallowing as a result of involvement of the mouth, larynx, and pharynx. Several types are incompatible with life.

Currently the various types are classified into three major groups based on the histological level of bulla formation and the molecular basis of the defect:

1. *Epidermolytic (simplex types)*. Separation occurs within the epithelium to produce intraepithelial bullae. This group results from mutation of the genes coding for keratins 5 and 14, expressed in basal keratinocytes.

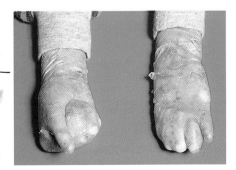

Fig. 12.27 Epidermolysis bullosa—scarring of hands.

2. *Junctional (gravis types).* Separation occurs within the lamina lucida to produce subepithelial bullae. This group is caused by mutations in the genes coding for a laminin associated with the anchoring filament–hemidesmosome complex of the basement membrane.

3. *Dermolytic (dystrophic types).* Separation occurs beneath the basal lamina to produce subepithelial bullae. Anchoring fibrils may be decreased in number and poorly developed. This group is due to mutation in the type VII collagen gene, the anchoring fibril collagen.

Classified in this way the different syndromes in each group tend to show similar clinical features and modes of inheritance (Table 12.6).

Oral lesions are seen mainly in the junctional and dermolytic types. Bullae may appear in neonates in response to suckling, and, later, minimal trauma from toothbrushing and routine dental treatment can cause serious consequences. The bullae rupture to leave painful erosions, and subsequent scarring can restrict the opening of the mouth, movement of lips and tongue, and cause obliteration of the sulci. Effective oral hygiene may be impossible and rampant caries and its sequelae add to the dental complications. Dental defects, especially enamel hypoplasia, have been described in some patients.

Epidermolysis bullosa acquisita

This is an uncommon, acquired blistering dermatosis characterized by subepithelial bullae. Oral bullae, ulceration, and scarring have been recorded in about half of the reported cases.

Separation occurs in or beneath the lamina densa and is associated with linear deposits of IgG and C3 in the basement membrane zone (see Table 12.5). Clinically, the disease has a wide range of presentations, but early stages may

Table 12.6 Principal modes of inheritance and main clinical features of the subgroups of epidermolysis bullosa

Type	Skin/general	Oral/mucosal	Inheritance
Epidermolytic (simplex)	Blisters present at birth Mild; no scarring Improvement at puberty	Absent or very mild Often abates Teeth normal	Autosomal dominant
Junctional (gravis)	Congenital blisters/ erosions Extensive, generalized, blistering, atrophy, prominent acral involvement Death common in infancy	Extensive involvement of all mucosae Severe dental abnormalities	Autosomal recessive
Dermolytic (dystrophic)	Congenital blisters/erosions Marked scarring, mitten deformity of hands, syndactyly, nail dystrophy	Oral and other mucosae often involved Hypoplastic teeth	Autosomal dominant

mimic pemphigoid while later it resembles the dermolytic type of epidermolysis bullosa.

Oral blood blisters (angina bullosa haemorrhagica)

Spontaneous blood-filled bullae (blisters) occasionally develop on the oral mucosa to which the term angina bullosa haemorrhagica has been applied. They may be up to 2–3 cm in diameter and occur on any part of the oral mucosa, although they are seen most commonly on the palate (Fig. 12.28). The patient may notice a pricking sensation when the blister arises and if large it may be uncomfortable. Early perforation is frequent, leaving an ulcer which heals uneventfully. Histology shows a subepithelial bulla with separation within the basement membrane zone (Fig. 12.29). Immunological findings are negative and no abnormalities in blood coagulation or in the tissues have been identified. The cause remains a mystery but it is probable that the bullae are related to trauma.

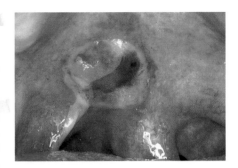

Fig. 12.28 Recently ruptured oral blood blister.

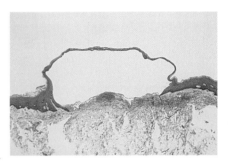

Fig. 12.29 Subepithelial bulla associated with oral blood blister

FURTHER READING

el-Mofty, S. K., Swanson, P. E., Wick, E. R., and Miller, A. S. (1993). Eosinophilic ulcer of the oral mucosa. Report of 38 new cases with immunohistochemical observations. *Oral Surgery, Oral Medicine, Oral Pathology*, **75**, 716–22.

Eversole, L. R. (1994). Immunopathology of oral mucosal ulcerative, desquamative, and bullous diseases. Selective review of the literature. *Oral Surgery, Oral Medicine, Oral Pathology*, **77**, 555–71.

Farthing, P. M., Maragou, P., Coates, M., Tatnall, F., Leigh, I. M., and Williams, D. M. (1995). Characteristics of the oral lesions in patients with cutaneous recurrent erythema multiforme. *Journal of Oral Pathology and Medicine*, **24**, 9–13.

Fraser, N. G., Kerr, N. W., and Donald, D. (1973). Oral lesions in dermatitis herpetiformis. *British Journal of Dermatology*, **89**, 439–50.

National Institutes of Health (1978). Aphthous stomatitis—Behçet's syndrome workshop. *Journal of Oral Pathology*, **7**, 341–440.

Nisengard, R. J. and Neiders, M. (1981). Desquamative lesions of the gingiva. *Journal of Periodontology*, **52**, 500–10.

Pearson, R. W. (1988). Clinicopathological types of epidermolysis bullosa and their non-dermatological complications. *Archives of Dermatology*, **124**, 718–25.

Pindborg, J. J. (1990). Diseases of the skin. In *Oral manifestations of systemic disease* (2nd edn) (ed. J. H. Jones and D. K. Mason), pp. 537–92. W. B. Saunders, London.

Rennie, J. S., Reade, P. C., and Scully, C. (1985). Recurrent aphthous stomatitis. *British Dental Journal*, **159**, 361–7.

Scully, C. and Porter, S. R. (1989). Recurrent aphthous stomatitis: current concepts of etiology, pathogenesis and management. *Journal of Oral Pathology and Medicine*, **18**, 21–7.

Scully, C. and Porter, S. R. (1994). Oral mucosal disease: a decade of new entities, aetiologies and associations. *International Dental Journal*, **44**, 33–43.

Ship, J. A. (1996). Recurrent aphthous stomatitis. An update. *Oral Surgery, Oral Medicine, Oral Pathology, Oral Radiology and Endodontics*, **81**, 141–7.

Vincent, S. D., Lilly, G. E., and Baker, K. A. (1993). Clinical, historic and therapeutic features of cicatricial pemphigoid, *Oral Medicine, Oral Surgery, Oral Pathology*, **76**, 453–9.

Williams, D. M. (1989). Vesiculobullous mucocutaneous disease: pemphigus vulgaris. *Journal of Oral Pathology and Medicine*, **18**, 544–53.

Williams, D. M. (1990). Vesiculobullous mucocutaneous disease: benign mucous membrane pemphigoid. *Journal of Oral Pathology and Medicine*, **19**, 16–23.

Williams, D. M. (1993). Non-infectious diseases of the oral soft tissue: a new approach. *Advances in Dental Research*, **7**, 213–19.

13 Miscellaneous disorders of oral mucosa

13 Miscellaneous disorders of oral mucosa

Fordyce's granules

Sebaceous glands in the oral mucosa are usually known as Fordyce's spots or granules, and are seen as separate small, yellowish bodies beneath the surface, although on occasions they may be so numerous as to form slightly raised confluent plaques. They are commonly seen in the mucosa of the upper lip, cheeks, and anterior pillar of the fauces, and usually have a symmetrical distribution. They rarely occur in the lower lip. The glands are present in about 60–75 per cent of adults, but the number of glands varies greatly between individuals. The prevalence and number in the upper lip increase at puberty, and there is an increase in the number of the glands in the cheeks in later life.

The glands lie quite superficially and consist of a number of lobules of sebaceous cells grouped around one or more ducts (Fig. 13.1). Sebaceous glands do not appear to have any function in the oral cavity, and no significant pathological changes are associated with them.

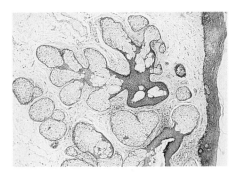

Fig. 13.1 Fordyce's granules—ectopic sebaceous glands.

Sublingual varices

The prevalence of varicosities of the lateral branches of the sublingual veins increases with age (Fig. 13.2). They have no relationship with systemic diseases. Histological investigation of the distribution of elastic tissue and fat in the supporting tissues has not revealed any morphological changes to account for their development. The varices have no clinical significance. Similar lesions are seen occasionally elsewhere in the mouth and on the lips.

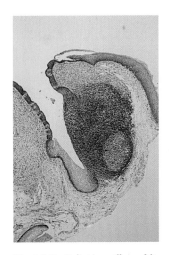

Fig. 13.2 Sublingual varicosities.

Lingual tonsil, foliate papillitis

Lingual tonsillar tissue is mainly located on the posterior part of the lateral aspect of the tongue and may be associated with vertical folds of mucosa, sometimes referred to as foliate papillae (Fig. 13.3). Small aggregates of subepithelial lymphoid tissue are occasionally found elsewhere in the oral cavity.

Diseases of lingual tonsillar tissue are uncommon, but they may become enlarged as a result of trauma from teeth or dentures, inflammation, or reactive hyperplasia of the lymphoid tissue. Inflammatory changes are sometimes referred to as foliate papillitis (Fig. 13.4). Occasionally, crypts may become obstructed and undergo cystic dilatation as a result of accumulation of squamous debris.

Median rhomboid glossitis

This condition is characteristically located in the midline of the dorsal surface of the tongue, just anterior to the foramen caecum. The lesion is roughly rhomboidal in shape and has a reddish surface, devoid of papillae, which may be

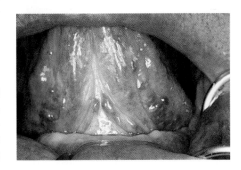

Fig. 13.3 Foliate papilla and lingual tonsillar tissue.

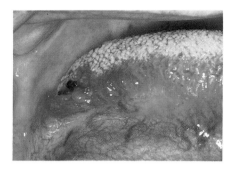

Fig. 13.4 Foliate papillitis associated with denture trauma.

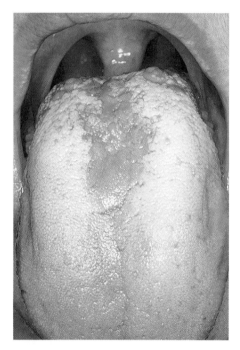

Fig. 13.5 Median rhomboid glossitis.

smooth, nodular, or fissured (Fig. 13.5). There may be slight induration on palpation. It is usually an asymptomatic condition.

Median rhomboid glossitis was for many years regarded as a developmental abnormality, due to persistence of the tuberculum impar on the dorsum of the tongue. The tuberculum impar is a small median elevation in the floor of the pharynx which appears by the fifth week of embryonic life, and is subsequently incorporated in the anterior part of the tongue. However, the condition appears to be exceedingly rare in children and young adults, and this has cast doubt on it being a developmental disorder.

In many cases candidal hyphae are present in the parakeratinized surface layers of the epithelium, suggesting the possibility of a peculiarly localized chronic candidosis. It is possible that in some patients trauma or local variation in the anatomy of the mid-dorsal surface of the tongue allows the proliferation of candidal hyphae with subsequent loss of the filiform papillae, but it is doubtful whether the clinical appearance can be altered by antifungal therapy. The candidosis may represent a secondary opportunistic infection of an already abnormal tissue. However, a palatal lesion in opposition to a tongue lesion is seen in some patients, generally heavy smokers, and the term multifocal candidosis has been used to describe this condition. Median rhomboid glossitis has also been reported in HIV-positive and other immunocompromised patients.

Histologically, the appearances are similar to those seen in other candidoses (see Chapter 11). The area is devoid of lingual papillae and is covered by parakeratotic, acanthotic squamous epithelium with neutrophil infiltration, and superficial microabscess formation associated with candida infection of the parakeratin. There is an associated chronic inflammatory cell infiltration in the lamina propria.

Geographic tongue (benign migratory glossitis)

This condition, of unknown aetiology, is seen clinically as irregular, partially depapillated, red areas on the anterior two-thirds of the dorsal tongue surface and is associated with loss of the filiform papillae, the fungiform papillae remaining as shiny, dark-red eminences (Fig. 13.6). The margins of the lesions are often outlined by a thin, white line or band and the disorder is frequently associated with fissured (scrotal) tongue (Fig. 13.7). The affected areas may begin as small lesions only a few millimetres in diameter which, after gradually enlarging, heal and then reappear in another location. The condition may regress for a period and then recur. It is usually symptomless but there may be some irritation associated with acid and spicy foods. The reported prevalence is approximately 1 per cent of the population and there is often a family history. The disorder occurs over a wide age range and presents both in children and adults.

Key points	Median rhomboid glossitis/geographic tongue

	• median rhomboid glossitis
	  —defined location
	  —associated with *Candida*
	• geographic tongue
	  —migratory lesions
	  —not associated with *Candida*

Similar lesions are seen occasionally affecting other areas of the oral mucosa, mainly lips and cheeks, and in these cases the condition may be referred to as migratory (or geographic) stomatitis or as erythema migrans (Fig. 13.8). An

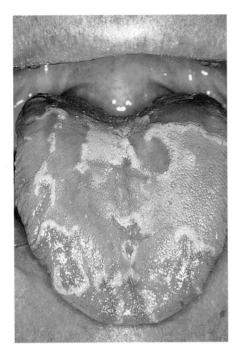

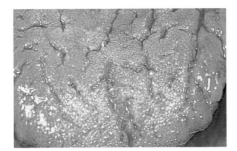

Fig. 13.7

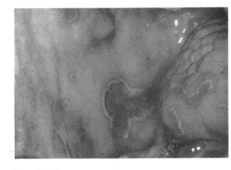

Fig. 13.6   Geographic tongue.

Fig. 13.7   Fissured (scrotal) tongue.

Fig. 13.8   Migratory stomatitis.

Fig. 13.6

Fig. 13.8

association with psoriasis has been suggested, but whether or not psoriasis has oral manifestations is unresolved.

Histological examination shows the epithelium at the edges of the lesions to be acanthotic with a dense, neutrophil leucocyte infiltration throughout the epithelium and the lamina propria. In the centres of the lesions, the loose desquamating cells on the surface have been lost and there is underlying chronic inflammatory cell infiltration.

Orofacial granulomatosis

Orofacial granulomatosis is not a disease entity but a term used to describe the common clinicopathological manifestations of a variety of different disorders. Typically, orofacial granulomatosis presents as recurrent or persistent diffuse enlargement of the lips and cheeks or as diffuse facial swelling, and is characterized histologically by non-caseating epithelioid cell granulomas with or without giant cells, and oedema of the tissues. The time of onset varies from infancy to old age.

Orofacial granulomatosis   **Key points**
- typical clinical features
- non-caseating granulomas
- several possible causes
    —Crohn's disease
    —sarcoidosis
    —infective granulomas
    —foreign bodies
    —Melkersson–Rosenthal syndrome
    —allergies
    —idiopathic

Orofacial granulomatosis should be regarded as a provisional diagnosis indicating the need for further investigation, since the condition includes localized disorders affecting the mouth and face as well as oral manifestations of systemic diseases. The latter include sarcoidosis and Crohn's disease (see later). (To avoid confusion the term orofacial granulomatosis should only be used until evidence of coexisting disease is found.) Orofacial granulomatosis also encompasses the disorders previously described as Melkersson-Rosenthal syndrome and its incomplete form, cheilitis granulomatosa. Classically, the Melkersson-Rosenthal syndrome consists of the triad of facial swellings, fissured tongue, and unilateral facial palsy. The full syndrome is rarely seen, and in all cases further investigation of the patient is indicated as some patients with the syndrome or its incomplete form may have underlying sarcoidosis, Crohn's disease, or allergies.

In all cases where the histopathological picture is characterized by granulomatous inflammation the possibility of infective granulomatous disease, such as tuberculosis (see Chapter 11), needs to be considered. Histological sections also need to be scrutinized carefully for foreign material to exclude foreign-body reactions.

The aetiology of orofacial granulomatosis in patients where no infective or underlying systemic cause can be found remains obscure. It is assumed that such cases represent a localized condition and there is evidence that allergic reactions to specific food substances, toothpastes, and occasionally dental materials are involved. Intolerance to specific foods, flavourings, or preservatives in the diet such as cinnamaldehyde, cocoa, and benzoates has been implicated most frequently.

Crohn's disease

This is a chronic granulomatous disease involving any part of the gastrointestinal tract, but most commonly the terminal ileum. Oral lesions may occur in patients with established Crohn's disease of the intestine or may be the presenting feature. The disease runs a chronic course, periods of quiescence being interrupted by episodes of varying severity and duration.

The aetiology is unknown, but some of the features suggest an unusual reaction to an extrinsic agent, possibly of infective origin. In some cases atypical mycobacteria have been implicated. Histological examination of affected tissues shows fibrosis and a dense, often focal, infiltration of the mucosa and submucosa with lymphocytes and plasma cells. Lymphoedema and dilated lymphatics may be a prominent feature. Non-caseating granulomas resembling those of sarcoidosis and consisting of macrophages, epithelioid cells, and occasional giant cells are present in about half of the cases and are often found in and around the dilated lymphatics (Figs 13.9, 13.10). Intestinal involvement usually causes recurrent episodes of abdominal pain, and nutritional deficiencies due to malabsorption are frequent.

The oral manifestations of Crohn's disease include:

1. Diffuse swellings of the lips and cheeks (Fig. 13.11). Crohn's disease is the most common systemic condition associated with orofacial granulomatosis.
2. Oedematous and hyperplastic thickening of the buccolabial mucosa together with fissuring, producing a 'cobble-stone' appearance (Fig. 13.12).
3. Oedematous and hyperplastic enlargements of the buccolabial mucosa, often involving the sulci, presenting as polypoid tag-like lesions or deep folds of mucosa that can mimic denture irritation hyperplasia (Fig. 13.13).
4. Aphthous (Fig. 13.14) or linear fissure-like ulcers involving any part of the mouth (Fig. 13.15).
5. Glossitis secondary to malabsorption of vitamin B_{12}.

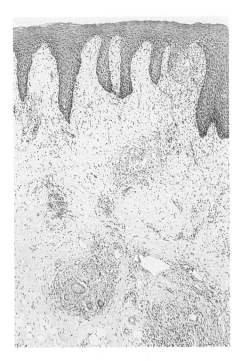

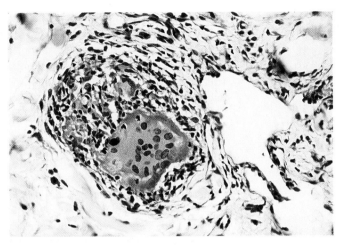

Fig. 13.10

Fig. 13.9

Figs 13.9, 13.10 Oedema of the lamina propria and granulomatous inflammation in oral Crohn's disease.

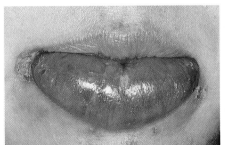

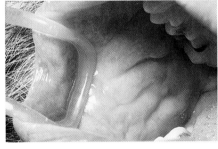

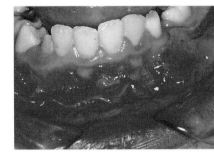

Fig. 13.11

Fig. 13.12

Fig. 13.13

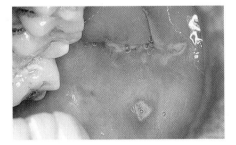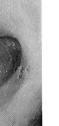

Fig. 13.14

Fig. 13.15

Figs 13.11–13.15 Oral manifestations of Crohn's disease presenting as orofacial granulomatosis showing (Fig. 13.11) diffuse swelling of lip; (Fig. 13.12) oedema and cobble-stone/fissured appearance of cheek; (Fig. 13.13) hyperplastic tags in the labial sulcus; (Fig. 13.14) aphthous-like ulcers; and (Fig. 13.15) linear, fissured ulcers.

Sarcoidosis

This systemic chronic granulomatous disorder of unknown aetiology most commonly affects young adults, and presents most frequently with bilateral hilar lymphadenopathy, pulmonary infiltration, and skin or eye lesions. Oral mucosal and gastrointestinal tract involvement is rare. Characteristically, the disease has an insidious onset. The signs and symptoms generally disappear in time but sometimes leave residual swelling.

Histological examination of affected tissue shows small tuberculoid granulomas consisting of macrophages and epithelioid cells, often with Langhans-type giant cells but with no caseous necrosis in the centre (Fig. 13.16). However, the lesions can only be distinguished histologically from tuberculosis by the absence of tubercle bacilli. The aetiology of sarcoidosis is unknown, but current evidence suggests that it is an unusual response to an exogenous agent acting as an antigen.

Blood examination usually shows a raised erythrocyte sedimentation rate (ESR), leucopenia, and hyperproteinaemia. The level of serum angiotensin-converting enzyme (SACE) is usually raised in active phases of the disease, the enzyme being synthesized by macrophages within the granulomas. Hypercalciuria is also common.

Sarcoid involvement of the oral mucosa is uncommon, but may present as submucosal, painless red nodules covered by normal mucosa and as erythema, granularity, or hyperplasia of the gingiva (Fig. 13.17). It may also present as orofacial granulomatosis. Salivary gland involvement (usually the parotid) may occur, and biopsy of palatal or labial mucous glands is sometimes helpful as a diagnostic procedure. The combination of uveitis, parotitis, and facial paralysis in sarcoidosis is known as uveoparotid fever, or Heerfordt syndrome.

Pyostomatitis vegetans

Pyostomatitis vegetans is a rare disorder associated with inflammatory bowel disease, especially ulcerative colitis. The lips and cheeks are diffusely inflamed with erosions, fissured ulcers, and pustules separating papillary projections and irregular outgrowths (vegetations) arising from the mucosal surface (Fig. 13.18). Cervical lymphadenitis and pyrexia are usual. The severity of the oral lesions tends to vary with the severity of the bowel involvement. Histological examination shows acanthosis and multiple microabscesses containing numerous

Fig. 13.16 Non-caseating granulomas in sarcoidosis.

Fig. 13.17 Sarcoidosis of the gingiva.

Fig. 13.18 Pyostomatitis vegetans.

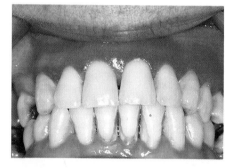

Fig. 13.17

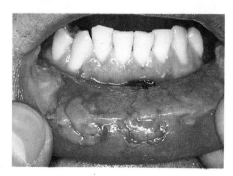

Fig. 13.18

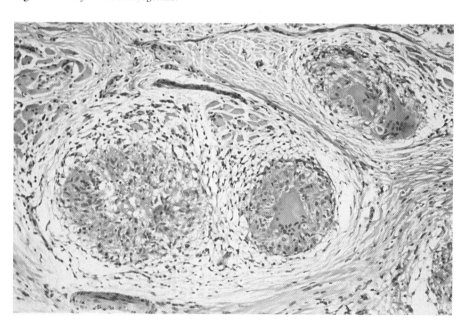

Fig. 13.16

eosinophils at the tips of the connective tissue papillae and within the epithelium. The lamina propria is densely inflamed.

Ulcerative colitis also predisposes to recurrent aphthous stomatitis (see Chapter 12).

Wegener's granulomatosis

This systemic disease is characterized by a necrotizing, destructive granulomatous inflammation principally involving the respiratory tract, and a generalized necrotizing vasculitis. The disease may occur at any age with a peak in the fourth and fifth decades. Many patients present with intractable rhinitis and sinusitis, cough, and haemoptysis. Oral lesions are common and may be the presenting feature. They include a characteristic hyperplastic type of gingivitis (strawberry gingivitis) (Fig. 13.19) with severe inflammation and multiple granular exophytic masses resembling pyogenic granulomas, palatal ulceration which may be followed by perforation, and delayed healing of extraction sockets.

Histological examination of the lesions shows granulation tissue with a very dense mixed inflammatory cell infiltrate comprising neutrophils, eosinophils, macrophages, lymphocytes, and plasma cells. Giant cells and areas of necrosis are frequently seen. Involved vessels characteristically show fibrinoid necrosis of their walls and intimal proliferation (Figs 13.20, 13.21). However, necrotizing vasculitis is not seen in gingival lesions, probably because the vessels are too small.

The aetiology of Wegener's granulomatosis is obscure. Autoantibodies directed against cytoplasmic constituents of neutrophils and monocytes are present in the serum of patients with Wegener's granulomatosis and may be involved in the pathogenesis of immune vascular injury. Levels of this antineutrophil-cytoplasmic antibody in the serum (ANCA test) can be used for diagnosis and as a marker of disease activity. The disease may be controlled with corticosteroids and cytotoxic drugs, otherwise it is rapidly fatal, usually following renal failure.

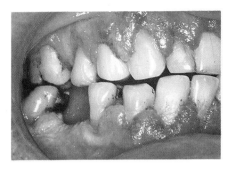

Fig. 13.19 Wegener's granulomatosis presenting as hyperplastic (strawberry) gingivitis.

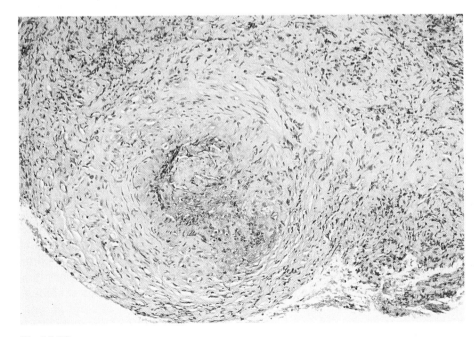

Fig. 13.20

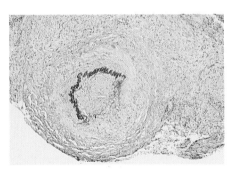

Fig. 13.21

Fig. 13.20 Necrotizing vasculitis in Wegener's granulomatosis showing fibrinoid necrosis (red) and intimal proliferation almost occluding the lumen.

Fig. 13.21 The corresponding field to that in Fig. 13.20 stained to demonstrate elastic tissue shows disruption of the internal elastic lamina associated with necrosis.

Progressive systemic sclerosis (scleroderma)

Progressive systemic sclerosis is a chronic multisystem disease characterized by diffuse fibrosis (sclerosis) of the skin with similar involvement of internal organs, such as the gastrointestinal tract, lungs, and kidney. The face may be involved with the sclerosis leading to restricted mouth opening, smoothing of the lines of facial expression, and an expressionless (mask-like) face. Widening of the periodontal ligament space, particularly on posterior teeth, is a characteristic radiological finding.

The disease most commonly affects females between the ages of 20 and 50 years. It is often associated with other connective tissue disease, such as systemic lupus erythematosus or rheumatoid arthritis and occasionally Sjögren syndrome, which suggests an immunological basis and possibly an auto-immune disorder.

Verruciform xanthoma

This is an uncommon disorder which occurs most frequently on the gingiva and alveolar mucosa. It presents as a flat or slightly raised, but otherwise symptomless, lesion with a papillary/warty (hence verruciform) surface. Histological examination shows hyperplastic epithelium thrown into papillary projections, but the characteristic feature is infiltration of the connective tissue papillae by lipid-containing foam cells. The infiltrate is sharply limited to the papillary lamina propria.

The aetiology of the disorder is unknown. It is not associated with HPV-infection or with disorders of lipid metabolism. It is probably a reactive inflammatory process associated with focal accumulation of foam cells in reaction to release of lipid from degenerating epithelial cells.

Oral submucous fibrosis

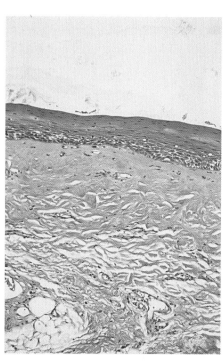

Fig. 13.22 Oral submucous fibrosis.

Oral submucuous fibrosis is an insidious chronic disease which may affect any part of the oral mucosa and occasionally may extend into the pharynx and oesophagus. It resembles scleroderma but is limited to the oral cavity; it is not a multisystem disease. Increasing stiffening of the oral mucosa associated with progressive underlying fibrosis leads to difficulty in opening the mouth and to a binding down of the tongue. Examination shows the mucosa to have a characteristic blanched, marble appearance, often with palpable bands of fibrous tissue. The disease occurs almost exclusively among Asiatic Indians. The aetiology is unknown, but is strongly linked to areca-nut chewing habits (betel quid, betel nut). Genetic susceptibility may also be involved, but the role of nutritional factors such as vitamin deficiency remains unclear.

Histological examination in an advanced case shows hyalinization of the subepithelial connective tissue with very few fibroblasts present and the blood vessels narrowed or totally obliterated by the fibrosis (Fig. 13.22). Lymphocytes and plasma cells are scattered throughout the hyalinized tissue. In the earlier stages the hyalinization is less intense, the vessels may be dilated, and the collagen bundles are partly separated by oedema. The overlying epithelium is generally atrophic with no rete ridges and the surface is keratinized or parakeratinized. Epithelial dysplasia has been found in up to 13 per cent of biopsies.

Oral submucous fibrosis can be regarded as a premalignant condition because it is often associated with epithelial atrophy and dysplasia. In addition, in geographical areas where oral submucous fibrosis is common, it is found in many patients with oral carcinoma.

Amyloidosis

Amyloidosis is a disease characterized by the extracellular deposition of fibrillar proteinaceous material—amyloid—in a wide variety of tissues. The chemical structure of amyloid is variable. In primary (idiopathic) amylodosis and amyloidosis associated with multiple myeloma it arises as a result of derangement of immunoglobulin synthesis and consists of fragments of immunoglobulin molecules. It is referred to as amyloid of immunoglobulin origin or AL type since the protein material in the amyloid fibril consists largely of fragments of immunoglobulin light (L) chains. Secondary or reactive amyloidosis occurs as a complication of a variety of other diseases, especially chronic destructive inflammatory lesions, such as rheumatoid arthritis, and certain malignant conditions. This type is chemically distinct from the AL type and does not contain light-chain fragments. In reactive amyloidosis the fibrils are composed of amyloid A protein (AA type), a polypeptide related to an acute-phase protein found in serum. Amyloid-like material is also a feature of the calcifying epithelial odontogenic tumour (see Chapter 15).

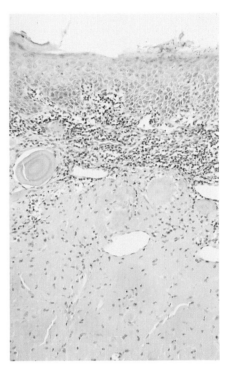

Fig. 13.23 Submucosal deposits of amyloid stained orange by Congo red.

Oral manifestations are described in primary amyloidosis, and macroglossia is the best known feature. This may occur in up to half of the patients but is usually a late event. The enlargement of the tongue is usually diffuse and symmetrical and the lateral borders may be indented by adjacent teeth. Mobility is diminished and the tongue is firm and indurated. Other oral manifestations include petechiae, ecchymoses, haemorrhagic bullae which rupture leaving shallow ulcers, and localized amyloid deposits in the form of yellowish macules or papules, but widespread symptomless infiltration of oral tissues also occurs. Involvement of salivary glands may result in xerostomia.

Where amyloidosis is suspected on clinical grounds, diagnosis must be confirmed by biopsy and the identification of deposits by various staining reactions. Classically, amyloid is positively stained by Congo red (Fig. 13.23), and when then viewed with polarized light produces a characteristic apple-green birefringence. Even in suspected cases, without apparent oral involvement, biopsy of the tongue or of gingival tissues may be a useful diagnostic test. The prognosis for most patients with primary, and many with secondary amyloidosis is poor; death is usually due to cardiac, hepatic, or renal failure.

Oral pigmentation

Oral pigmentation may result from the localization of exogenous substances on or within the mucosa, or may be due to deposition in the tissues of endogenous pigments (i.e. substances produced by the body), of which melanin is the most common.

The main causes of oral mucosal pigmentation are listed in Table 13.1. Some of the conditions are described elsewhere in this book.

Superficial staining of the mucosa

This may be caused by a great variety of foods, drinks, and topical medicaments, as well as habits such as chewing betel nut or betel quid, and smoking or chewing tobacco.

Black hairy tongue

This is a condition in which there is marked hyperplasia of filiform papillae, sometimes up to about 1 cm in length, and discoloration associated with overgrowth of

Table 13.1   Causes of oral mucosal pigmentation

I *Exogenous pigmentation*

    Superficial staining of the mucosa

    Black hairy tongue

    Foreign bodies
        amalgam tattoo
        miscellaneous

    Heavy metal salts

II *Endogenous pigmentation due to melanin*

    Developmental causes

        Racial pigmentation

        Pigmented naevi

        Peutz-Jeghers syndrome

    Acquired causes

        Associated with systemic disease
          Addison's disease
          pulmonary disease
          HIV infection

        Associated with hyperkeratosis, chronic inflammation, and lichen planus

        Drug-induced

        Idiopathic oral melanotic macule (oral freckle)

        Lentigo simplex

    Neoplastic causes
        Malignant melanoma *in situ*
        Malignant melanoma

III *Other endogenous pigments*

    Blood breakdown products and disturbances of iron metabolism

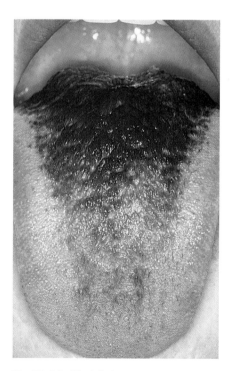

Fig. 13.24   Black hairy tongue.

pigment-producing bacteria and fungi (Fig. 13.24). The aetiology is unknown but smoking may be a factor, and in some patients the disorder follows antibiotic therapy suggesting that disturbance of the normal oral flora is also involved. The condition is usually symptomless but 'tickling' of the soft palate may cause gagging and nausea. Black hairy tongue should be distinguished from a simple staining where there is no associated overgrowth of filiform papillae.

Foreign bodies

A variety of foreign substances may be implanted in the oral mucosa giving rise to localized areas of pigmentation. Amalgam is the commonest and best known example but other materials include road grit following road traffic accidents and traumatic implantation of graphite in lead-pencil chewers. Some individuals may even have artistic tattooing of the mucosa (Fig. 13.25).

Amalgam tattoo

This is a relatively common, often incidental clinical finding, which rarely produces symptoms other than that of an area of discoloration. It manifests as a localized blue/black or greyish area (Fig. 13.26) and is due to the introduction of amalgam into the soft tissues during such dental procedures as the insertion or removal of restorations, the extraction of teeth when portions of fractured

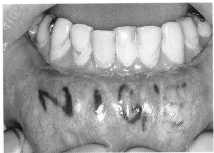

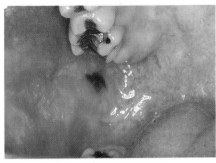

Fig. 13.25

Fig. 13.26

Fig. 13.25 Tattooing of the oral mucosa.

Fig. 13.26 Amalgam tattoo of the buccal mucosa.

restorations may fall into sockets, and retrograde filling of a root canal after apicectomy. The tattoos may be found in any part of the mouth but are most common in mandibular gingival or alveolar mucosa (Figs 13.27, 13.28). Histologically, the pigment is present as widely dispersed, fine brownish or blackish granules, or as solid fragments of varying size which when large may be detected on radiographs. The pigment granules may be scattered haphazardly but are often associated with collagen and elastic fibres and basement membranes, and may be seen intracellularly within fibroblasts, endothelial cells, macrophages, and occasional foreign-body giant cells (Fig. 13.29). Apart from the macrophages and giant cells there is little or no tissue reaction. Ultrastructural and analytical studies have shown that the amalgam is slowly corroded and that mercury, together with some tin, is lost leaving silver residues. The silver released by corrosion may become associated with sulphur and be picked up by various cells and fibres in the connective tissue.

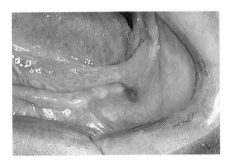

Fig. 13.27

Heavy metal salts

Deposits of metallic sulphides in the marginal gingiva may follow absorption of bismuth, lead, or mercuric salts either as a result of environmental or occupational exposure or, rarely these days, following therapeutic administration. The salts are present in crevicular fluid and are precipitated as sulphides by the action of hydrogen sulphide released as a waste product from plaque organisms. The precipitates cause linear grey or blue/black lines of pigmentation which follow the gingival contour around the necks of the teeth. Faint purplish discoloration of the gingiva may also follow prolonged therapeutic administration of gold compounds, the pigmentation being due mainly to deposition of colloidal metal itself rather than gold salts.

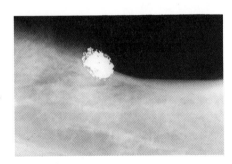

Fig. 13.28

Figs 13.27, 13.28 Amalgam tattoo associated with a large fragment of a restoration detectable on radiograph.

Melanin pigmentation—developmental causes

Melanin is the commonest of the endogenous pigments in skin and oral mucosa, and is produced by melanocytes present in the basal layer of the epithelium. These specialized dendritic cells are of neural crest origin. Melanin is formed in melanosomes within the cytoplasm of melanocytes, the melanin then passing into the dendritic processes to be injected into, or ingested by, neighbouring keratinocytes.

There is no difference in the number of melanocytes between fair- and dark-skinned individuals, the variation in skin and mucosal pigmentation between racial groups being related to differences in activity of the melanocytes. The intensity and distribution of racial pigmentation of the oral mucosa is very variable not only between races but also between different individuals of the same

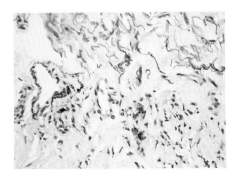

Fig. 13.29 Finely dispersed pigmented silver residues in an amalgam tattoo.

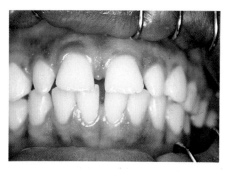

Fig. 13.30 Racial pigmentation.

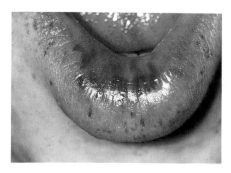

Fig. 13.31 Pigmentation of the lip in Peutz-Jeghers syndrome.

race and within different areas of the same mouth. Pigment may be found in any part of the mucosa but the gingiva is the most common site (Fig. 13.30).

Pigmented naevi are the commonest cause of abnormal melanin pigmentation of skin and every person has a variable number of such lesions, between 20 and 30 on average. However, they are relatively rare in oral mucosa (see Chapter 10).

Hypermelanic pigmentation of skin and/or oral mucosa is also associated with various other developmental conditions which are not primarily disorders of the melanocyte system.

Peutz-Jeghers syndrome is transmitted through an autosomal dominant gene and is characterized by mucocutaneous pigmentation and gastrointestinal polyposis. The polyposis chiefly affects the small intestine and the lesions are not generally considered as premalignant. However, malignant gastrointestinal tract disease has been reported in a minority of cases and a guarded prognosis should be adopted in patients with Peutz-Jeghers syndrome. The melanic pigmentation resembles freckling and appears in infancy. In the mouth the buccal mucosa and lips (Fig.13.31) are usually affected and skin pigmentation occurs rather characteristically around the mouth, nostrils, and eyes. Other areas of the skin and other mucosae may be affected. There is a tendency for the skin pigmentation to fade in adult life but the mucosal pigmentation persists.

Melanic pigmentation of skin, described as *café-au-lait* spots because of their light brown colour, is also seen in some cases of polyostotic fibrous dysplasia and in patients with neurofibromatosis. Pigmentation of the oral mucosa is absent or has only rarely been recorded.

Melanin pigmentation—acquired causes

Acquired melanosis of the oral mucosa may be a manifestation of systemic disease, malignancy, or of a simple local disorder. It is an important sign indicating the need for careful investigation of the patient.

Key points	**Abnormal melanin pigmentation**
	• underlying local and/or systemic factors must be considered
	• may precede malignant melanoma

The association of oral pigmentation with Addison's disease is well recognized and may be the initial manifestation of adrenal insufficiency. Adrenal insufficiency results in elevated secretion of adrenocorticotrophic hormone (ACTH) by the pituitary, the melanocyte-stimulating properties of the heptapeptide core probably being responsible for the pigmentation. The pigmentation is most common in areas subjected to masticatory trauma, especially the cheeks, but can involve any part of the oral mucosa.

An association between smoking, pigmentation of the soft palate, and pulmonary disease, especially bronchogenic carcinoma, has also been demonstrated. The mechanism underlying the melanic pigmentation is uncertain, but it is interesting to note that some bronchogenic carcinomas may be associated with ectopic ACTH production. Oral hypermelanosis may also be seen in patients with HIV infection (see Chapter 11).

Melanic pigmentation is an occasional feature of some hyperkeratoses giving the lesions a dusky or greyish hue, and less commonly of some other chronic inflammatory mucosal diseases. A link with cigarette smoking has been suggested in some patients. The pigmentation is presumably a reaction of melanocytes to chronic irritation and there may also be some associated dysfunction in the transfer and/or uptake of melanin from melanocytes to keratinocytes. This is suggested since much of the melanin in these lesions is present in subepithelial macrophages having apparently leaked out of melanocytes and/or basal cells (melanin incontinence) (Fig. 13.32). However, as far as is known this pigmentation has no diagnostic or prognostic significance. Similar changes may be seen in lichen planus as a result of basal cell degeneration and may persist after the lesions have healed.

Drug-induced melanic pigmentation of the oral mucosa is rare, but may be seen in some patients taking various cytostatic agents and may also be produced by progestogens in oral contraceptives. Pigmentary changes, especially of the hard palate, may be seen in patients taking antimalarial drugs. The nature of this pigment is uncertain but melanin may be involved. Oral pigmentation has also been reported in patients taking minocycline, a tetracycline derivative widely used for the treatment of acne. As with other tetracyclines the drug may also be incorporated in and cause discoloration of bones and teeth (see Chapter 3).

Occasionally, patients present with single, or less frequently multiple, pigmented macules of the oral mucosa which cannot be classified histologically into any of the recognized types of melanotic lesion and for which no local or systemic cause can be found. They occur more often in women than in men and usually present around 40 years of age. The vermilion border of the lower lip, gingiva, and buccal mucosa are the commonest sites. Histological examination shows a localized area of increased melanin pigment in the basal cell layer, with or without melanin incontinence. The term 'idiopathic oral melanotic macule' (Figs 13.33, 13.34) has been applied to this lesion but it is also referred to as an oral ephelis (freckle).

Primary malignant melanoma of the oral mucosa is rare (see Chapter 10) and metastatic melanoma is exceptional.

Other endogenous pigments

Oral pigmentation due to other endogenous substances is uncommon apart from transitory discoloration caused by blood breakdown products in a haematoma and the yellowish hue produced by bilirubin in patients with jaundice (Fig. 13.35).

Pigmentation associated with disturbances of iron metabolism is seen in the rare disorder, haemochromatosis. Haemosiderin is deposited in many organs and tissues and there is also pigmentation of the skin and oral mucosa. Classically, the pigmentation produces coppery or bronze discoloration and is chiefly due to melanin, although haemosiderin is also deposited. The serious manifestations are due to deposition of haemosiderin in the myocardium, liver, and pancreas. Pancreatic involvement may result in diabetes which, because of the associated skin pigmentation, may be referred to as bronze diabetes.

Age changes in the oral mucosa

Although a variety of changes may occur in the oral mucosa of the elderly, distinguishing those attributable to ageing from those due to systemic disease, nutritional deficiencies, or the side-effects of medication can be difficult. Atrophic changes have been reported in lingual mucosa related to an almost linear reduction in epithelial thickness with increasing age, by about 30 per cent of the initial thickness around 85 years of age. However, this may not apply to other oral mucosal surfaces. The question of whether increased keratinization of the oral mucosa occurs in old age has not been resolved.

Oral mucosal connective tissues become more fibrosed, less vascular, and less cellular with age. Atherosclerotic changes are also seen in arteries of the oral

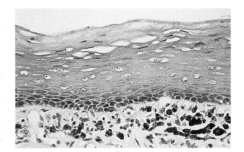

Fig. 13.32 Incontinence of melanin associated with hyperkeratosis showing melanin pigment in subepithelial macrophages.

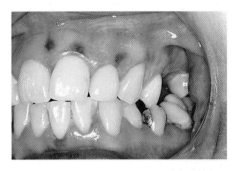

Fig. 13.33 Idiopathic oral melanotic macules.

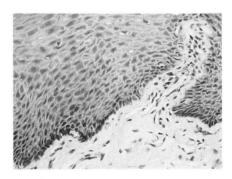

Fig. 13.34 Histological appearances of a melanotic macule showing hypermelanosis in the basal layer.

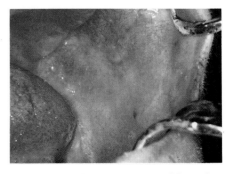

Fig. 13.35 Yellow pigmentation of the oral mucosa in a patient with jaundice.

mucosa, and a progressive, partial ischaemia may contribute to some of the atrophic changes.

Certain local oral mucosal lesions are reported to occur more frequently in the elderly, examples being sublingual varices, increased prominence of Fordyce's granules, and inflammatory enlargement of foliate papillae, but supportive evidence is often lacking.

FURTHER READING

Basu, M. K. and Chesner, I. M. (1990). Diseases of the gastrointestinal tract. In *Oral manifestations of systemic disease* (2nd edn) (ed. J. H. Jones and D. K. Mason), pp. 783–99. W. B. Saunders, London.

Editorial (1991). Orofacial granulomatosis. *The Lancet*, **338**, 20–1.

Field, E. A. and Tyldesley, W. R. (1989). Oral Crohn's disease revisited—a 10-year-review. *British Journal of Oral and Maxillofacial Surgery*, **27**, 114–23.

Handlers, J. P., Waterman, J., Abrams, A. M., and Melrose, R. J. (1985). Oral features of Wegener's granulomatosis. *Archives of Otolaryngology*, **111**, 267–70.

Harrison, J. D., Rowley, P. S. A., and Peters, P. D. (1977). Amalgam tattoos: light and electron microscopy and electron-probe microanalysis. *Journal of Pathology*, **121**, 83–92.

Healy, C. M., Farthing, P. M., Williams, D. M., and Thornhill, M. H. (1994). Pyostomatitis vegetans and associated systemic disease. *Oral Surgery, Oral Medicine, Oral Pathology*, **78**, 323–8.

Hume, W. J. (1975). Geographic stomatitis: a critical review. *Journal of Dentistry*, **3**, 25–43.

Israelson, H., Binnie, W. H., and Hurt, W. C. (1981). The hyperplastic gingivitis of Wegener's granulomatosis. *Journal of Periodontology*, **52**, 81–7.

Kaugars, G. E., Heise, A. P., Riley, W. T., Abbey, L. M., and Svirsky, J. A. (1993). Oral melanotic macules. A review of 353 cases. *Oral Surgery, Oral Medicine, Oral Pathology*, **76**, 59–61.

Murti, P. R., Bhonsle, R. B., Gupta, P. C., Daftary, D. K., Pinborg, J. J., and Mehta, F. S. (1995). Etiology of oral submucous fibrosis with special reference to the role of areca nut chewing. *Journal of Oral Pathology and Medicine*, **24**, 145–52.

Neville, B. W. and Weathers D. R. (1980). Verruciform xanthoma. *Oral Surgery, Oral Medicine, Oral Pathology*, **49**, 429–34.

Pillai, R., Balaram, P., and Reddiar, K. S. (1992). Pathogenesis of oral submucous fibrosis. Relationship to risk factors associated with oral cancer. *Cancer*, **69**, 2011–20.

Sainsbury, C. P. Q., Dodge, J. A., Walker, D. M., and Aldred, M. J. (1987). Orofacial granulomatosis in childhood. *British Dental Journal*, **163**, 154–7.

Scott, J. and Baum, B. J. (1990). Oral effects of Ageing. In *Oral manifestations of systemic disease* (2nd edn) (ed. J. H. Jones and D. K. Mason), pp. 311–38. W. B. Saunders, London.

Scully, C. and Porter, S. R. (1994). Oral mucosal disease: a decade of new entities, aetiologies and associations. *International Dental Journal*, **44**, 33–43.

Smith, A. and Speculand, B. (1985). Amyloidosis with oral involvement. *British Journal of Oral and Maxillofacial Surgery*, **23**, 435–44.

Van Maarsseveen, A. C. M. Th., Van Der Waal, I., Stam, J., Veldhuizen, R. W., and Van Der Kwast, W. A. M. (1982). Oral involvement in sarcoidosis. *International Journal of Oral Surgery*, **11**, 21–9.

Weisenfeld, D., Ferguson, M. M., Mitchell, D. N., Macdonald, D. G., Scully, C., Cochran, K., and Russell, R. I. (1985). Oro-facial granulomatosis—a clinical and pathological analysis. *Quarterly Journal of Medicine, New Series*, **54**, No. 213, 101–13.

Wray, D. (1984). Pyostomatitis vegetans. *British Dental Journal*, **157**, 316–18.

14 Diseases of salivary glands

14 Diseases of salivary glands

The salivary glands consist of three paired major glands, parotid, submandibular, and sublingual, and the countless minor salivary glands found in almost every part of the oral cavity, except the gingiva and anterior regions of the hard palate. The secretion of saliva is essential for the normal function and health of the mouth, and disorders of salivary gland function, which affect the composition and secretion of saliva, predispose to oral disease. Functional disorders in salivary secretion and composition may be associated with organic disease of the salivary glands, but in other cases are caused by systemic factors, such as neurological disease, drug therapy, and endocrine disturbances. This chapter is only concerned with organic salivary gland diseases; for further discussion of functional disorders, the reader is referred to texts in oral medicine.

DEVELOPMENTAL ANOMALIES

Developmental anomalies of the salivary glands are rare. Aplasia of one or more major glands and atresia of one or more major salivary gland ducts have been reported. Congenital aplasia of the parotid gland may be associated with other facial abnormalities, for example mandibulofacial dysostosis, aplasia of the lacrimal glands, and hemifacial microsomia.

Heterotopic salivary tissue has been reported from a variety of sites in the head and neck, the most frequent being its inclusion at the angle or within the body of the mandible, presenting as Stafne's idiopathic bone cavity (see Chapter 6). Accessory parotid tissue within the cheek or masseter muscle is relatively common and is subject to the same diseases that may affect the main gland.

SIALADENITIS

Inflammatory disorders of the major salivary glands are usually the result of bacterial or viral infection but occasionally sialadenitis is due to other causes, such as trauma, irradiation, and allergic reactions.

Bacterial sialadenitis

Bacterial sialadenitis may present as an acute or chronic condition.

Acute bacterial sialadenitis

This uncommon disorder principally involves the parotid gland. Acute parotitis is an ascending infection, that is, the bacteria reach the gland from the mouth by

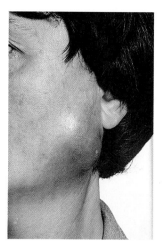

Fig 14.1

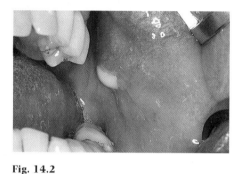

Fig. 14.2

Figs 14.1, 14.2 Acute bacterial sialadenitis of the parotid gland with pus being expressed from the duct.

ascending the ductal system, the main organisms involved being *Streptococcus pyogenes* and *Staphylococcus aureus*. Less commonly, *Haemophilus* species or members of the 'black-pigmented bacteroides' group may be isolated. It was once a common postoperative complication in debilitated and dehydrated patients, particularly following abdominal surgery, but is a rare complication nowadays. Reduced salivary flow is the major predisposing factor, and acute parotitis may occur in patients with Sjögren syndrome or following the use of drugs with xerostomic side-effects. Acute infection may also arise in immunocompromised patients or as a result of acute exacerbation in a previously chronic sialadenitis. The latter is usually the cause when acute sialadenitis involves the submandibular gland.

The onset of acute sialadenitis is rapid. Clinically, it presents as swelling of the involved gland accompanied by pain, fever, malaise, and redness of the overlying skin. Pus may be expressed from the affected duct (Figs 14.1, 14.2).

Chronic bacterial sialadenitis

Chronic sialadenitis of the major salivary glands is usually a non-specific inflammatory disease associated with duct obstruction (discussed later in this chapter) and low-grade ascending infection. The submandibular gland is much more commonly involved than the parotid gland. In cases where no cause of obstruction can be identified, the predisposing factor may be a disorder of secretion resulting in decreased salivary flow. The sialadenitis is usually unilateral, and the symptoms of recurrent tender swelling of the affected gland are mainly related to the associated obstruction. The duct orifice may appear inflamed and in acute exacerbations there may be a purulent or salty-tasting discharge. Histological examination shows varying degrees of dilatation of the ductal system, hyperplasia of duct epithelium, periductal fibrosis, acinar atrophy with replacement fibrosis, and chronic inflammatory cell infiltration (Figs 14.3, 14.4). The duct obstruction, destruction of glandular tissue, and duct dilatation (sialectasia) may be demonstrated by sialography.

In the submandibular gland, progressive chronic inflammation may result eventually in almost complete replacement of the parenchyma by fibrous tissue (Fig. 14.4) producing a firm mass that may be mistaken clinically for a neoplasm. This type of inflammatory reaction may be referred to as chronic sclerosing sialadenitis.

Recurrent parotitis

Recurrent parotitis is a rare disorder which can affect children or adults. Rarely the adult form may follow on from the childhood type, but in most cases it is

Fig. 14.3 Chronic bacterial sialadenitis showing early periductal inflammation.

Fig. 14.4 Destruction of glandular tissue and replacement fibrosis in long-standing chronic bacterial sialadenitis.

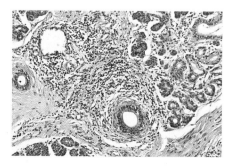

Fig. 14.3

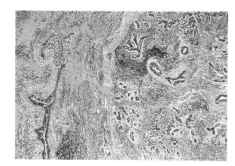

Fig. 14.4

probably due to persistence of factors, such as calculi or duct strictures, leading to recurrent attacks of low-grade ascending infection.

The aetiology of the childhood type is unclear but an abnormally low secretion rate predisposing to ascending infection and immaturity of the immune response in infants may be involved. Congenital abnormalities of the ductal system have also been suggested and almost all cases show sialectasia or some other duct abnormality on sialography. The condition may be unilateral or bilateral and is associated with recurrent painful swelling of the gland. Pus may be expressed from the duct orifice. In most cases the condition resolves spontaneously by the time the patient reaches early adult life, but repeated infection may result in irreversible damage to the main duct predisposing to duct obstruction. This may lead to further episodes of ascending infection and damage and to recurrent parotitis in adult life.

Bacterial sialadenitis   **Key points**
- ascending infections associated with decreased salivary flow
- acute suppurative, mainly parotid
- chronic, mainly submandibular, and associated with duct obstruction

Viral sialadenitis

Mumps (epidemic parotitis)

Mumps is an acute, contagious infection which often occurs in minor epidemics and is caused by a paramyxovirus. It is the commonest cause of parotid enlargement and the commonest of all the salivary gland diseases. Although infection can occur at any age, it is most common in childhood. The virus is transmitted by direct contact with infected saliva and by droplet spread, and has an incubation period of 2–3 weeks. Non-specific prodromal symptoms of fever and malaise are followed by painful swelling of sudden onset involving one or more salivary glands. The parotid glands are almost always involved, bilaterally in about 70 per cent of cases, and occasionally the submandibular and sublingual glands may be affected, but rarely without parotid involvement also. The salivary gland enlargement gradually subsides over a period of about 7 days. The virus is present in the saliva 2–3 days before the onset of sialadenitis and for about 6 days afterwards.

Occasionally in adults other internal organs are involved, such as testes, ovaries, central nervous system, and pancreas. Orchitis is the most common complication, occurring in about 20 per cent of cases of mumps in adult males.

The diagnosis of mumps is usually made on clinical grounds, but in atypical cases can be confirmed by the detection of IgM class antibodies and by the rise in serum antibody titre to mumps virus antigens which occurs within the first week. After an attack immunity is long-lasting and so recurrent infection is rare.

Cytomegalic inclusion disease (salivary gland inclusion disease)

Infection with cytomegalovirus, a member of the herpesvirus group, is common in humans and endemic worldwide. Most primary infections are asymptomatic, but the virus can cause severe disseminated disease in neonates and in immunocompromised hosts such as transplant patients and HIV-infected patients (see Chapter 11). Salivary gland involvement is usually an incidental histological finding, the characteristic feature being the presence of large, doubly contoured 'owl-eye' inclusion bodies within the nucleus or cytoplasm of duct cells of the parotid gland. It may be associated with xerostomia in HIV-infection. In disseminated disease similar inclusions frequently occur in the kidneys, liver, lungs, brain, and other organs.

Postirradiation sialadenitis

The effects of radiation on oral mucosa are discussed in Chapter 12. Radiation sialadenitis is a common complication of radiotherapy and there is a direct correlation between the dose of irradiation and the severity of the damage. The latter is often irreversible leading to fibrous replacement of the damaged acini and squamous metaplasia of ducts, but with less severe damage some degree of function may return after several months. Serous acini are more sensitive to radiation damage than mucous acini.

Sarcoidosis

Sarcoidosis (see Chapter 13) may affect the parotid and minor salivary glands. Parotid involvement presents as persistent often painless, enlargement and may be associated with involvement of the lacrimal glands in Heerfordt syndrome.

Sialadenitis of minor glands

Sialadenitis of minor glands is often an incidental and insignificant finding although it may be of diagnostic significance, for example in sarcoidosis and Sjögren syndrome. However, it is seen most frequently in association with mucous extravasation cysts and stomatitis nicotina of the palate.

Very rarely, sialadenitis of minor glands may present with multiple mucosal swellings associated with cystic dilatation of ducts and chronic suppuration. This condition may be referred to as stomatitis glandularis. It occurs most commonly on the lips, and probably represents an acute exacerbation of a previously chronic sialadenitis associated with obstruction, for example from denture trauma, or reduction in salivary flow.

OBSTRUCTIVE AND TRAUMATIC LESIONS

Duct obstruction and trauma are important factors in the aetiology of a number of salivary gland diseases, such as chronic sialadenitis in major glands and mucoceles in minor glands (salivary cysts are discussed in Chapter 6). Duct obstruction may be due to a blockage within the lumen or result from disease in or around the duct wall, such as fibrosis or neoplasia. Obstruction to the duct orifice is usually due to chronic trauma, for example from sharp cusps or overextended dentures, resulting in fibrosis and stenosis.

Salivary calculi (sialoliths)

Salivary calculi cause obstruction within the duct lumen and can occur at any age, but are most common in middle-aged adults. Calculi may form in ducts within the gland or in the main excretory duct. Data on their distribution vary considerably but the submandibular gland is most frequently involved, accounting for about 70–90 per cent of cases (Fig. 14.5). The parotid gland is the next

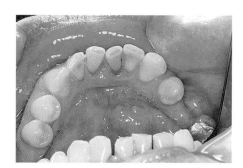

Fig. 14.5 Swelling of the floor of the mouth associated with a calculus in the submandibular duct.

most commonly involved, whereas sialolithiasis in sublingual and minor glands is uncommon and generally accounts for only about 2 per cent of cases. Calculi are usually unilateral, although multiple stones in the same gland are not uncommon. The typical signs and symptoms of calculi associated with major glands are pain and sudden enlargement of the gland, especially at meal times when salivary secretion is stimulated. The reduction in salivary flow predisposes to ascending infection and chronic sialadenitis. The calculi may be detected by palpation and on radiographs, and may be round or ovoid, rough or smooth, and vary considerably in size. They are usually yellowish in colour and comprise mainly calcium phosphates with smaller amounts of carbonates (Fig. 14.6). On section, they may be homogeneous but many have a lamellated structure (Fig. 14.7).

Salivary calculi   **Key points**

- mainly submandibular gland or duct
- recurrent swelling related to gustatory stimuli
- predispose to ascending infection and chronic sialadenitis

The aetiology and pathogenesis of salivary calculi are largely unknown. It is generally thought that they form by deposition of calcium salts around an initial organic nidus which might consist of altered salivary mucins together with desquamated epithelial cells and microorganisms. Successive deposition of inorganic and organic material would produce a lamellated calculus. Ultrastructural studies have also shown that microcalculi form in acinar cells and stagnant secretions of the submandibular gland, especially during periods of secretory inactivity. Although in the normal gland these microcalculi are eliminated, if there is disturbed secretion they could accumulate and lead to the formation of calculi.

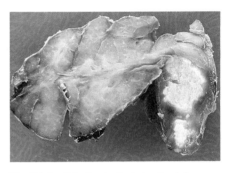

Fig. 14.6 Calculus in the intraglandular portion of the submandibular duct.

Necrotizing sialometaplasia

Necrotizing sialometaplasia is a relatively uncommon disorder which clinically and on histological examination may be mistaken for malignant disease. It occurs most frequently on the hard plate in middle-aged patients and is about twice as common in men as women. It presents most commonly as a deep crater-like ulcer which may mimic a malignant ulcer and which may take up to eight weeks to heal. In some cases the ulcer may be preceded by an indurated swelling.

Histopathological examination shows lobular necrosis of salivary glands, squamous metaplasia of ducts and acini, mucous extravasation, and prominent inflammatory cell infiltration (Fig. 14.8). The surrounding palatal mucosa shows pseudoepitheliomatous hyperplasia and the histopathological features may be mistaken for either squamous cell carcinoma or mucoepidermoid carcinoma.

The aetiology of the condition is unknown, but ischaemia leading to infarction of salivary lobules is the most widely accepted theory. In some patients there may be a history of trauma or of previous surgery at the site.

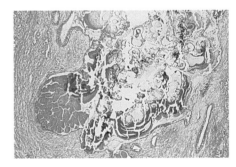

Fig. 14.7 Decalcified section showing a lamellated calculus in dilated submandibular duct.

SJÖGREN SYNDROME AND RELATED DISORDERS

Historically, several somewhat confusing terms and eponyms have been applied to this group of disorders. Sjögren syndrome is now a well-documented and defined entity which is classified into two groups (see later). The term myo-epithelial sialadenitis (or benign lymphoepithelial lesion) is used to denote a condition of bilateral or occasionally unilateral salivary gland enlargement, the

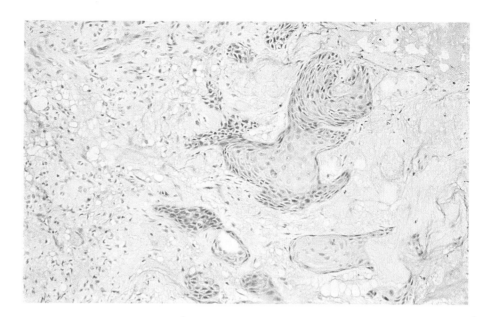

Fig. 14.8 Necrosis of salivary tissue and squamous metaplasia of ducts in necrotizing sialometaplasia.

histopathological features of which appear identical to those in Sjögren syndrome. However, the condition lacks the widespread systemic involvement and immunological derangement of Sjögren syndrome. Although it probably represents a variant of Sjögren syndrome, some cases have been followed for long periods and the salivary lymphoepithelial lesion has remained the only manifestation of disease. The benign lymphoepithelial lesion has also been referred to as Mikulicz *disease*. Mikulicz *disease* must be distinguished from Mikulicz *syndrome*, a term which has been used to describe bilateral salivary and lacrimal gland enlargement occurring as a manifestation of some other generalized disease, such as tuberculosis, sarcoid or malignant lymphoma. Mikulicz syndrome describes a clinical presentation; it is not a pathological diagnosis. The terms only serve to confuse and their use should be abandoned.

Sjögren syndrome

Sjögren syndrome is an immune-mediated chronic inflammatory disease characterized by lymphocytic infiltration and acinar destruction of lacrimal and salivary glands. It is classified into two groups:

1. *Primary Sjögren syndrome*—the association of dry mouth (xerostomia) and dry eyes (xerophthalmia or keratoconjuctivitis sicca);
2. *Secondary Sjögren syndrome*—the triad of xerostomia, xerophthalmia, and a connective tissue disease (usually rheumatoid arthritis) (Figs 14.9–14.11).

Primary Sjögren syndrome is also known as the sicca syndrome and accounts for about half of the cases. Rheumatoid arthritis is the most commonly associated connective tissue disease in secondary Sjögren syndrome. Other autoimmune diseases that may be associated include systemic lupus erythematosus, systemic sclerosis, primary biliary cirrhosis, and mixed connective tissue disease.

Although primary and secondary types are related they can be separated on clinical and immunological grounds. Both exhibit a spectrum of clinical features, in addition to xerostomia and xerophthalmia, associated with widespread involvement of other exocrine glands and a variety of extraglandular manifestations (Table 14.1). The most common symptoms are severe tiredness (patients may rest or sleep 10–15 hours a day or more) and those related to xeroph-

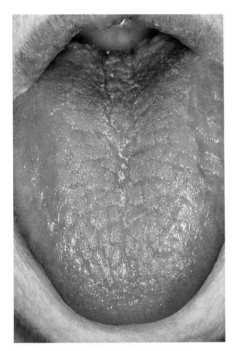

Fig. 14.9.

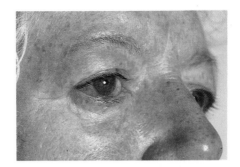

Fig. 14.10

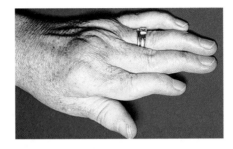

Fig. 14.11

Figs 14.9–14.11 Secondary Sjögren syndrome showing lingual changes associated with xerostomia (Fig. 14.9), xerophthalmia (Fig. 14.10), and rheumatoid arthritis (Fig. 14.11).

thalmia, xerostomia, and arthralgia. In general, the ocular and oral manifestations are more severe in primary Sjögren syndrome and this type is more likely to be complicated by lymphomatous change.

Unless otherwise specified, the general term Sjögren syndrome is used to encompass both types.

Sjögren syndrome predominantly affects middle-aged females (the female:male ratio is about 9:1), and symptoms related to dryness and soreness of the mouth and eyes are common presentations. Xerostomia may be associated with difficulty

Table 14.1   Manifestations of Sjögren syndrome

Glandular (exocrine glands)	
Salivary	—xerostomia
Lacrimal	—xerophthalmia
Skin	—xeroderma
Respiratory tract	—nasal dryness, sinusitis, tracheitis
Pharynx and GI tract	—dysphagia, atrophic gastritis, pancreatitis
Reproductive system	—vaginal dryness
Extraglandular	
Joints	—arthritis
Skin	—purpura, Raynaud's phenomenon
Liver	—primary biliary cirrhosis
Renal	—renal tubular defects
Endocrine	—thyroiditis
Neurological	—central and peripheral neuropathies
Haematological	—anaemia, leucopenia, thrombocytopenia
Immunological	—autoantibodies, hypergammaglobulinaemia

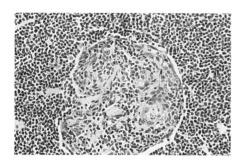

Fig. 14.12 Acinar destruction, dense lymphocytic infiltration and epimyoepithelial islands in parotid gland in Sjögren syndrome.

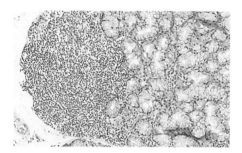

Fig. 14.13 Focal lymphocytic sialadenitis of minor glands in Sjögren syndrome.

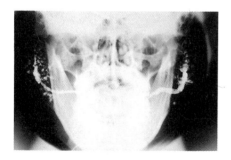

Fig. 14.14 Cavitary sialectasia in Sjögren syndrome.

in swallowing and speaking, increased fluid intake, and disturbances of taste. In addition, it predisposes to oral candidosis, which is found in about 70 per cent of patients and accounts for the soreness and redness of the mucosa, to acute bacterial sialadenitis, and in dentate patients to rapidly progressive dental caries. The oral mucosa appears dry, smooth, and glazed. lingual changes may be prominent, the dorsum of the tongue often appearing red and atrophic and showing varying degrees of fissuring and lobulation (see Fig. 14.9). Keratoconjuctivitis sicca manifests as dryness of the eyes with conjunctivitis, and causes a gritty, burning sensation (see Fig. 14.10).

Salivary gland enlargement is very variable. Although approximately 30 per cent of patients may give a history of such enlargement it is only clinically apparent in about half that number. The enlargement is usually bilateral, predominantly affects the parotid glands, and is seldom painful. Lacrimal gland enlargement is uncommon.

Histopathological examination of involved major glands shows lymphocytic infiltration, initially around intralobular ducts, which eventually replaces the whole of the affected lobules. The infiltration is accompanied by acinar atrophy but, in contrast, the ductal epithelium may show proliferation. The hyperplasia of ductal epithelium eventually obliterates the duct lumen and leads to the formation of islands of epithelial tissue, termed epimyoepithelial islands (Fig. 14.12). Thus, the fully developed lesion typically consists of sheets of lymphoid cells surrounding epimyoepithelial islands and replacing entire salivary gland lobules. This appearance is described as myoepithelial sialadenitis. As noted previously, it may occur in the absence of the characteristic clinical features listed above, which, by definition, are required to make the diagnosis of Sjögren syndrome. The lymphoid infiltrate does not cross the interlobular connective tissue septa and this helps in differentiating the lesion from the diffuse infiltration of malignant lymphoma, when the connective tissue septa are obliterated.

Although clinical involvement of the minor salivary glands is uncommon, they are often involved at the microscopic level. The glands show focal collections of lymphoid cells related to blood vessels adjacent to the ducts, and the number of such foci reflects the overall severity of the disease. The infiltrate is associated with acinar atrophy (Fig. 14.13). Labial salivary gland biopsy is a simple technique and the semi-quantitative assessment of focal lymphocytic sialadenitis is a useful investigation in helping to establish a diagnosis of Sjögren syndrome. However, the appearances are non-specific and are seen in other diseases and as incidental findings. They must be interpreted in the light of the clinical features and results of other investigations.

Other investigations useful in assessing the degree of salivary gland involvement include estimation of parotid salivary flow rates, which are usually reduced, and sialography which shows varying degrees of sialectasis (Fig. 14.14) often producing a 'snowstorm', or 'cherry tree in blossom'—like appearance. Salivary scintiscanning using [^{99}Tc^{m}]pertechnetate is also of value. The radioisotope is concentrated in salivary glands and its uptake is reduced in patients with Sjögren syndrome.

Key point

Oral manifestations of Sjögren syndrome

- xerostomia, predisposing to
  —candidosis
  —caries
  —sialadenitis
  —oral dysfunction

The aetiology and pathogenesis of Sjögren syndrome are uncertain although there is strong evidence that it is an autoimmune disease. A variety of circulating autoantibodies of both organ-specific and non-organ-specific type may be demonstrated, together with other serological changes (Table 14.2). Rheumatoid factor, which is associated with a variety of other autoimmune diseases, is present in most patients with primary or secondary Sjögren syndrome, as are a variety of antinuclear factor antibodies. These include autoantibodies to the nuclear antigens known as Ro and La, also referred to as SS-A and SS-B, respectively (SS for Sjögren syndrome). Anti-Ro precipitating antibodies are found in about 75 per cent of patients with primary Sjögren syndrome. Anti-La antibodies can also be detected in about 40 per cent of patients with Sjögren syndrome. Although neither anti-Ro nor anti-La is specific for the disease, the antibodies are diagnostically helpful, since they may be detected some time before the development of the full clinical picture. Various other autoantibodies are less frequently detected, including salivary duct autoantibody in about 50 per cent of patients. However, the latter does not appear to correlate with the severity of the disease and there is no evidence that any of the autoantibodies that have been detected are directly involved in damage to the affected organs.

Sjögren syndrome—investigations
Key points

- labial gland biopsy
- serology
- sialography/other imaging techniques
- salivary flow rates

Although the immunological and histopathological findings in Sjögren syndrome support an autoimmune pathogenesis, characterized by hyperactivity of B lymphocytes and the production of multiple autoantibodies, little is known about the aetiological factors underlying the disturbances in immunoregulation. Polyclonal B-cell expansion occurs in Sjögren syndrome which may be related to loss of regulatory T-cell activity.

Sjögren syndrome—pathology
Key points

- autoimmune disease
- multisystem involvement
- myoepithelial sialadenitis
- may progress to lymphoma

A viral aetiology has also been suggested, and raised titres of serum antibodies to cytomegalovirus (CMV) have been found in some patients. However, similar changes have been reported in other connective tissue diseases and it is likely that any association of Sjögren syndrome with CMV is of no aetiological significance.

More recent studies have concentrated on a possible role for the Epstein-Barr virus (EBV). Following primary infection EBV remains latent in the oropharynx and salivary glands and is excreted in saliva. Salivary excretion of EBV is increased in patients with rheumatoid arthritis. In addition, EBV antigens have been detected in parotid tissue in patients with Sjögren syndrome. However, as with CMV, it is probable that the underlying immune defect simply allows reactivation of latent viral infection rather then the viral infection being the causal factor. Recently, a possible role for human herpesvirus-6 (HHV-6) has been

Table 14.2   Approximate frequencies of serological abnormalities and autoantibodies in primary and secondary Sjögren syndromes

Serological abnormalities	Primary (per cent)	Secondary (per cent)
Elevated ESR	50–100	50–100
Hypergammaglobulinaemia	50–90	50–90
Immune complexes	85	up to 50
Elevated β_2 microglobulin (increased in exacerbations)	30–50	30–50
Autoantibodies		
Rheumatoid factor	40–60	75–100
Antinuclear antibody	40–70	up to 100
Anti-Ro/Anti-La	80–90	20–60
Gastric parietal cell		
Thyroid	variable	variable
Mitochondrial	5–30	5–30
Smooth muscle		

investigated. The virus has been identified in salivary glands, but since HHV-6 products can be detected in the saliva of healthy individuals its role, if any, remains speculative. The evidence for a viral aetiology in Sjögren syndrome must be regarded, at present, as inconclusive.

In both primary and secondary Sjögren syndrome, and in patients with myoepithelial sialadenitis (benign lymphoepithelial lesion) without other features of Sjögren syndrome, there is a risk of B-cell malignant lymphoma arising within an affected gland estimated to be 44 times that of the general population. The level of risk varies in different series from less than 1 per cent, to about 6 per cent of patients, and may be slightly greater in primary compared to secondary Sjögren syndrome. Malignant change usually occurs late in the course of the disease and may be associated with increased swelling of the affected gland. The lymphomas share many similarities with those derived from MALT (see Chapter 8). They tend to pursue an indolent course and remain localized until late in their natural history. The development of lymphoma is associated with proliferation of atypical lymphoid cells around the epimyoepithelial islands. As the malignant population expands there is destruction of the islands, replacement of the inflammatory lymphoid infiltrate, and obliteration of interlobular septa leading to diffuse infiltration of the gland by neoplastic cells.

More rarely, malignant change occurs in the epithelial component with squamous cell carcinoma or adenocarcinoma developing.

SIALADENOSIS

Sialadenosis (or sialosis) is a condition characterized by non-inflammatory, non-neoplastic, recurrent bilateral swelling of salivary glands. The parotid glands are most commonly affected. It is probably due to abnormalities of neurosecretory control and has been reported in association with diverse conditions such as hormonal disturbances, malnutrition, liver cirrhosis, chronic alcoholism, and following the administration of various drugs. The histology of sialadenosis is characterized by hypertrophy of serous acinar cells to about twice their normal size. The cytoplasm is often densely packed with secretory granules.

HIV-ASSOCIATED SALIVARY GLAND DISEASE

As mentioned in Chapter 11, salivary gland disease may be a feature in a small proportion of adults with HIV infection. The prevalence may be higher in infected children. HIV-associated salivary gland disease is characterized by xerostomia and/or swelling of the major glands, almost invariably the parotid. The xerostomia may be caused by a Sjögren syndrome-like disease associated with a myoepithelial sialadenitis, but the patients do not show the autoantibody profile commonly seen in Sjögren syndrome. Parotid swelling may be due to enlargement of intraparotid nodes as part of persistent glandular lymphadenopathy (PGL, see Chapter 11) or be due to the development of multiple lymphoepithelial cysts of varying size within the nodes, similar to those seen in non-HIV infected patients (see Chapter 6).

SALIVARY GLAND TUMOURS

Salivary gland tumours are relatively uncommon, comprising about 3 per cent of all tumours, although there is some geographical variation. For example, there is an unusually high prevalence in Inuit and in parts of Scotland. Tumours of the major glands are far more common than those of the minor glands which account for only about 15–20 per cent of all salivary tumours. Of the tumours in major glands about 90 per cent occur in the parotid gland and about 10 per cent in the submandibular gland, sublingual gland tumours being rare. About 55 per cent of minor salivary gland tumours arise in the palate and about 20 per cent of cases in the upper lip, with the remainder scattered throughout the mouth. Tumours of the lower lip are rare. Although the minority of salivary tumours occur in the minor glands the proportion of carcinomas in these glands is higher than in major glands. Exceptionally rare examples of salivary neoplasms arising as central intraosseous lesions of the jaws (mainly the mandible) have also been reported. They may be derived from ectopic entrapped salivary glands or from mucous metaplasia in the lining of odontogenic cysts.

Very little is known about the genetic alterations that occur in salivary tumours, but elevated expression of various oncogenes including *ras*, c-*myc*, and *erb* B-2 have been reported, as have a variety of structural abnormalities of chromosomes.

Classification

A great variety of salivary gland tumours are now recognized and their nomenclature and classification have recently been reviewed by the World Health Organization (WHO, 1991). The classification and nomenclature used in this chapter (Table 14.3) is based on that proposed by the WHO (1991). The list presented in Table 14.3 is not comprehensive; some of the recently described tumours are exceedingly rare and it is not yet clear whether they are distinct clinicopathological entities or histological varieties of already known types. This chapter is only concerned with primary neoplasms of epithelial origin, which account for nearly all salivary tumours, but it should be remembered that other neoplasms, such as malignant lymphomas, connective tissue, and metastatic tumours, may occasionally involve salivary glands.

Table 14.3 Classification of salivary tumours

Adenomas
Pleomorphic adenoma
Warthin tumour (adenolymphoma)
Basal cell adenoma
Oncocytoma
Canalicular adenoma
Ductal papillomas

Carcinomas
Mucoepidermoid carcinoma
Acinic cell carcinoma
Adenoid cystic carcinoma
Carcinoma arising in pleomorphic adenoma
Polymorphous low-grade adenocarcinoma
Other carcinomas

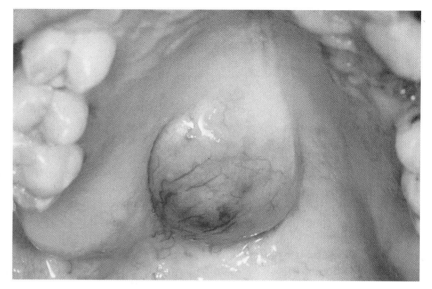

Fig. 14.15 Pleomorphic adenoma of the palate.

Adenomas

Pleomorphic adenoma

The pleomorphic adenoma is by far the commonest type of salivary gland tumour and accounts for 60–65 per cent of all tumours of the parotid gland and for about 45 per cent of all tumours of the minor glands. Approximately 7 per cent of cases originate in minor glands, the palate being the site of predilection. The tumour can occur at all ages but the majority of patients are in the fifth and sixth decades of life and there is a preponderance of women (about 60 per cent of cases). The tumour is usually solitary, although recurrences may be multifocal, and presents as a slowly growing, painless, rubbery swelling that the patient may have been aware of for several years (Fig. 14.15). The overlying skin or mucosa is usually intact.

Pleomorphic adenomas show a great variety of histological appearances with complex intermingling of epithelial components and mesenchymal-like areas. The diversity and complexity of appearances account for the term pleomorphic; the term does not imply cellular pleomorphism. In the same way the term 'mixed tumours', which has been used as a synonym for pleomorphic adenoma, described the varied appearances of the lesion rather than implying a dual origin from epithelium and mesenchyme. The tumour is composed of cells of epithelial and myoepithelial origin.

The pleomorphic adenoma is a benign tumour, although a connective tissue capsule does not always envelop the lesion completely. The capsule may also show variation in thickness and density, but regardless of its completeness or not, the tumour is clearly demarcated (Fig. 14.16). Apparently isolated nodules of tumour may also be seen within or even outside the capsule giving the impression of invasive growth, but serial sections show that these are outgrowths of the main mass (Fig. 14.17) and should not be taken as an indicator of malignancy nor of malignant potential. An important aspect of the deficient encapsulation and of intra- and extracapsular nodules is that they influence the surgical management of the tumour. Simple enucleation could establish a plane of cleavage within or just below the capsule, leaving behind islands of neoplastic tissues in the tumour bed which could give rise to uni- or multifocal recurrence. For these reasons the tumour is usually excised with a margin of surrounding normal tissue.

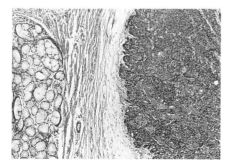

Fig. 14.16 Encapsulated pleomorphic adenoma clearly demarcated from surrounding minor salivary glands.

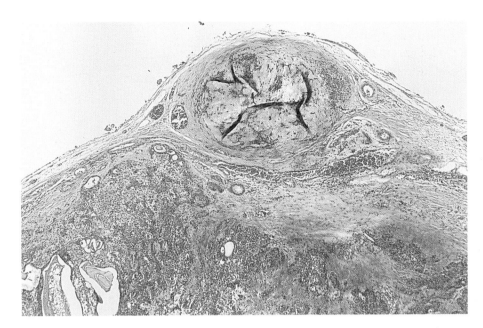

Fig. 14.17 Pleomorphic adenoma showing tumour nodule within the capsule.

Microscopically, there is considerable variation in the arrangement of the epithelial and stromal components between different tumours and within different areas of the same tumour. The epithelial component may be arranged in duct-like structures or as sheets, clumps, and interlacing strands (Fig. 14.18). Both epithelial-duct cells and myoepithelial-type cells are present. The epithelial-duct cells line the duct-like structures which vary in size, shape, number, and distribution. They often contain brightly eosinophilic, PAS positive, epithelial mucins. The sheets, clumps, and strands of epithelium, which usually form the bulk of the epithelial component consist of polygonal, spindle or stellate-shaped cells, many of which are considered to be derived from myoepithelium. Occasionally, groups of ovoid cells with eccentric nuclei and abundant hyaline cytoplasm are seen. These plasmacytoid or hyaline cells are thought to represent modified myoepithelial cells. Areas of squamous metaplasia and epithelial pearl formations may also be present.

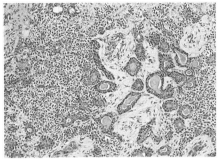

Fig. 14.18 Epithelial sheets and ductal structures in a pleomorphic adenoma.

The intercellular material varies in quantity and quality but is generally abundant. It may be predominantly fibrous, consisting of a delicate network or of dense bundles of collagen which can undergo hyalinization to form an apparently structureless eosinophilic material. In addition to sheaves of collagen fibres, these hyaline areas often contain elastic tissue. However, the most characteristic feature of the stroma is the presence of myxoid and/or chondroid areas, the appearances of which are associated with the accumulation of abundant connective tissue mucins. In myxoid areas, single epithelial cells or strands and clumps of cells are widely separated and surrounded by mucoid material. The separated epithelial cells have long stellate processes and often appear to melt into the mucinous background. In chondroid areas, isolated epithelial cells appear as rounded cells lying in lacunae within the mucoid material so that the tissue comes to resemble hyaline cartilage (Figs 14.19, 14.20). The mucoid material in the myxochondroid area is composed of glycosaminoglycans and consists mainly of chondroitin sulphates. It is generally regarded as being a product of the myoepithelial cells within the tumour. Tumours rich in mucoid material tend to rupture more readily during surgical removal allowing spillage and implantation of tumour into surrounding tissues, giving rise to multifocal recurrences.

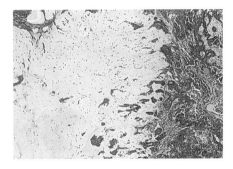

Fig. 14.19 Myxoid and chondroid areas (myxochondroid tissue) in a pleomorphic adenoma.

Malignant transformation can occur, usually in tumours that have been present for many years (see later).

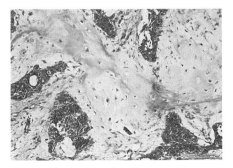

Fig. 14.20 High-power view of myxochondroid tissue in a pleomorphic adenoma.

Warthin tumour (adenolymphoma, papillary cystadenoma lymphomatosum)

Warthin tumour occurs almost exclusively in the parotid gland and is a slow-growing lesion which may arise multifocally. Bilateral parotid tumours occur in 5–10 per cent of cases and most patients are over 50 years of age. Although a striking predominance of males over females (about 5:1) has been reported in the past, recent series have demonstrated a change in incidence pattern and the male: female ratio is now 1.5:1.

On section, the tumour characteristically has a papillary cystic structure and shows multiple, irregular cystic spaces containing mucoid material separated by papillary projections of tumour tissue (Fig. 14.21). Microscopically, the tumour consists of epithelial and lymphoid elements. The epithelial component which clothes the papillary processes is double-layered and comprises a basal layer of roughly cuboidal cells surmounted by columnar cells. The epithelial cells have markedly eosinophilic granular cytoplasm, are rich in abnormal mitochondria, and resemble oncocytes. The stroma contains a variable amount of lymphoid tissue which often includes numerous germinal centres (Fig. 14.22).

The histogenesis of the tumour is uncertain, but it most likely arises from residues of salivary duct epithelium entrapped within lymph nodes during development.

Basal cell adenoma

This tumour accounts for about 1–2 per cent of all salivary tumours, of which about 70 per cent occur in the parotid gland and 20 per cent in the upper lip. It consists of cytologically uniform basaloid cells arranged in a variety of patterns (Fig. 14.23). The tumour is well encapsulated and the peak incidence is in the 7th decade of life.

Oncocytoma

The oncocytoma is a rare tumour usually arising in the parotid gland and occurring in patients over 60 years of age. It is usually surrounded by a thin capsule and consists of oncocytes, large cells with granular eosinophilic cytoplasm rich in mitochondria, many of which are abnormal. Hyperplasia of oncocytes also occurs and may be difficult to distinguish from oncocytoma.

Canalicular adenoma

This tumour occurs mainly in patients over 50 years of age and almost all cases are located in the upper lip. It consists of anastamosing strands of epithelial cells and may be partly or grossly cystic due to degeneration of its loose vascular stroma.

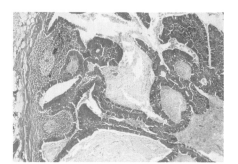

Fig. 14.21 Warthin tumour showing papillary-cystic pattern.

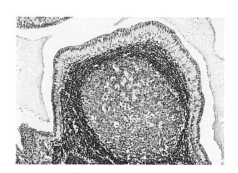

Fig. 14.22 Lymphoid tissue with germinal centres in Warthin tumour.

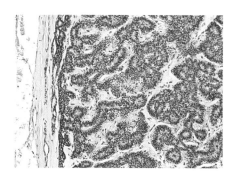

Fig. 14.23 Tubular/trabecular basal cell adenoma.

Ductal papillomas

Ductal papillomas are rare tumours most of which have a papillary structure projecting into the ductal system. Several subtypes are recognized.

Carcinomas

Malignant tumours of the salivary glands are relatively uncommon, accounting for about 1 per cent or less of all malignancies. Although carcinomas of salivary glands arise most frequently in the major glands, especially the parotid, the proportion of malignant to benign tumours is higher in minor glands. There are also differences in the incidence of the various types of carcinomas between major and minor glands. For example, the adenoid cystic carcinoma accounts for between 10 and 15 per cent of tumours of the minor salivary glands but only for about 3 per cent of parotid neoplasms.

Mucoepidermoid carcinoma

Mucoepidermoid carcinoma accounts for about 5 per cent of all salivary gland tumours and most arise in the parotid gland. However, their relative incidence is higher in the minor salivary glands where they may account for 10–15 per cent of tumours, the palate being the site of predilection.

Mucoepidermoid carcinoma may occur at any age but the highest incidence is during the fourth and fifth decades of life. There is a slight female predominance. The tumour often presents clinically in a similar manner to a pleomorphic adenoma, but grossly cystic tumours may be fluctuant and the more aggressive ones may be accompanied by pain and ulceration.

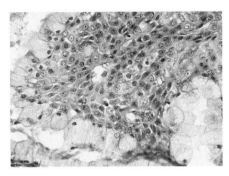

Fig. 14.24 Mucus-secreting, epidermoid, and intermediate cells in mucoepidermoid carcinoma.

Microscopically, the tumours are characterized by the presence of squamous cells, mucus-secreting cells, and cells of intermediate types which have the potential for further differentiation towards mucous or squamous cells (Fig. 14.24). The relative proportions of individual cell types and their arrangements vary from lesion to lesion, but it is customary to distinguish between well-differentiated (low-grade) and poorly differentiated (high-grade) tumours. They are non-encapsulated and invasive. Some (mainly low-grade types) may appear to advance on a broad 'pushing' front, whilst others (mainly high-grade types) are ill-defined, highly infiltrative growths (Fig. 14.25).

In well-differentiated tumours, mucus-secreting and epidermoid cells predominate and there is no cellular pleomorphism. Such tumours are often cystic, either wholly or in part, the cysts being lined mainly by mucus-secreting cells (Fig. 14.26). The epidermoid cells are usually present in the form of clumps or strands which may show keratinization but may also partially line the cysts. Discharge of mucus into the cysts can lead to their distension, coalescence, or rupture, in which case the release of mucus into the stroma is accompanied by reactive inflammation.

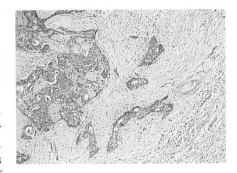

Fig. 14.25 Mucoepidermoid carcinoma showing infiltrative growth.

In poorly differentiated tumours, epidermoid and intermediate cells predominate and there is nuclear and cellular pleomorphism and nuclear hyperchromatism. Cystic spaces are not prominent and may be absent. In some cases differentiation from squamous cell carcinoma is difficult.

Although well-differentiated tumours rarely metastasize, the behaviour of a mucoepidermoid carcinoma cannot be predicted with any degree of certainty from its histology. The overall 5-year survival rate is about 70 per cent. However, well-differentiated, low-grade tumours have a local recurrence rate of less than 10 per cent and a 5-year survival of about 95 per cent. In contrast, poorly differentiated (high-grade) tumours have been reported to have local recurrence rates of 80 per cent and 5-year survival rates of only 30–40 per cent.

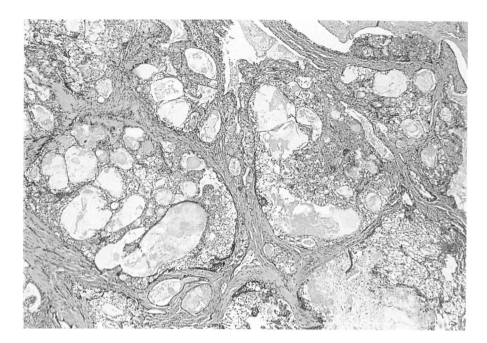

Fig. 14.26 Well-differentiated mucoepidermoid carcinoma showing multiple mucin-filled cysts.

Key points	**Mucoepidermoid carcinoma**
	• mucous, epidermoid, and intermediate cells
	• well differentiated
	—>50 per cent mucous cells
	—cystic
	—good prognosis
	• poorly differentiated
	—<10 per cent mucous cells
	—solid/infiltrative
	—poor prognosis

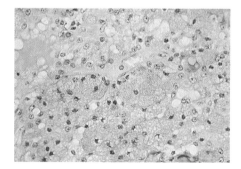

Fig. 14.27 Acinic cell carcinoma.

Acinic cell carcinoma

The acinic cell carcinoma is an uncommon neoplasm, the great majority arising in the parotid gland. It accounts for about 2–3 per cent of all parotid tumours and up to 20 per cent of malignant parotid neoplasms. It is more common in women and may present as an apparently encapsulated tumour that cannot be distinguished clinically from an adenoma.

Microscopically, the tumour is non-encapsulated and many show a 'pushing' margin or frankly infiltrative pattern of growth. It presents a spectrum of histological appearances, but typically consists of sheets or acinar groupings of large, polyhedral cells which have basophilic, granular cytoplasm, similar in appearance to the serous acinar cells of salivary glands (Fig. 14.27). Other tumours may show a papillary cystic pattern and contain other cell types, including duct cells and clear cells. Less well-differentiated lesions may show obvious cytological features of malignancy.

As with the mucoepidermoid carcinoma it is difficult to predict the behaviour of acinic cell carcinomas on the basis of their histological features. However acinic cell carcinoma is regarded as a low-grade malignancy. Five-year survival rates of 80–100 per cent have been reported for well-differentiated tumours and 65 per cent (or better) for poorly differentiated types.

Key points

Acinic cell carcinoma

- mainly parotid
- low-grade malignancy
- good prognosis

Adenoid cystic carcinoma

Adenoid cystic carcinomas usually arise in middle-aged or elderly patients. They account for up to 30 per cent of minor salivary gland tumours but only for about 6 per cent of parotid tumours. Clinically, they may present as slowly enlarging tumours indistinguishable from pleomorphic adenoma, but pain and ulceration of the overlying skin or mucosa are much more common than in pleomorphic adenoma (Fig. 14.28). Parotid tumours may also present with facial palsy. The neurological manifestations are a reflection of the predilection of the tumour to infiltrate and spread along nerve pathways.

The tumour has a wide spectrum of histological appearances, but most commonly the neoplastic epithelium is arranged as ovoid and irregularly shaped islands or as anastomosing strands lying in a scanty connective tissue stroma. The characteristic feature of the tumour is the presence of numerous microscopic cyst-like spaces within the epithelial islands, producing a cribriform, lace-like or 'Swiss-cheese' pattern (Figs 14.29, 14.30). The spaces are formed by partial enclavement of areas of stroma or of mucoid materials produced by the tumour epithelium which are deposited adjacent to the stroma. Partial enclavement means that the contents of the spaces are still in continuity with the stroma; the appearances of microcysts apparently enclosed by epithelium is a plane of section artefact. They contain acellular basophilic or occasionally hyaline substances rich in glycosaminoglycans and basement membrane-like material.

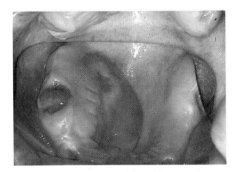

Fig. 14.28 Ulcerated adenoid cystic carcinoma of the palate (mirror view).

Key points

Adenoid cystic carcinoma

- proportionally more common in minor glands
- cribriform pattern is commonest type
- perineural invasion
- poor long-term prognosis

In tumours showing the characteristic cribriform pattern the epithelial components consists predominantly of small, rather uniform polygonal cells with basophilic cytoplasm. Mitoses are rarely seen. Less frequently the tumour shows a tubular or solid pattern.

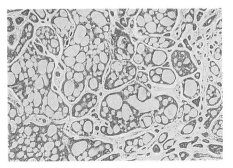

Fig. 14.29

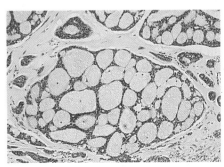

Fig. 14.30

Figs 14.29, 14.30 Adenoid cystic carcinoma showing characteristic cribriform pattern and uniform small basaloid cells.

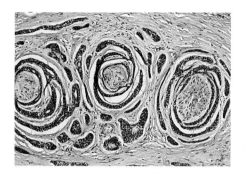

Fig. 14.31 Adenoid cystic carcinoma showing prominent perineural infiltration.

Infiltration of adjacent tissues and spread along and around nerves are often prominent features and may be extensive (Fig. 14.31). In addition, in the maxilla the tumour may infiltrate extensively along marrow spaces with little or no evidence of bone destruction, and these factors must be borne in mind in the surgical treatment of adenoid cystic carcinoma. Radiotherapy may be used to obtain palliation in inoperable cases, but does not result in a permanent cure. The disease runs a prolonged clinical course and metastases are usually a late finding. However, the long-term prognosis is grave and patients must be followed for much longer than 5 years before assuming that a permanent cure has been obtained. For example, survival rates for adenoid cystic carcinoma of the parotid are about 75 per cent at 5 years, about 40 per cent at 10 years, but less than 15 per cent at 20 years. Cribriform and tubular types have a better prognosis than the solid type. The prognostic outcome for patients with primary tumours of the minor salivary glands appears less favourable.

Carcinoma arising in pleomorphic adenoma

Carcinoma arising in pleomorphic adenoma is relatively uncommon and accounts for about 3 per cent of salivary tumours, although the true incidence is difficult to establish. Almost all arise in the parotid in adenomas that have usually been present for many years. The histological diagnosis requires evidence of a pre-existing pleomorphic adenoma, but in some tumours this may be difficult to identify and only hyaline scar-like tissue may remain. The malignant component is usually an adenocarcinoma or undifferentiated carcinoma but may assume the features of any of the types of salivary carcinomas. In some tumours more than one morphological type of carcinoma may be present. Whilst the malignant component is confined to areas still within the pre-existing adenoma ('non-invasive' stage) the tumour has a good prognosis. However, when there is infiltration of surrounding tissues the tumour carries a poor prognosis. Five-year survival rates of about 55 per cent falling to about 30 per cent at 10 years have been reported.

Polymorphous low-grade adenocarcinoma

This carcinoma occurs almost exclusively in minor salivary glands. Most have presented in the palate. As its name implies it is a tumour that shows a variety of growth patterns within the same lesion, including solid, tubular, papillary, and cribriform areas. Cytologically, the tumour appears bland; mitotic figures are infrequent and nuclear atypia is lacking. The tumour has a good prognosis. Although it has an infiltrative pattern of growth, local recurrence is uncommon and metastatic spread to regional nodes is rare.

Other carcinomas

A variety of other histological types of salivary carcinomas are described, including adenocarcinoma (not otherwise specified), squamous cell carcinoma, basal cell adenocarcinoma, sebaceous carcinoma, and undifferentiated carcinomas.

AGE CHANGES IN SALIVARY GLANDS

Age changes can be detected in both major and minor salivary glands.

Reduction in the weights of submandibular and parotid glands have been reported with increasing age associated in the submandibular gland with an age-dependent reduction in flow rates. In contrast, several studies have demonstrated that there is no significant reduction in parotid flow rates in the elderly. In both glands the reduction in weight is related to atrophy of secretory tissue and replacement by fibro-fatty tissue. The adiposity of the glands tends to increase linearly with age, and in both there is a reduction in the volume of acinar tissue of about 30–35 per cent from approximately 20 years to 75 years of age. Similar changes, amounting to about 45 per cent loss of acinar tissue, have been reported in minor glands in the lower lip.

In both major and minor salivary glands oncocytic change is a prominent feature in ductal epithelium with ageing.

FURTHER READING

Anneroth, G. and Hansen, L. S. (1982). Necrotising sialometaplasia. *International Journal of Oral Surgery*, **11**, 283–91.

Batsakis, J. G. (1980). Salivary gland neoplasias: an outcome of modified morphogenesis and cytodifferentiation. *Oral Surgery, Oral Medicine, Oral Pathology*, **49**, 229–32.

Cannell, H., Kerawala, C., and Farthing, P. (1997). Stomatitis glandularis—two confirmed cases of a rare condition, *British Dental Journal*, **182**, 222–5.

Caselitz, J., Schulze, I., and Seifert, G. (1986). Adenoid cystic carcinoma of the salivary glands: an immunohistochemical study. *Journal of Oral Pathology*, **15**, 308–18.

Dardick, I., Byard, R. W., and Carnegie, J. A. (1990). A review of the proliferative capacity of major salivary glands and the relationship to current concepts of neoplasia in salivary glands. *Oral Surgery, Oral Medicine, Oral Pathology*, **69**, 53–67.

Evans, H. L. and Batsakis, J. G. (1984). Polymorphous low-grade adenocarcinoma of minor salivary glands. *Cancer*, **53**, 935–42.

Eveson, J. W. and Cawson, R. A. (1985). Tumours of the minor (oropharyngeal) salivary glands: a demographic study of 336 cases. *Journal of Oral Pathology*, **14**, 500–9.

Eveson, J. W. and Cawson, R. A. (1985). Salivary gland tumours: a review of 2410 cases with particular reference to histological types, site, age and sex distribution. *Journal of Pathology*, **146**, 51–8.

Hamper, K., Lazar, F., Dietel, M., Caselitz, J., Berger, J., Arps, H., Falkmer, U., Auer, G., and Seifert, G. (1989). Prognostic factors for adenoid cystic carcinoma of the head and neck: a retrospective evaluation of 96 cases. *Journal of Oral Pathology and Medicine*, **19**, 101–7.

Imbery, T. A. and Edwards, P. A. (1996). Necrotizing sialometaplasia: literature review and case reports. *Journal of the American Dental Association*, **127**, 1087–92.

Jordan, R. C. K. and Speight, P. M. (1996). Lymphoma in Sjögren's syndrome. *Oral Surgery, Oral Medicine, Oral Pathology, Oral Radiology and Endodontics*, **81**, 308–20.

Mandel, L. and Reich, R. (1992). HIV parotid gland lymphoepithelial cysts. *Oral Surgery, Oral Medicine, Oral Pathology*, **74**, 273–8.

Mintz, G. A., Abrams, A. M., and Melrose, R. J. (1982). Monomorphic adenomas of the major and minor salivary glands. Report of 21 cases and review of the literature. *Oral Surgery, Oral Medicine, Oral Pathology*, **53**, 375–86.

Pape, S. A., MacLeod, R. I., McLean, N. R., and Soames, J. V. (1995). Sialadenosis of the salivary glands. *British Journal of Plastic Surgery*, **48**, 419–22.

Schiødt, M. (1992). HIV-associated salivary gland disease: a review. *Oral Surgery, Oral Medicine, Oral Pathology*, **73**, 164–7.

Scott, J. (1986). Structure and function in ageing human salivary glands. *Gerodontology*, **5**, 149–58.

Scully, C. S. (1986). Sögren's syndrome: Clinical and laboratory features, immunopathogenesis and management. *Oral Surgery, Oral medicine, Oral Pathology*, **62**, 510–23.

Seifert, G. (1992). Histopathology of malignant salivary gland tumours. *Oral Oncology, European Journal of Cancer*, **28B**, 49–56.

Seifert, G. and Sobin, L. H. (1991). *Histological typing of salivary gland tumours* (2nd edn). World Health Organization International Classification of Tumours. Springer-Verlag. Berlin.

Spiro, R. H., Huvos, A. G., and Strong, E. W. (1978). Acinic cell carcinoma of salivary origin. A clinicopathological study of 67 cases. *Cancer*, **41**, 924–35.

Vincent, S. D., Hammond, H. L., and Finkelstein, M. W. (1994). Clinical and therapeutic features of polymorphous low-grade adenocarcinoma. *Oral Surgery, Oral Medicine, Oral Pathology*, **77**, 41–7.

Waldron, C. A., El-Mofty, S. K., and Gnepp, D. R. (1988). Tumours of intraoral minor salivary glands: A demographic and histological study of 426 cases. *Oral Surgery, Oral Medicine, Oral Pathology*, **66**, 323–33.

15 Odontomes and odontogenic tumours

15 Odontomes and odontogenic tumours

CLASSIFICATION

Odontomes and odontogenic tumours form a complex group of lesions derived from the dental formative tissues. The term odontome is used to designate a non-neoplastic, developmental anomaly or malformation that contains fully formed enamel and dentine. Odontomes can, therefore, be considered as dental hamartomas containing the calcified dental tissues. The latter is an important qualification since odontogenic hamartomas that do not contain both enamel and dentine should not be designated as odontomes. Although this use of the term is generally accepted, there is no consensus as to which dental anomalies and malformations should be included under this heading, with the exception of the complex and compound odontomes. Nevertheless, it does permit the grouping of several related disorders. Lesions that can be considered as odontomes are listed in Table 15.1. Geminated odontomes are discussed in Chapter 1.

The odonotogenic tumours are uncommon lesions, some of them exceedingly so, and the status of many is unknown. Some are truly neoplastic but others are probably hamartomatous, and for this reason the term 'tumour' in this context indicates a localized non-inflammatory swelling without any implication regarding neoplasia. The nomenclature and classification used in this chapter (Table 15.2) are based on that recommended by the World Health Organization (1992). Another two lesions of debatable origin are appended to the classification. (The WHO classification also includes the complex and compound odontomes in the group of benign epithelial lesions with odontogenic mesenchyme.)

ODONTOMES

Invaginated odontome

Invaginated odontomes (dens invaginatus) arise as a result of invagination of a portion of the enamel organ into the dental papilla at an early stage in odontogenesis, before the formation of calcified dental tissues. The majority of invaginations originate in the coronal part of the tooth but radicular invaginations also occur (see later).

Clinical and radiological features

Although coronal invaginations may involve any type of tooth, including supernumerary teeth, the permanent maxillary lateral incisors are the teeth most frequently affected. The anomaly is often bilateral. The condition is uncommon in mandibular teeth and cases reported involving the primary dentition are exceedingly rare.

In the permanent maxillary lateral incisors the degree of invagination varies from accentuation of the cingulum pit to deep infoldings arising from the crown and extending into the root, some reaching the apical foramen. The invagination in pegshaped lateral incisors often arises from the incisal tip. Where the invagination is of a minor degree the tooth may be of normal appearance, but with the more extensive forms the crown, and particularly the root, may be considerably dilated. The terms dilated or gestant odontome are sometimes applied to describe such anomalies (Figs 15.1, 15.2). Although severe degrees of invagination are rare, minor invaginations are not uncommon and if all grades of invagination are included the incidence in permanent maxillary lateral incisors may be as high as 5 per cent of all patients examined. Some invaginations may be discovered on clinical examination, particularly if there is gross disturbance in tooth morphology, or on routine radiographs, but many are undetected until the patient presents with symptoms of pulpitis and its sequelae which are common complications of invagination.

Radiographs reveal an invagination lined by enamel which is continuous with the normal enamel covering of the tooth (Fig. 15.3). The appearances may resemble a tooth within a tooth, hence the term dens-in-dente.

Histopathology and pathogenesis

Ground sections show an invagination of enamel and dentine arising from the crown and sometimes extending into the root (Fig. 15.4). The invagination cavity opens on the surface of the tooth, and the enamel lining the invagination is continuous with that covering the external surfaces of the tooth. The enamel lining the invagination is often defective and may be poorly mineralized or absent in areas, particularly near the bottom of the cavity. The dentine of the invagination is also commonly defective and may show abnormalities in calcification and fine channels or cracks running between the invagination and the pulp. Because

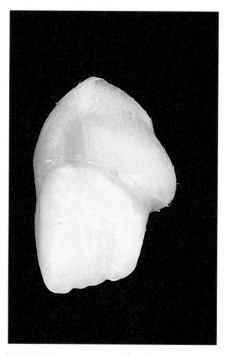

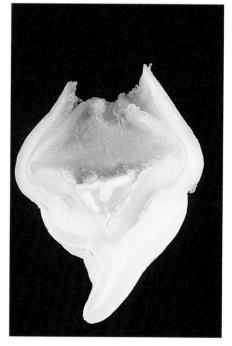

Figs 15.1 and 15.2 Dilated invaginated odontome involving a permanent maxillary incisor; macroscopic and bisected appearances.

Fig. 15.1   **Fig. 15.2**

Table 15.1 Odontomes

Invaginated odontone (dens invaginatus, dens-in-dente)

Evaginated odontome

Enamel pearl (enameloma)

Geminated odontome

Complex odontome

Compound odontome

Table 15.2 Classification of odontogenic tumours

Benign odontogenic tumours

Epithelial lesions

(1) Without odontogenic mesenchyme
  Ameloblastoma
  Squamous odontogenic tumour
  Calcifying epithelial odontogenic tumour
  Clear-cell odontogenic tumour

2) With odontogenic mesenchyme
  Ameloblastic fibroma
  Ameloblastic fibrodentinoma and fibro-odontoma
  Odontoameloblastoma
  Adenomatoid odontogenic tumour
  Calcifying odontogenic cyst
  Complex odontome
  Compound odontome

Mesenchymal lesions
  Odontogenic fibroma
  Myxoma
  Benign cementoblastoma

Malignant odontogenic tumours

Odontogenic carcinomas
  Malignant ameloblastoma
  Primary intraosseous carcinoma
  Malignant variants of other epithelial tumours
  Malignant change in odontogenic cysts
Odontogenic sarcomas
  Ameloblastic fibrosarcoma
  Ameloblastic fibro-odontosarcoma

Tumours of debatable origin

Melanotic neuroectodermal tumour of infancy

Congenital gingival granular cell tumour (congenital epulis)

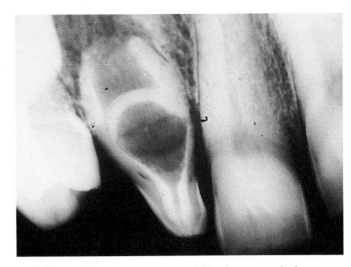

Fig. 15.3 Radiographic appearances of dilated invaginated odontome associated with peg-shaped lateral incisor.

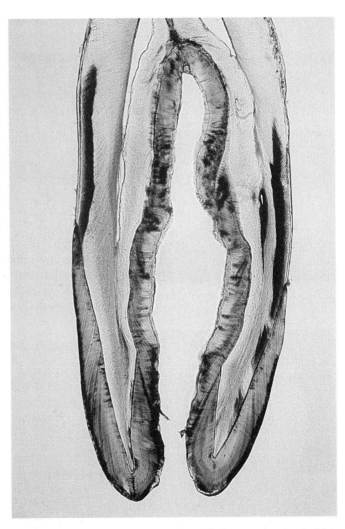

Fig. 15.4 Ground section of an invaginated odontome associated with a peg-shaped lateral incisor.

the invagination encroaches upon the pulp cavity the latter may be reduced to slit-like spaces around the sides of the invagination. In rare cases, both enamel and dentine may be absent in the base of the invagination and so the cavity communicates directly with the pulp. Whilst the tooth is unerupted the invagination cavity contains connective tissue continuous with the dental follicle, within which islands of bone are occasionally formed. On eruption this connective tissue undergoes necrosis. Once the invagination is exposed to the oral environment food debris and bacteria come to occupy the cavity and the various defects in the lining of the invagination may permit ready access of bacteria to the pulp. This accounts for the frequency with which the anomaly presents with pulpits and its sequelae even though the tooth may appear clinically sound.

The pathogenesis of the invagination is unknown. The milder forms probably represent exaggeration of the normal process involved in the formation of the cingulum pit, and it may be that the more severe infoldings represent a more pronounced disturbance of the same process. Although the causes of such a disturbance have yet to be determined, invagination could be the result either of active proliferation of an area of the enamel organ with infolding of the proliferating cells into the dental papilla, or of displacement of part of the enamel organ into the papilla as a result of abnormal pressure from the surrounding tissue.

Key points	Invaginated odontome
	• mainly permanent maxillary lateral incisors
	• enamel-lined invagination on radiograph
	• pulpitis and sequelae common
	• abnormalities of crown/root morphology

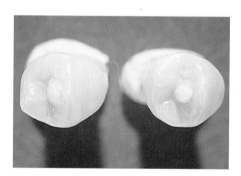

Fig. 15.5

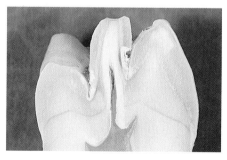

Fig. 15.6

Figs 15.5 and 15.6 Evaginated odontomes associated with premolar teeth; macroscopic and bisected appearances.

Radicular invaginations

Radicular invaginations are uncommon and are of two distinct types. The first type is represented as an axial infolding of the root, which is lined by cementum. It is an exaggeration of the grooving normally present on the roots of some teeth, notably mandibular first premolars, and indicates an incomplete attempt at root bifurcation.

The second type is rare and presents as an enamel-lined, saccular invagination originating from the surface of the root. Presumably this type arises as a result of invagination of the epithelial root sheath of Hertwig into the dental papilla followed by differentiation of ameloblasts and subsequent amelogenesis (cf. the formation of the enamel pearl).

Evaginated odontome

The evaginated odontome (dens evaginatus) occurs predominantly in people of Mongoloid stock; it is very rare in other racial groups. The anomaly presents as an enamel-covered, teat-like tubercle projecting from the occlusal surface of an otherwise normal premolar (Figs 15.5, 15.6). The evagination is easily fractured resulting in exposure of the pulp and its sequelae.

Enamel pearl (enameloma)

The enamel pearl presents as a small droplet of enamel on the root of a tooth and is found most frequently near or in the furcation of the roots of maxillary permanent molar teeth. Most arise close to the amelocemental junction but they are occasionally found near the root apex.

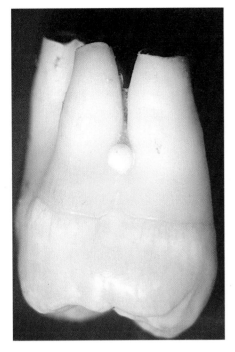

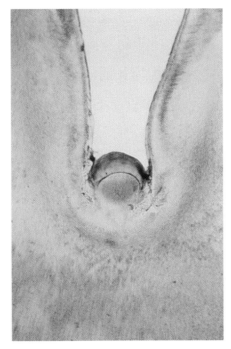

Fig. 15.7   **Fig. 15.8**

Fig. 15.7 and 15.8 Enamel pearl; macroscopic appearance and ground section, respectively.

The lesion is symptomless and is discovered as an incidental finding on radiographs or when the tooth is extracted. Microscopically, some consist entirely of enamel but others contain a core of dentine and even a small amount of pulp tissue (Figs 15.7, 15.8). The anomaly is thought to arise as a result of a growth disturbance of Hertwig's sheath resulting in budding of the sheath followed by differentiation of ameloblasts and amelogenesis.

Complex and compound odontomes

The complex and compound odontomes are closely related malformations. The complex odontome consists mainly of a mass of haphazardly arranged enamel, dentine, and cementum, whereas the compound odontome consists of collections of numerous small, discrete, tooth-like structures. All gradations between these two extremes may be encountered and the distinction between complex and compound odontomes is somewhat arbitrary, being based on the preponderance in the lesion of either discrete denticles or a disorganized mass of dental tissues. Both are hamartomatous lesions with limited growth potential.

Clinical and radiographic features

Complex and compound odontomes are most often diagnosed in the second decade of life but may also be seen in older individuals. The complex odontome is located most frequently in the premolar and molar regions of the jaws and is slightly more common in the mandible. Most compound odontomes arise in the intercanine area, particularly of the maxilla (Figs 15.9, 15.10). The majority of odontomes are small and arise in association with the permanent dentition. Often they are discovered as incidental findings when investigating a patient with a tooth missing from the dental arch, but occasionally the odontomes are sufficiently large to produce expansion of bone. In some cases, this is associated with cystic change around the odontome. The majority of odontomes are associated with the crowns of

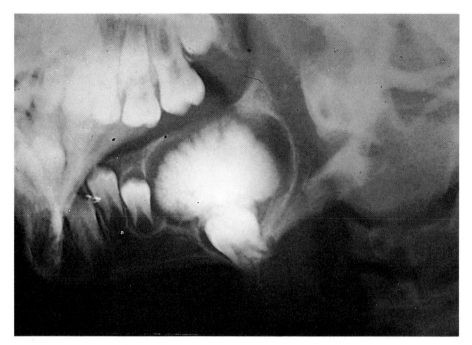

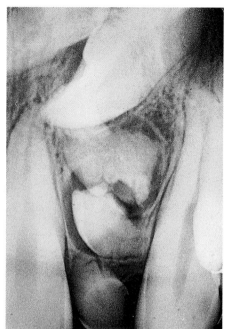

Fig. 15.9

Fig. 15.10

Fig. 15.9 Complex odontome overlying a first permanent molar showing radiolucent zone analogous to the pericoronal space and radiopaque mass with radiating structure.

Fig. 15.10 Compound odontome overlying the crown of an impacted maxillary canine.

unerupted teeth and occasionally they take the place of a missing tooth. Lesions that have remained undetected in the jaws for many years may appear to erupt following resorption of overlying alveolar bone and this may lead to secondary infection and pain. Multiple odontomes are rare.

Radiographically, fully formed complex and compound odontomes appear as radiopaque lesions, but the developing stages show a well-defined radiolucency in which there is deposition of radiopaque material as calcification proceeds. The mature lesions are also surrounded by a narrow radiolucent zone analogous to the pericoronal space around unerupted teeth. The complex odontome appears as a radiopaque mass which sometimes has a radiating structure; the compound odontome shows numerous small denticles and resembles a bag of teeth.

Key points	**Complex and compound odontomes**
	• structure
	—complex: disorganized mass of dental tissues
	—compound: separate denticles
	• site
	—complex: usually posterior mandible
	—compound: usually anterior maxilla
	• clinical presentation
	—missing tooth
	—variable expansion

Histopathology

Microscopically, the fully developed complex odontome consists mainly of a mass of irregularly arranged, but well-formed enamel, dentine, and cementum surrounded by a fibrous capsule. Dentine forms the bulk of the lesion and, on surfaces not covered by enamel or cementum, is in contact with connective tissue similar in appearance to normal pulp. Much of the enamel is fully calcified so

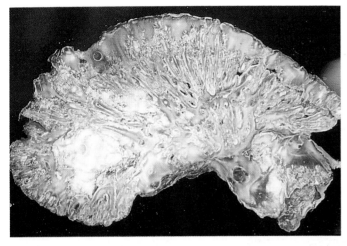

Fig. 15.11

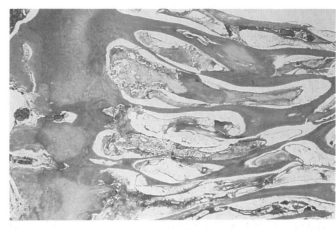

Fig. 15.12

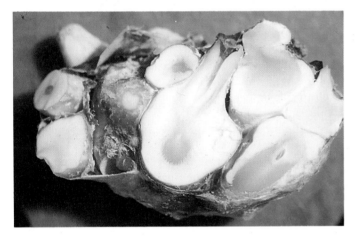

Fig. 15.13

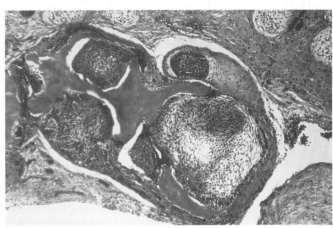

Fig. 15.14

that in sections of decalcified specimens its participation in the lesion is indicated by empty spaces (Figs 15.11, 15.12). In areas where enamel maturation is incomplete, some of the spaces contain remnants of enamel matrix, recognized by its fibrillar appearance.

The fully developed compound odontome consists of a number of separate denticles embedded in fibrous tissue (Fig. 15.13). Although morphologically most of the denticles do not resemble the teeth of the normal dentition, in each one enamel, dentine, cementum, and pulp are arranged as in a normal tooth.

Developing complex and compound odontomes contain appreciably more soft tissue which includes varying amounts of odontogenic epithelium and structures resembling enamel organs (Fig. 15.14). Indeed, developing lesions show histological features of all stages in odontogenesis and they may be difficult to differentiate from ameloblastic fibroma and ameloblastic fibro-odontoma.

Figs 15.11 and 15.12 Ground and decalcified sections of a complex odontome.

Fig. 15.13 Macroscopic appearances of the cut surface of a compound odontome showing separate denticles embedded in fibrous tissue.

Fig. 15.14 Developing odontome showing structures resembling enamel organs and early dentine formation.

ODONTOGENIC TUMOURS

Ameloblastoma

The ameloblastoma is a benign but locally invasive neoplasm derived from odontogenic epithelium. It is the commonest of the odontogenic tumours but, even so,

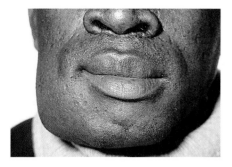

Fig. 15.15 Facial deformity associated with ameloblastoma at angle of mandible.

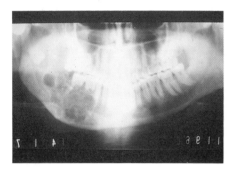

Fig. 15.16 Radiographic appearances of lesion in Fig. 15.15 showing multilocular radiolucency and root resorption.

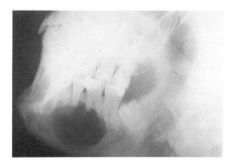

Fig. 15.17 Radiographic appearance of unilocular ameloblastoma showing resorption of roots of involved teeth.

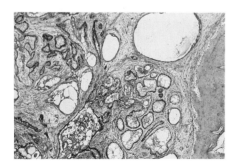

Fig. 15.18 Follicular ameloblastoma showing islands of neoplastic epithelium in mature fibrous stroma.

in most series only accounts for approximately 1 per cent of all oral tumours. However, it is more common in black Americans and in West Africans, in particular, where it accounts for 6 per cent or more of oral tumours. Two variants, the unicystic ameloblastoma and the peripheral ameloblastoma, are sufficiently distinct to merit separate mention later in this chapter.

Clinical and radiographic features

Ameloblastomas present over a wide age range but in industrialized countries are usually diagnosed in the fourth and fifth decades of life, although they can occur in children or the elderly. In developing countries, ameloblastoma tends to present about 10-15 years earlier. About 80 per cent of tumours occur in the mandible, of which some 70 per cent arise in the molar region and ascending ramus, 20 per cent in the premolar region, and 10 per cent in the incisor region. In the maxilla, most also occur in the molar region but about 15 per cent involve the antrum.

The tumour is slow-growing and in the early stages may be asymptomatic and be discovered as an incidental finding. As the tumour enlarges the patient may become aware of a gradually increasing facial deformity and expansion of the jaw-bone (Fig. 15.15). The enlargement is usually bony hard, non-tender, and ovoid or fusiform in outline but in advanced cases, egg-shell crackling may be elicited due to thinning of the overlying bone. However, perforation of bone and extension of the tumour into soft tissues are late features. In the maxilla, even large tumours may produce little expansion as the lesion can extend into the sinus and beyond. Teeth in the area of the tumour may become loosened, but pain is seldom a feature.

Radiographically, the ameloblastoma appears most commonly as a multiloculated radiolucency. Roots of teeth involved by the tumour show varying degrees of resorption (Fig. 15.16). As the tumour enlarges it may become associated with an unerupted tooth, particularly an impacted third molar, and the appearances may mimic those of a dentigerous cyst. Less frequently, ameloblastomas present as a single unilocular radiolucency indistinguishable from an odontogenic cyst (Fig. 15.17). The unicystic ameloblastoma has distinct features and is considered separately in this chapter.

Histopathology

There is considerable variation in the histopathology of ameloblastomas but two main patterns, the follicular and plexiform, are described depending on the arrangement of the neoplastic epithelium. In some tumours both patterns coexist.

The tumour epithelium in the follicular pattern is arranged into more or less discrete, rounded islands or follicles, each one resembling the enamel organ of the developing tooth germ (Fig. 15.18). The follicles each consist of a central mass of loosely connected, angular cells resembling the stellate reticulum of the normal enamel organ, surrounded by a layer of cuboidal or columnar cells resembling ameloblasts. The nuclei of the latter are situated away from the basal ends of the cells, and this is described as reversed polarity (Fig. 15.19). The follicles are separated by varying amounts of fibrous connective tissue stroma.

A variety of changes can occur within the stellate area of the follicles and these include cystic breakdown, squamous metaplasia, and granular cell change (Figs 15.20-15.22). Microcyst formation is common and by coalescence of these small cysts larger areas of cystic change can occur within the tumour. Small areas of squamous metaplasia are not infrequent, although extensive change of

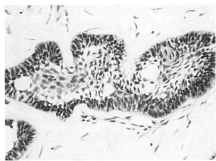
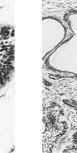

Fig. 15.19

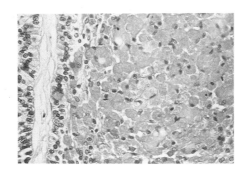

Fig. 15.20

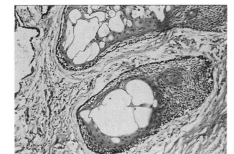

Fig. 15.21

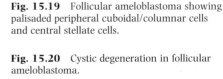

Fig. 15.22

Fig. 15.19 Follicular ameloblastoma showing palisaded peripheral cuboidal/columnar cells and central stellate cells.

Fig. 15.20 Cystic degeneration in follicular ameloblastoma.

Fig. 15.21 Squamous metaplasia in follicular ameloblastoma.

Fig. 15.22 Granular cell change in follicular ameloblastoma.

this type is uncommon. In those tumours that show extensive squamous metaplasia the term acanthomatous ameloblastoma is usually applied. Granular cell change is uncommon. The cells are large, eosinophilic, and their cytoplasm contains prominent PAS-positive granules. Electron microscopy has shown that these represent complex lysosomes and residual bodies.

The tumour epithelium in the plexiform type is arranged as a tangled network of anastomosing strands and irregular masses each of which shows the same cell layers as for the follicular pattern (Fig. 15.23). Thus each strand or mass is bounded by columnar or cuboidal cells resembling ameloblasts, whilst the central area is occupied by stellate reticulum-like cells (Fig. 15.24). Cyst formation is common but, in contrast to the follicular type, is usually due to stromal degeneration rather than to cystic change within the stellate areas of the epithelium. Again, large areas of cystic change can occur within the tumour by coalescence of stromal cysts.

Pathogenesis

The pathogenesis of the tumour and origin of the neoplastic epithelium have been the subject of much debate but remain largely unresolved, although the histological similarities between the tumour epithelium and the normal enamel organ support an odontogenic origin. However, unlike the normal enamel organ, enamel is not formed in ameloblastomas. It will be recalled that in normal odontogenesis the differentiation of the inner enamel epithelium into ameloblasts and the formation of enamel occurs only after the differentiation of odontoblasts and the beginning of dentinogenesis. Odontoblasts are not present in ameloblastomas and so this inductive effect is absent and mature ameloblasts do not differentiate. For this reason the cuboidal or columnar cells bounding the neoplastic epithelium are thought to represent preameloblasts. Enamel and dentine are not formed in ameloblastomas.

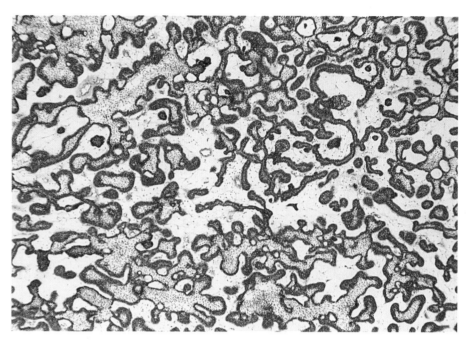

Fig. 15.23 Plexiform ameloblastoma showing complex pattern of interconnecting epithelial strands.

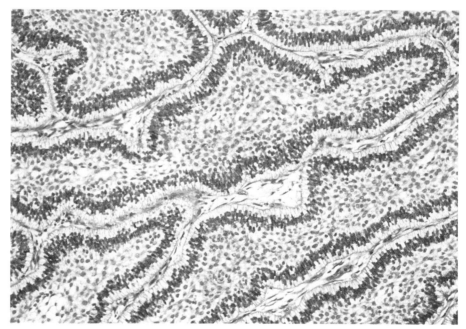

Fig. 15.24 Plexiform ameloblastoma showing peripheral columnar/cuboidal and central stellate cells.

Possible origins of the neoplastic epithelium are the dental lamina or its residues, the enamel organ, Hertwig's root sheath or its residues (cell rests of Malassez), the epithelial lining of odontogenic cysts, and the basal layer of the oral epithelium. General opinion supports an origin from the dental lamina or its residues.

Behaviour

The typical intraosseous ameloblastoma is locally invasive and islands of tumour may infiltrate the cancellous marrow spaces without initially causing bone destruction (Fig. 15.25). These would not be eliminated by simple curettage and such treatment of an ameloblastoma is associated with a high recurrence rate (50-90 per cent). Surgical resection with a margin of normal bone is the preferred treatment. Although it is generally accepted that there are no consistent differences in clinical behaviour between the two main histological types, significantly lower recurrence rates have been reported for some variants, for example the acanthomatous type. Rare reports of pulmonary metastases of typical ameloblastoma are probably the result of aspiration of tumour cells associated with surgery, particularly in cases that have required multiple operations because of recurrences. Truly malignant ameloblastomas are very rare and are discussed later with the other odontogenic carcinomas.

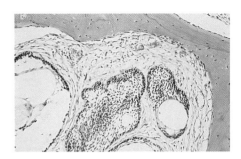

Fig. 15.25 Follicular ameloblastoma infiltrating mandibular marrow spaces.

Ameloblastoma	**Key points**
• molar region mandible is commonest site	
• multilocular/unilocular radiolucency	
• follicular/plexiform patterns on histology	
• does not contain enamel or dentine	
• locally invasive	

Unicystic ameloblastoma

This type of ameloblastoma typically presents in a younger age group than other variants of ameloblastoma (second to third decade) and occurs predominantly in the mandibular third molar region. Radiographically, it appears as a well-defined unilocular radiolucency, usually associated with an unerupted tooth, and is indistinguishable from a dentigerous cyst (Fig. 15.26). The diagnosis is made only after histopathological examination.

Histologically, the lesion presents as a cyst lined by ameloblastomatous epithelium comprising a basal layer of columnar cells with polarization of the hyperchromatic nuclei away from the basal lamina, covered by a loose, vacuolated layer of stellate epithelial cells. In some cases, there is a localized nodular proliferation of typical plexiform ameloblastomatous tissue into the cyst lumen (Fig. 15.27). A third pattern is identified where ameloblastomatous tissue infiltrates the wall of the cyst. This type is important to distinguish since, whilst the first two variants may be treated by simple enucleation and curettage, the third is likely to behave as a typical intraosseous lesion and requires to be treated as such.

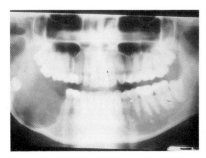

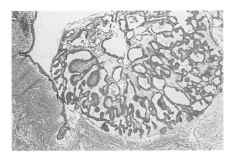

Fig. 15.26 Radiographic appearances of a unicystic ameloblastoma presenting as a dentigerous cyst.

Fig. 15.27 Unicystic ameloblastoma with proliferation into the cyst lumen.

Fig. 15.26

Fig. 15.27

Peripheral (extraosseous) ameloblastoma

Rarely, ameloblastomas present in the gingival or alveolar soft tissues without involving bone. Such lesions may arise from the basal cell layer of the oral epithelium or from extraosseous rests of the dental lamina. They are much less invasive than intraosseous tumours and less drastic surgery is required for their treatment. Histologically, they may resemble intraosseous types or consist mainly of basaloid cells.

Squamous odontogenic tumour

The squamous odontogenic tumour is a rare lesion presenting with few symptoms except for local tenderness and tooth mobility. Radiographically, the lesion usually presents as a well-circumscribed, often semilunar or triangular-shaped radiolucency with a sclerotic border associated with the roots of teeth.

Histologically, the tumour consists of irregularly-shaped islands of well-differentiated squamous epithelium in a stroma of mature fibrous tissue. The islands lack the peripheral palisaded and polarized basal cells typical of ameloblastoma. It is thought to be derived from the rests of Malassez.

Although some lesions may be locally aggressive, curettage is the treatment of choice.

Calcifying epithelial odontogenic tumour

The calcifying epithelial odontogenic tumour is a rare, benign but locally invasive epithelial neoplasm. It occurs over a wide age range and is about twice as common in the mandible as in the maxilla. Most of the tumours arise in the molar or premolar area and about half are associated with the crown of an unerupted tooth. Although most tumours arise within bone, extraosseous lesions have been reported.

Radiographs of intraosseous tumours show an irregular radiolucent area which may or may not be clearly demarcated from the surrounding normal bone. The radiolucency contains varying amounts of radiopaque bodies due to calcification within the tumour.

Histologically, the tumour consists of sheets and strands of polyhedral epithelial cells with abundant eosinophilic cytoplasm lying in a fibrous stroma. The epithelial cells often show prominent intercellular bridges and marked nuclear pleomorphism but the latter is not indicative of malignancy (Fig. 15.28). A characteristic feature is the presence within the sheets of epithelial cells of homogeneous, amyloid-like material which may become calcified. The calcifications are concentric laminated structures that may fuse into complex masses. The nature of the amyloid-like material is uncertain but is probably derived from products synthesized by the epithelial cells.

Although the tumour is locally invasive it appears to be less aggressive than the ameloblastoma.

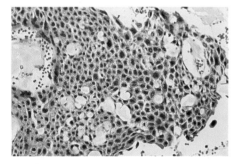

Fig. 15.28 Sheets of polyhedral epithelial cells with prominent intercellular bridges and nuclear pleomorphism in a calcifying epithelial odontogenic tumour.

Clear-cell odontogenic tumour

The clear-cell odontogenic tumour is a very rare intraosseous tumour that can occur in either the mandible or the maxilla. Few cases have been reported but most have presented in females over 50 years of age. Histologically, it is a poorly circumscribed tumour composed of sheets of cells with clear cytoplasm rich in glycogen lying in a fibrous stroma. It may be difficult to distinguish from other primary or metastatic clear-cell tumours. It behaves as a locally aggressive tumour with a high rate of recurrence.

Ameloblastic fibroma, ameloblastic fibrodentinoma, and fibro-odontoma

The ameloblastic fibroma is a rare benign tumour in which both the epithelial and mesenchymal elements are neoplastic. In ameloblastomas only the epithelium is neoplastic. It is important to differentiate the lesion from ameloblastoma since, unlike the latter, it does not exhibit a locally invasive growth pattern. It is a well-circumscribed lesion and does not require the radical excision that may be necessary to effect cure with the ameloblastoma. However, recurrence rates of about 18 per cent have been reported.

The ameloblastic fibroma usually occurs in a younger age-group than ameloblastoma and is uncommon over 21 years of age. It presents as a slowly enlarging painless swelling and arises most frequently in the premolar or molar region of the mandible. Radiographically, the tumour appears as a well-defined, usually unilocular, radiolucency.

Histologically, the tumour consists of proliferating strands and clumps of odontogenic epithelium lying in highly cellular fibroblastic tissue resembling the dental papilla of the developing tooth (Fig. 15.29). The epithelial component shows a peripheral layer of cuboidal or columnar cells which encloses a few stellate reticulum-like cells. The appearances are similar to ameloblastoma but the stellate cells are much less abundant and cyst formation is unusual. The richly cellular mesenchymal component is markedly different from the fibrous stroma of ameloblastoma. There may be a narrow cell-free zone of hyaline connective tissue bordering the epithelial component.

In some lesions dentine may be present and such tumours may be designated ameloblastic fibrodentinoma. The dentine is usually poorly formed and includes entrapped cells. Tubular dentine is rare. Tumours previously classified as dentinomas are now thought to be examples of the ameloblastic fibrodentinoma. In some tumours further inductive changes occur leading to the differentiation of ameloblasts and the formation of enamel. Such tumours may be designated ameloblastic fibro-odontoma but are extremely difficult to distinguish from developing complex odontomes.

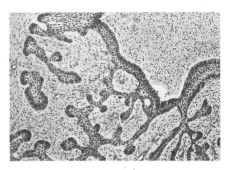

Fig. 15.29 Ameloblastic fibroma showing epithelial component resembling ameloblastoma and cellular mesenchymal component resembling dental papilla.

Ameloblastic fibroma and related lesions **Key points**
- clinically and histologically distinct from ameloblastoma
- odontogenic epithelium and cellular mesenchyme
- may include dentine and enamel
- well-circumscribed, non-invasive

Odontoameloblastoma

The odontoameloblastoma is an exceedingly rare tumour characterized by the combination of ameloblastoma-like tissue with enamel and dentine as irregular masses or small denticles. The lesion appears to behave as an ameloblastoma.

Adenomatoid odontogenic tumour

The adenomatoid odontogenic tumour usually presents during the second and third decades of life. The majority of tumours arise in the anterior part of the maxilla, especially in the canine areas, and there are usually few symptoms apart from a slowly enlarging swelling. On radiographs it usually appears as a well-defined radiolucency but in some cases calcification within the tumour may produce faint radiopacities. The lesion is often associated with an unerupted

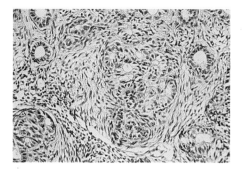

Fig. 15.30 Adenomatoid odontogenic tumour showing duct-like structures.

tooth and may simulate a dentigerous cyst. Very rare extraosseous lesions have been reported, most located in the anterior maxillary gingiva.

Histologically, the lesion is well encapsulated and may be solid or partly cystic; in some cases the tumour is almost entirely cystic. It consists of sheets, strands, and whorled masses of epithelium which in places differentiates into columnar, ameloblast-like cells. The columnar cells form duct or tubule-like structures (hence adenomatoid) with the central spaces containing homogenous eosinophilic material (Fig. 15.30). However, serial sections show that these structures are blind-ending; they are thought to represent abortive attempts at enamel organ formation. There is very little supporting stroma. Small foci of calcification are scattered throughout the tumour and occasionally tubular dentine and enamel matrix may be seen.

The nature of the lesion is uncertain and it may be hamartomatous rather than truly neoplastic. It must be differentiated from ameloblastoma. The adenomatoid odontogenic tumour is readily enucleated and does not recur: it does not require radical excision.

Calcifying odontogenic cyst

Despite the terminology applied to this uncommon lesion it is customary to group it with the odontogenic tumours rather than with the odontogenic cysts. Indeed, the term is not altogether appropriate since some lesions are solid and not cystic.

Clinically, the lesion occurs over a wide age range but is usually seen below 40 years of age. About 75 per cent are intraosseous and either jaw may be involved. The majority, including those located in the gingival or alveolar soft tissues, arise anteriorly to the first permanent molar tooth. The lesion usually presents as a slowly enlarging but otherwise symptomless swelling.

Radiographically, the lesion appears as a well-defined unilocular or multilocular radiolucent area containing varying amounts of radiopaque, calcified material. It may be associated with the crown of an unerupted tooth.

Histologically, the lesion is often cystic but may be solid. The cyst cavity (or potential cavity) is lined by epithelium which shows a well-defined basal layer of columnar, ameloblast-like cells and overlying layers of more loosely arranged cells that may resemble stellate reticulum. A characteristic feature (Fig. 15.31) is

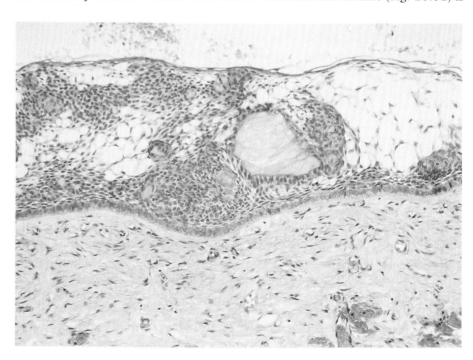

Fig. 15.31 Calcifying odontogenic cyst showing palisaded basal layer, stellate cells, and keratinized ghost cells.

the presence within the lining of masses of swollen and keratinized epithelial cells which are usually referred to as 'ghost' cells since the original cell outlines can still be discerned (Fig. 15.32). The 'ghost' epithelial cells may calcify. Breakdown of the epithelium may release keratinous debris into the supporting connective tissue resulting in a prominent foreign-body, giant-cell reaction. Irregular masses of dentine-like matrix material are frequently found in the supporting fibrous tissue in direct contact with the basal layer of the epithelium (Fig. 15.33). Less commonly, more extensive formation of dental hard tissues is seen, including enamel, producing a structure similar to a complex or compound odontome as an integral part of the lesion Calcifying odontogenic cysts associated with odontomes tend to occur in a younger age group and most have presented in the anterior maxilla.

The nature of the calcifying odontogenic cyst is uncertain but the great majority respond well to conservative treatment, such as enucleation and curettage. However, some appear to pursue a more aggressive course. It has been suggested that lesions designated as calcifying odontogenic cysts may represent two entities, one predominantly cystic and probably non-neoplastic, and the other a more solid and potentially aggressive neoplasm for which the term dentinogenic ghost-cell tumour has been proposed.

Odontogenic fibroma and myxoma

The odontogenic fibroma and myxoma of the jaws are derived from mesenchymal dental tissues. They may arise in relation to the root of a tooth, to the crown of an unerupted tooth, or may take the place of a tooth missing from the arch. These different presentations reflect the different mesenchymal tissues that may give rise to the tumours—periodontal ligament, dental follicle, and dental papilla.

The odontogenic fibroma, as defined by the WHO (1992), is a relatively uncommon, well-demarcated and readily enucleated benign fibroblastic neoplasm comprising mature collagenous tissue containing varying amounts of apparently inactive odontogenic epithelium. Foci of cementum-like material and dentine-like matrix may also be present. Other authors have also included the loose, thickened fibrous and myxoid tissues surrounding the crowns of some unerupted teeth under this heading. However, it is likely that such lesions represent thickened dental follicle rather than an odontogenic tumour.

A peripheral odontogenic fibroma is also recognized which may be indistinguishable clinically from a fibrous epulis. Histologically, it comprises fibrous or fibromyxoid tissue containing varying amounts of odontogenic epithelium and sometimes cementum or dentinoid material.

Myxoma of the jaws is a benign but locally invasive neoplasm and is more common than the odontogenic fibroma. Radiographically, it appears typically as a multilocular radiolucency (soap-bubble appearance) often with a well-defined margin, although, histologically, the lesion is non-encapsulated and has an infiltrative pattern of growth (Fig. 15.34). Roots of teeth involved by the tumour may show resorption.

Histologically, the tumour consists of stellate, fibroblast-like cells with long anastomosing processes, separated by abundant connective tissue ground substances, predominantly glycosaminoglycans (Fig. 15.35). Some cases contain a few strands of odontogenic epithelium. Variable amounts of collagen may be present and, in some cases, it is difficult to distinguish between myxoid change in a fibroma and fibrous change in a myxoma, hence such terms as myxofibroma and fibromyxoma.

Unlike the fibroma which is readily enucleated, the locally invasive growth of a myxoma makes complete removal difficult and predisposes to local recurrence.

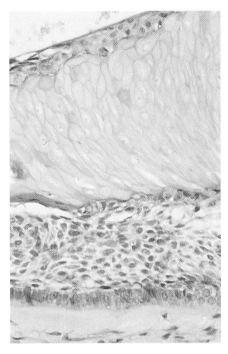

Fig. 15.32 High-power view of keratinized ghost cells in a calcifying odontogenic cyst.

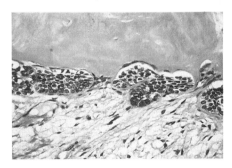

Fig. 15.33 Dentine-like matrix in a calcifying odontogenic cyst.

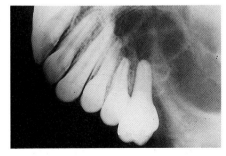

Fig. 15.34 Odontogenic myxoma presenting as a multilocular radiolucency.

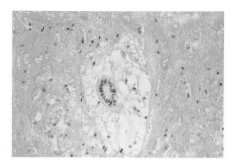

Fig. 15.35 Odontogenic myxoma stained by Alcian blue to show abundance of glycosaminoglycans in the stroma.

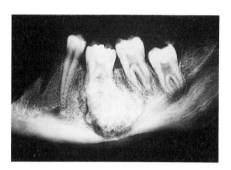

Fig. 15.36 Radiographic appearances of benign cementoblastoma.

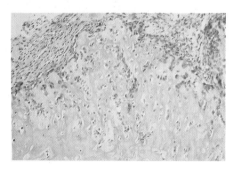

Fig. 15.37 Benign cementoblastoma showing central calcified material rimmed by cementoblasts.

Cementum-containing lesions

Lesions containing cementum or cementum-like tissue form a complex group with ill-defined characteristics. Several share similarities with primary diseases of bone and, since cementum-like material can be found in bone lesions in other parts of the skeleton they cannot be considered as unique odontogenic tumours. Because of this the WHO (1992), when revising the classification of the odontogenic tumours grouped lesions containing mixtures of bone and cementum-like tissue (cemento-ossifying fibroma, periapical cemental dysplasia, and florid cemento-osseous dysplasia) with neoplasms and other lesions related to bone, and they are discussed in Chapters 16 and 17. However, for the time being, at least, the benign cementoblastoma is still considered as an odontogenic tumour of cemental origin because of its unique association with the root of a tooth. Lesions which are not connected with a tooth are indistinguishable from osteoblastoma of bone.

Benign cementoblastoma (true cementoma)

This is a true benign neoplasm most frequently seen in patients under 25 years of age. It usually arises in the molar or premolar area of the mandible and is attached to the root of a tooth. Most cases involve the mandibular first permanent molar. It presents as a slowly enlarging swelling which sometimes gives rise to pain, but the involved tooth is vital. Radiographs show a well-demarcated, mottled or dense radiopaque mass with a radiolucent margin, attached to the root of a tooth which usually shows resorption (Fig. 15.36). Histologically, the tumour consists of a mass of calcified cementum-like tissue showing numerous criss-crossing reversal lines and containing scattered cells lying in lacunae. Around the periphery and in other actively growing parts of the lesion, extensive sheets of uncalcified matrix formed by plump, deeply staining cementoblasts may be seen (Fig. 15.37).

Malignant ameloblastoma

Exceedingly rarely, an ameloblastoma shows true malignant behaviour with development of metastases. In some instances, both the primary and metastatic deposits show histological features typical of ameloblastoma, and in such cases the possibility of seeding rather than of true metastatic spread has to be considered. Seeding, including aspiration into the lung, follows inappropriate surgical management, particularly in cases associated with repeated operations for multiple local recurrences. In other instances, the tumours show mitotic activity and varying degrees of cellular and nuclear atypia, and such lesions are sometimes referred to as ameloblastic carcinomas.

Primary intraosseous carcinoma

Carcinomas arising as primary growths within the jaws, unless related to a pre-existing cyst, are presumed to arise from residues of odontogenic epithelium and as such may also be referred to as odontogenic carcinomas. Tumours of this type are rare.

Malignant change in odontogenic cysts

Cases have been reported describing lesions which clinically and radiologically were diagnosed as odontogenic cysts (radicular, residual, dentigerous, and keratocysts) but which were found to be carcinomas on histological examination.

Such lesions could have resulted from malignant change in a cyst, but the possibilities of cystic degeneration in an existing carcinoma or of an existing carcinoma involving an otherwise unrelated cyst may be difficult to exclude.

Odontogenic sarcomas

The odontogenic sarcomas are exceedingly rare lesions, and are essentially fibrosarcomas containing non-neoplastic odontogenic epithelium and occasionally dental hard tissues.

TUMOURS OF DEBATABLE ORIGIN

Melanotic neuroectodermal tumour of infancy

This rare tumour occurs in infants usually between 1 and 3 months of age. It arises much more frequently in the maxilla than the mandible. The lesion may also be referred to as the pigmented tumour of the jaw of infants, although similar tumours have been reported from other sites in the body. It usually presents as an otherwise symptomless mass expanding the bone. Radiographically, the lesion is usually well defined and displaces the associated developing teeth.

Histologically, the lesion consists of varying proportions of epithelium-like cells containing melanin and small darkly staining round cells lying in a fibrous stroma.

The histogenesis of the tumour is uncertain, but there is good evidence that the lesion is derived from cells of neural crest origin. It is benign and recurrence is rare following conservative excision.

Congenital gingival granular cell tumour (congenital epulis)

This rare lesion occurs in new-born infants (Fig. 15.38) and is usually located in the incisor region of the maxilla. Females are affected about ten times more frequently than males.

Histologically, the lesion consists of large, closely packed granular cells and resembles the granular cell tumour (see Chapter 8) except that the covering epithelium does not show pseudo-epitheliomatous hyperplasia. Its nature and origin are unknown but it is probably reactive rather than truly neoplastic, and odontogenic, fibroblastic, neurogenic, and vascular origins have all been suggested. In any event, it is benign and does not recur following excision.

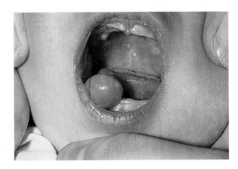

Fig. 15.38 Congenital gingival granular cell tumour (congenital epulis)

FURTHER READING

Ackermann, G. L., Altini, M., and Shear, M. (1988). The unicystic ameloblastoma: a clinicopathological study of 57 cases. *Journal of Oral Pathology*, **17**, 541–6.

Buchner, A. and Sciubba, J. J. (1987). Peripheral epithelial odontogenic tumours: a review. *Oral Surgery, Oral Medicine, Oral Pathology*, **63**, 688–97.

Budnick, S. D. (1976). Compound and complex odontomas. *Oral Surgery, Oral Medicine, Oral Pathology*, **42**, 501–6.

Daley, T. D. and Wysocki, G. P. (1994). Peripheral odontogenic fibroma. *Oral Surgery, Oral Medicine, Oral Pathology*, **78**, 329–36.

Fanibunda, K. and Soames, J. V. (1995). Malignant and premalignant change in odontogenic cysts. *Journal of Oral and Maxillofacial Surgery*, **53**, 1469–72.

Gardner, D. G. (1996). Some current concepts on the pathology of ameloblastomas. *Oral Surgery, Oral Medicine, Oral Pathology, Oral Radiology and Endodontics*, **82**, 660–9.

Goldblatt, L. I., Brannon, R. B., and Ellis, G. L. (1982). Squamous odontogenic tumour. *Oral Surgery, Oral Medicine, Oral Pathology*, **54**, 187–96.

Hansen, L. S., Eversole, L. R., Green, T. L., and Powell, N. B. (1985). Clear cell odontogenic tumour—a new histological variant with aggressive potential. *Head and Neck Surgery*, **8**, 115–23.

Hirshberg, A., Kaplan, I., and Buchner, A. (1994). Calcifying odontogenic cyst associated with odontoma. *Journal of Oral and Maxillofacial Surgery*, **52**, 555–8.

Kramer, I. R. H., Pindborg, J. J., and Shear, M. (1992). *Histological typing of odontogenic tumours* (2nd edn). World Health Organization International Classification of Tumours. Springer-Verlag, Berlin.

Leider, A. S., Eversole, L. R., and Barkin, M. E. (1985). Cystic ameloblastoma. *Oral Surgery, Oral Medicine, Oral Pathology*, **60**, 624–30.

Petola, J., Magnusson, B., Happonen, R.-P., and Borman, H. (1994). Odontogenic myxoma—a radiographic study of 21 tumours. *British Journal of Oral and Maxillofacial Surgery*, **32**, 298–302.

Philipson, H. E., Samman, N., Ormiston, I. W., Wu, P. C., and Reichart, P. A. (1992). Variants of the adenomatoid odontogenic tumour with a note on tumour origin. *Journal of Oral Pathology and Medicine*, **21**, 348–52.

Reichart, P. A., Philipsen, H. P., and Sonner, S. (1995). Ameloblastoma: biological profile of 3677 cases. *Oral Oncology, European Journal of Cancer*, **31B**, 86–99.

Slootweg, P. J. (1981). An analysis of the interrelationship of the mixed odontogenic tumours—ameloblastic fibroma, ameloblastic fibro-odontoma and the odontomes. *Oral Surgery, Oral Medicine, Oral Pathology*, **51**, 226–76.

Stirling, R. W., Powell, G., and Fletcher, C. D. M. (1988). Pigmented neuroectodermal tumour of infancy: an immunohistochemical study. *Histopathology*, **12**, 425–35.

Ulmansky, M., Hjørting-Hansen, E., Praetorius, F., and Hague, F. (1994). Benign cementoblastoma. A review and five new cases. *Oral Surgery, Oral Medicine, Oral Pathology*, **77**, 48–55.

Waldron, C. A. and El-Mofty, S. K. (1987). A histopathologic study of 116 ameloblastomas with special reference to the desmoplastic variant. *Oral Surgery, Oral Medicine, Oral Pathology*, **63**, 441–51.

16 Inherited, developmental, inflammatory, and metabolic disorders of bone

16 Inherited, developmental, inflammatory, and metabolic disorders of bone

The diagnosis of diseases of bone is often difficult and is established by a combination of clinical, radiological, histological, and biochemical investigations. The estimation of serum levels of calcium, phosphorous, and alkaline phosphatase are the principal biochemical investigations required.

INHERITED AND DEVELOPMENTAL DISORDERS OF BONE

Patients with inherited or developmental disorders of bone are infrequently seen in dental practice, partly because the disorders are uncommon and partly because jaw involvement may only be a minor feature or be absent altogether. Four of the more common inherited developmental disorders of bone are described in this chapter together with the fibro-osseous lesions. In addition, there are many types of developmental malformations of the head and jaws in which the structure of the bone is normal, for example those associated with cleft palate, but description of these is outside the scope of the book.

Osteogenesis imperfecta

This hereditary disease consists of a heterogeneous group of related disorders characterized by generalized osteoporosis with slender bones and a marked tendency for the bones to fracture on slight provocation. The slender long bones have narrow, poorly formed cortices composed of immature, woven bone, but fractures usually heal without trouble although exuberant callus may be formed. The skull is thin and tends to bulge over the ears but the jaws are seldom severely affected. The sclerae may appear blue because they are so thin that the pigmented choroid shines through (Fig. 16.1), and there is sometimes a family history of deafness caused by distortion of the ossicles in the ears. Other abnormalities which may be present are joint hypermobility with lax ligaments, thin translucent skin, and heart valve defects. Osteogenesis imperfecta is often associated with dentinogenesis imperfecta especially in the deciduous dentition (see Chapter 1) (Fig. 16.2), and it is thought the two defects are carried by separate but related genes. Recent findings confirm the idea that the basic biochemical abnormality is a defect in collagen synthesis involving type 1 collagen.

Four main types of osteogenesis imperfecta have been described (Table 16.1). Those inherited as autosomal dominant traits are the most common, but severe recessive forms and sporadic cases due to spontaneous mutation also occur. Type I is dominant and the commonest form, presenting with bone fragility, blue sclerae, and deafness. Marked long bone deformity is uncommon and affected infants rarely have multiple fractures. Type II is recessive and the most severe form. Multiple fractures occur *in utero* or during parturition and this type is

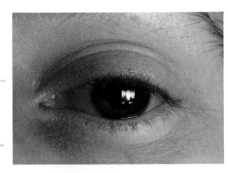

Fig. 16.1 Blue sclera in osteogenesis imperfecta Type I.

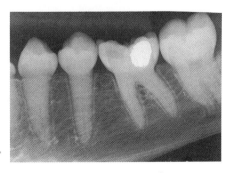

Fig. 16.2 Dentinogenesis imperfecta associated with osteogenesis imperfecta.

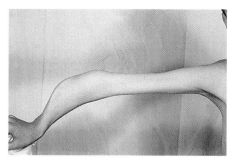

Fig. 16.3 Osteogenesis imperfecta associated with severe deformity of long bones.

Table 16.1 Subtypes of osteogenesis imperfecta

Type I	Childhood (tarda) type Blue sclera, autosomal dominant
Type II	Congenital/perinatal type Lethal, autosomal recessive
Type III	Progressive deformation trunk and long bones Autosomal recessive
Type IV	Similar to Type I White sclera, autosomal dominant

usually fatal within a few hours of birth. Type III is also recessive with fractures present either at birth or in the first year of life. The long bones are particularly affected and multiple fractures lead to progressive deformity (Fig. 16.3). Blue sclerae are present which become paler in adolescence. Type IV is dominant and resembles Type I, apart from the colour of the sclera. (White Sclera)

Osteopetrosis (marble bone disease)

This disease is characterized by excessive density of all bones with obliteration of marrow cavities and the development of a secondary anaemia. There appears to be a defect in osteoclastic activity and, as normal bone formation relies on the interdependence of deposition and resorption, there is a failure in the remodelling of the developing bone. There is, therefore, an excessive formation of bone which is mechanically weak and so fractures are common. The jaws are composed of dense bone with greatly reduced medullary spaces. Delayed eruption of teeth may occur and osteomyelitis is a common complication of tooth extraction.

There are two basic patterns of the disease. A malignant and progressive type is inherited as an autosomal recessive and occurs early in life with severe bone fragility and malformations resulting from multiple fractures. Death usually occurs before puberty. A benign autosomal dominant type also occurs in which the bone changes are less severe and the diagnosis may not be made until late in life. There may be repeated fractures following minor trauma, but in some patients the diagnosis is only made during the investigation of intercurrent illness.

Radiographic examination shows an increased density of the whole skeleton with no distinction between cortical and medullary bone. The base of the skull shows marked radiopacity whereas the vault is generally less dense. Jaw involvement is variable, the mandible being more frequently affected than the maxilla, and the density of the bone may render the roots of the teeth almost invisible on radiographs.

Histological examination of affected bones shows thickened cortices and reduced marrow cavities. There is a persistence of woven bone and a marked lack of mature, lamellar bone. The shapes of the trabeculae follow no specific arrangement.

Cleidocranial dysplasia (cleidocranial dysostosis)

This disease is transmitted as an autosomal dominant trait. It is characterized by abnormalities of many bones, but particularly of the skull, jaws, and clavicle. Dental anomalies are also common. A variety of abnormalities of the skull may be present, the fontanelles and sutures tend to remain open and the skull appears flat with prominent frontal, parietal, and occipital bones. The nasal bridge is also depressed. Partial or complete absence of the clavicles allows the shoulders to be brought forwards until they meet in the midline (Fig. 16.4). The maxilla may be

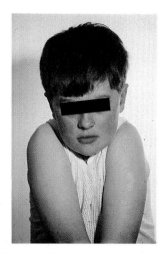

Fig. 16.4 Absence of clavicles in cleidocranial dysplasia.

underdeveloped with a high, narrow arched palate. The deciduous dentition tends to be retained with delayed or non-eruption of the permanent dentition because of multiple impactions (Figs 16.5, 16.6). Supernumerary teeth and dentigerous cysts are also common. The roots of the teeth tend to be thinner than normal and secondary, cellular cementum is either absent or sparsely present on both deciduous and permanent teeth.

Achondroplasia

This disorder may be inherited as an autosomal dominant trait, but many cases have no family history and appear to be due to spontaneous mutations. It is the most common form of dwarfism and is associated with an abnormality in endochondral ossification. There is an absence or a defect in the zone of provisional calcification of the cartilage in the epiphyses and in the base of the skull. The trunk and head are of normal size but the limbs are excessively short. The middle third of the face is retrusive due to defective growth of the base of the skull (Fig. 16.7) and severe malocclusion is common.

Inherited disorders of bone   **Key points**

- uncommon diseases
- jaw involvement variable
- orofacial manifestations include:
  —abnormalities in number, form, and structure of teeth
  —malocclusion
  —abnormal facial appearances

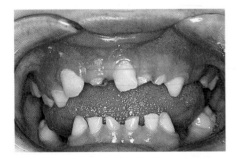

Fig. 16.5

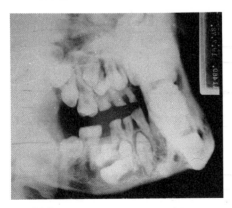

Fig. 16.6

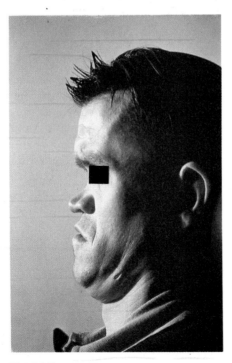

Fig. 16.7

Fig. 16.5 and 16.6 Retention of deciduous teeth with multiple impactions of permanent teeth in cleidocranial dysplasia.

Fig. 16.7 Retrusive middle third of the face in achondroplasia.

Table 16.2 Fibro-osseous lesions

A. *Non-neoplastic lesions*
Fibrous dysplasia
—monostotic
—polyostotic

Periapical cemental dysplasia
(periapical fibrous dysplasia)

Florid cemento-osseous dysplasia
(gigantiform cementoma)

B. *Fibro-osseous neoplasms*
Ossifying/cemento-ossifying fibroma

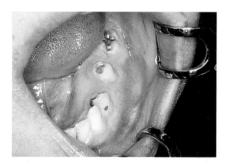

Fig. 16.8 Buccal expansion of the maxilla in fibrous dysplasia.

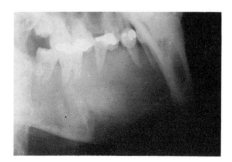

Fig. 16.9 Fibrous dysplasia of the mandible showing fusiform expansion.

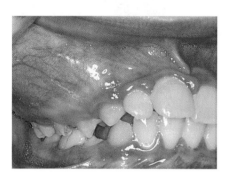

Fig. 16.10 Radiograph of the mandible in Fig. 16.9 showing increase in depth of the jaw and ground-glass appearance of bone.

Fibro-osseous lesions

The term fibro-osseous lesion is used to describe a variety of disorders which, histologically, are characterized by the replacement of normal bone by cellular fibrous tissue within which islands and trabeculae of metaplastic bone develop. They cannot be distinguished by histology alone and in their diagnosis the clinical and radiographic features must also be considered.

There is no general agreement on the number of pathological entities within this group or on their classification. The diseases included range from those associated with disorganized development (dysplasia) of bone through to benign neoplasms. In addition, as discussed in Chapter 15, some of the lesions previously placed within the cementoma group are now classified with the fibro-osseous lesions of bone. The main disorders are listed in Table 16.2. The non-neoplastic lesions are discussed in this chapter; fibro-osseous neoplasms are described in Chapter 17.

Fibrous dysplasia of bone

Fibrous dysplasia of bone may involve one or several bones in the body, and the terms monostotic and polyostotic are applied to these different forms of the disease.

Monostotic fibrous dysplasia

Monostotic fibrous dysplasia is much more common than polyostotic forms. Virtually any bone may be involved but the lesion arises most frequently in a limb bone, rib, or skull bone, particularly the jaws. Jaw lesions are more common in the maxilla than mandible. When the maxilla is affected, adjacent bones such as the zygoma and sphenoid may also be involved and the disease is then not strictly monostotic. However, since the distribution is restricted to contiguous bones within a defined anatomical area the pattern is not that typically associated with polyostotic disease. For these reasons, it has been suggested that the term craniofacial fibrous dysplasia is appropriate in such circumstances.

The majority of patients with monostotic fibrous dysplasia present in childhood or adolescence, but occasionally the disease is not diagnosed until adult life. Patients presenting in adult life may have been aware of a quiescent bony enlargement for some years and may give a history of recent expansion of the lesion which has prompted them to seek advice. Reactivation of quiescent lesions may occur for unknown reasons and has been reported in pregnancy.

In either jaw the first sign of the disease is a gradually increasing painless swelling which is not well circumscribed and which causes a gradually increasing facial asymmetry. The enlargement is usually smooth, often fusiform in outline, and is more pronounced buccally than lingually or palatally. When the maxilla is involved there is usually increased prominence of the cheek and buccal expansion distal to the canine, which may extend to involve the tuberosity (Fig. 16.8). The canine fossa is obliterated. Maxillary lesions commonly extend locally to involve the sinus, zygomatic process, and floor of orbit, and the orbital contents may be displaced. In some cases where growth is more rapid and extensive, there may be marked swelling of the cheek with exophthalmos and proptosis. Mandibular lesions occur most frequently in the molar and premolar regions and if the lower border is involved there may be an obvious protruberance and increase in depth of the jaw (Figs 16.9, 16.10). In either jaw there may be some malalignment, tipping, or displacement of teeth and in children any teeth involved by the lesion may fail to erupt.

Radiographically, the jaw lesions are variable in appearance and their borders are often difficult to define because of the gradual transition to a normal, uninvolved bone pattern. The variable appearances reflect differing amounts of metaplastic bone formed within the fibrous tissue of the lesions. The lesions may resemble cyst-like radiolucencies containing faint bony trabeculae but as the degree of trabeculation increases they become mottled and eventually opaque, the many delicate trabeculae giving a ground-glass or orange-peel-stippling effect on intraoral radiographs (Fig. 16.11). In some lesions there may be coarse mottling of smoke-screen pattern produced by irregular radiopaque masses lying in a radiolucent background. In the maxilla, lesions may extend up to and distort, but do not cross the suture lines.

Roots of teeth in the involved areas may be separated and the teeth may be displaced, but root resorption is exceptional.

Polyostotic fibrous dysplasia

Polyostotic fibrous dysplasia is two to three times as common in females as males and the distribution of lesions is very variable. They frequently occur in the bones of one limb, especially the lower, but the skull (Fig. 16.12), vertebrae, ribs, and pelvis are also often involved. Although almost any combination can occur there is a tendency for the lesions to arise segmentally and to be localized in one limb or on one side of the body.

Patients with severe polyostotic disease are usually diagnosed in childhood because of the associated bony deformities and pathological fractures. The disorder may be accompanied by patchy melanic pigmentation of the skin (*café-au-lait* spots). The polyostotic form may also present as Albright syndrome in which the bone lesions are accompanied by skin pigmentation, precocious puberty in females, and occasionally other endocrine abnormalities and premature skeletal maturation. Pigmentation of the oral mucosa has also been reported. The syndrome is very uncommon. A similar syndrome in males may occur without precocious puberty.

Pathology

Microscopically, the lesions show replacement of normal bone by fibrous tissue containing islands and trabeculae of metaplastic bone (Fig. 16.13), but the histological appearances of fibrous dysplasia of the jaws are more variable than in other bones.

The fibrous tissue may be richly cellular and show a whorled pattern or consist mainly of thick, interlacing collagen bundles.

Typically, the newly formed trabeculae of bone are delicate and of irregular shape resembling Chinese characters, and consist of immature, coarse-fibred woven bone (Fig. 16.14). In jaw lesions the trabeculae may be thicker and blunter than in long bones, and spheroidal areas of calcification resembling cementum may also be present. Osteoblastic and osteoclastic activity may be seen in relationship to some trabeculae and collections of osteoclast-like cells may also be present in the fibrous tissue at some distance from the bone, although these are seldom prominent. At the margins of the lesion the lesional bone fuses with that of the surrounding normal bone and it is this feature in particular which distinguishes the lesion from ossifying fibroma (see Chapter 17). It is suggested that with increasing age of the lesions the amount and cellularity of the fibrous tissue decreases whilst the amount of bone increases, although these are not constant features. As the lesion matures there is progressive remodelling of the woven bone to lamellar bone. Occasionally, the lesion may also be associated with the development of aneurysmal bone cyst (see Chapter 6).

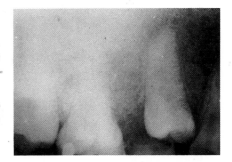

Fig. 16.11 Intraoral radiograph of fibrous dysplasia of the maxilla showing ground-glass/orange-peel stippling of bone.

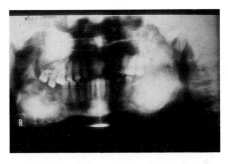

Fig. 16.12 Polyostotic fibrous dysplasia involving the skull with bilateral mandibular and right maxillary lesions.

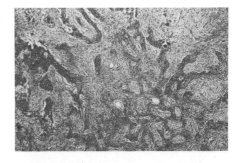

Fig. 16.13 Delicate trabeculae of metaplastic woven bone forming in fibrous tissue in fibrous dysplasia. The pattern of the trabeculae may resemble Chinese letters.

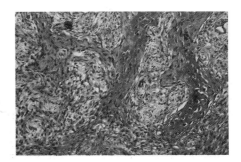

Fig. 16.14 Trabeculae of metaplastic, coarse-fibred woven bone forming in cellular fibrous tissue in fibrous dysplasia.

Key points	**Fibrous dysplasia**
	• more common in maxilla than mandible
	• lesions merge with surrounding normal bone
	• radiographic appearances reflect histological features
	• expansion stops with skeletal maturation
	• lesions tend to mature with increasing age

There are no consistent changes in blood chemistry, although the serum alkaline phosphatase level may be elevated in the polyostotic form depending on the severity of the disease.

Aetiology and behaviour

The aetiology of fibrous dysplasia is unknown. The disorder is not inherited but it is generally regarded as a developmental defect. This is supported by the age incidence, segmental distribution in the polyostotic form, and the natural history of the lesions, most of which expand during the period of active skeletal growth and become inactive in adult life. Occasionally, quiescent lesions become reactivated in adults for unknown reasons. The relationship of the monostotic to the polyostotic form is unclear but it is generally accepted that the former does not progress to the latter.

A few cases of malignant transformation of fibrous dysplasia have been reported, usually to fibrosarcoma, some of which have followed radiotherapy. However, the lesions of fibrous dysplasia are not radiosensitive and radiotherapy, which may increase the risk of malignant change, is not an acceptable treatment. The majority of cases are treated by conservative surgical removal of sufficient of the lesion to reduce deformity.

Periapical cemental dysplasia (periapical fibrous dysplasia)

This condition arises most frequently in the incisor region of the mandible in females over the age of 30 years and often involves several teeth. It is usually symptomless and is discovered as an incidental finding on routine radiographs. The disease closely resembles fibrous dysplasia of bone and is sometimes referred to as periapical fibrous dysplasia. Initially, there is a replacement of bone by cellular fibrous tissue around the apices of the involved teeth resulting in ill-defined radiolucent areas which must be distinguished from periapical granulomas. Periapical cemental dysplasia is of unknown aetiology; chronic inflammation is not implicated and the involved teeth remain vital. As the lesions mature cementum-like tissue and trabeculae of bone are deposited in the fibrous tissue resulting in increasing radiopacity. No treatment is required.

Florid cemento-osseous dysplasia (gigantiform cementoma)

The lesions of florid cemento-osseous dysplasia are often multiple and symmetrically distributed in the jaws, although solitary lesions may occur. The condition arises most frequently in middle-aged Negro females and there may be a family history. The usual complaint is of a painless swelling, slowly increasing in size. Radiographs show poorly demarcated, dense, lobular, radiopaque masses (Fig. 16.15), and histologically the lesions consist of dense, highly calcified, and almost acellular cementum (Fig. 16.16). The condition is referred to as 'florid' because of its extent and it may represent a florid variant of periapical cemental

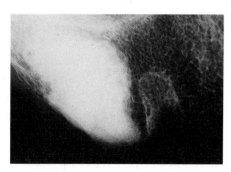

Fig. 16.15 Radiographic appearances of florid cemento-osseous dysplasia.

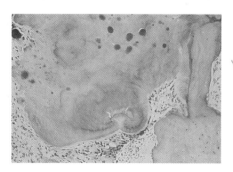

Fig. 16.16 Florid cemento-osseous dysplasia comprising mainly masses of acellular cementum.

dysplasia. It is likely that some cases previously reported as multiple enostoses or as diffuse chronic osteomyelitis are examples of florid cemento-osseous dysplasia.

Cherubism (Clinical appearance)

Cherubism is a rare dysplasia of bone inherited as an autosomal dominant character with variable expressivity. Males are affected about twice as frequently as females. The descriptive term cherubism relates to the unusual clinical appearance and facial deformity of patients with this disease. The condition is also known under a variety of synonyms, including familial multilocular cystic disease of the jaws which was applied on the basis of the radiographic appearance; the lesions themselves are not cystic.

Clinical and radiographic features

Children with cherubism appear normal at birth but painless swellings of the jaws appear between the ages of 2 and 4 years. The swellings are usually symmetrical and always involve the mandible either alone or in combination with the maxilla. They enlarge rather rapidly up to the age of about 7 years but then become static and begin to regress, with progressive reduction in the facial deformity, as the patient passes from puberty into adult life. The characteristic facial deformity is a fullness of the cheeks and jaws producing a typical chubby face (Fig. 16.17). There is often a rim of sclera visible beneath the iris due to stretching of the skin over the swellings or to upward displacement of the orbit by maxillary lesions, so that the eyes appear upturned to heaven. The chubby face and upturned eyes produce a cherubic appearance and the chubbiness is enhanced by fullness of the submandibular space due to enlargement of the submandibular lymph nodes. (Histologically, the nodes show reactive hyperplasia; they subside completely during adolescence.) Abnormalities of the dentition include premature loss of deciduous teeth and displacement, lack of eruption, and failure of development of many permanent teeth.

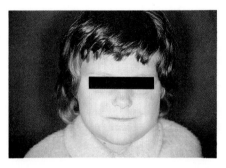

Fig. 16.17   Chubby face of cherubism.

Radiological examination shows sharply defined, multilocular radiolucencies (Fig. 16.18) with expansion and severe thinning of the cortical plates which may even be perforated. Mandibular lesions appear to begin near the angle and then spread to involve the body and ramus of the bone, although the condyle is spared. Maxillary lesions are often confined to the tuberosities but the sinus may be obliterated.

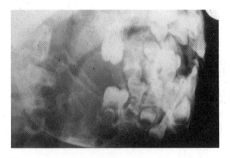

Fig. 16.18   Multilocular radiolucency of the mandible in cherubism.

Pathology and behaviour

Microscopically, the lesions consist mainly of cellular and vascular fibrous tissue containing varying numbers of multinucleate giant cells (Fig. 16.19). The giant cells resemble those found in other giant-cell lesions of bone and these conditions cannot be differentiated on the basis of histology alone. However, cherubism is unlikely to be confused with the others when the characteristic history and clinical features are taken into consideration. Hyperparathyroidism can be excluded by serum biochemistry, which in cherubism is normal, although serum alkaline phosphatase may be slightly raised during periods of rapid expansion of the lesions. The giant cells are distributed as focal collections, often around thin-walled vascular channels. In addition, many vessels are surrounded by a cuff of hyaline, eosinophilic collagen. Extravasated red blood cells and deposits of haemosiderin are common in the intercellular stroma. As the activity of the lesions decreases they become progressively more fibrous, the number of giant cells diminishes, and varying amounts of metaplastic bone are laid down.

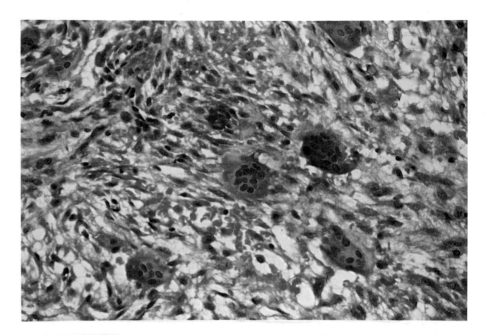

Fig. 16.19 Multinucleated giant cells in a vascular spindle cell stroma in cherubism.

Key points	**Cherubism**
	● family history
	● distinct clinical features
	● bilateral, symmetrical, multilocular radiolucencies
	● one of the giant-cell lesions of bone

As noted above, cherubism is a self-limiting condition and there is progressive improvement in facial appearance from about puberty onwards, but conservative cosmetic surgery is often required. Radiographically, the improvement in appearance may be accompanied by some bony infilling of the lesions but residual radiolucent areas can remain into old age.

HEALING OF BONE

Healing of an extraction socket

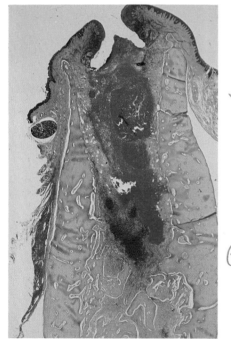

Fig. 16.20 Healing socket 7 days after extraction.

Following extraction of a tooth, the socket rapidly fills with extravasated blood which then clots. The blood clot is organized to form granulation tissue which consists of proliferating fibroblasts and endothelial cells derived from remnants of the periodontal membrane, the surrounding alveolar bone, and the gingival mucosa. Osteoclastic resorption of the crestal bone and small spicules of bone detached during the extraction also commences at this time. Gingival epithelial migration and regeneration occur across the defect, the epithelium migrating between the blood clot and the proliferating granulation tissue (Fig. 16.20). Epithelial continuity is restored 10–14 days after the extraction, the epithelium at first being thin with an irregular surface. Osteoblasts usually first appear in the granulation tissue towards the base of the socket and the granulation tissue is gradually replaced by woven bone. After approximately 6 weeks the regenerated epithelium over the socket appears normal, the supra-alveolar connective tissues have healed by repair, and the socket is filled with woven bone. However, the outline of the socket can still be discerned both histologically and radiologically (Fig. 16.21). Subsequently, this woven bone is remodelled with the formation of cortical and cancellous bone and disappearance of the lamina dura. Remodelling also includes a reduction in the height of the alveolar bone in the area of the extraction. Radiographically, the socket is generally obliterated between 20 and 30 weeks after the extraction.

Osseointegrated implants

Osseointegration has been defined as a direct, structural and functional connection between ordered, living bone and the surface of a load bearing implant. However, no implant has total surface contact with bone since varying amounts of bone marrow and other soft tissue may be interposed between the bone and the implant. In addition, electron microscopy has shown that even when bone and implant appear in direct apposition at the light microscope level, they are usually separated by an electron-dense, non-mineralized layer. For an implant to be successful it must be biocompatible; both titanium and ceramic implants are currently in use. The implant surface can also have a significant effect on bone apposition, a roughened surface, for example, having more bone contact and requiring greater forces to be displaced than a smoother surface.

In the preparation of the implant site, overheating of the bone must be avoided. Temperatures above 47°C increasingly lead to bone tissue damage which interferes with healing. Once the implant has been inserted into the bone, a healing period of up to 3 months is required, during which no load should be applied to the implant. As healing takes place, compact and cancellous bone forms around the implant together with a variable amount of fibrous marrow.

Osseointegrated implants penetrate the alveolar mucosa, and the interface between the implant and the soft tissues serves a similar barrier function to the dentogingival tissues around a tooth. In a successful implant, the alveolar connective tissue is in intimate contact with the implant post. Dense bundles of collagen fibres run predominantly parallel to the long axis of the implant. The gingival epithelium is arranged as a collar around the implant post, and is attached to the implant surface by a basal lamina and hemidesmosomes similar to that seen in normal junctional epithelium. The epithelium does not migrate apically along the post surface.

Plaque accumulation can lead both to inflammatory changes around the implant and to alveolar bone loss similar to that seen in chronic periodontal disease, especially if there is excessive implant load. Microbiological examination of plaque associated with implants shows a similar range of organisms to that found in plaque associated with chronic periodontal disease.

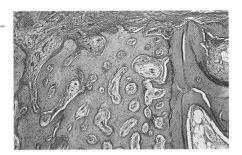

Fig. 16.21   Healing socket 6 weeks after extraction.

INFLAMMATORY DISEASES OF BONE

Inflammatory diseases of bone can be divided into three broad but overlapping categories depending largely on the extent of involvement of the bone. The term osteitis is generally used to describe a localized inflammation of bone with no progression through the marrow spaces, particularly that associated with infected sockets following removal of teeth (dry socket, see later). Osteomyelitis is a more extensive inflammation of the interior of the bone involving, and typically spreading through, the marrow spaces. Periostitis means inflammation of the periosteal surface of the bone and may or may not be associated with osteomyelitis.

Alveolar osteitis (dry socket)

This unpredictable complication in the healing of extraction wounds follows between 1 and 3 per cent of all extractions. It occurs most commonly following the extraction of a molar, particularly a lower molar, the incidence then decreasing when premolar and incisor teeth are extracted. It also occurs more commonly with difficult extractions, and the highest incidence of dry socket follows the extraction of impacted lower third molars. Tobacco use by the patient has also been identified as a risk factor.

Key points	**Alveolar osteitis**
	• incidence after surgical removal of impacted third molars 20–30 per cent
	• loss of protection by blood clot:
	—failure to form clot
	—dislodgement of clot
	—breakdown of clot

A dry socket is a localized inflammation of the bone following either the failure of a blood clot to form in the socket, or the premature loss or disintegration of the clot. Failure of a clot to form may be due to a relatively poor blood supply to the bone such as that found in osteopetrosis, Paget's disease of bone, or following radiotherapy, or it might result from the excessive use of vasoconstrictors in local anaesthetics. In cases where an adequate blood clot forms, the latter may be washed away by excessive mouth rinsing, or may disintegrate prematurely due to fibrinolysis of the clot most likely as a result of infection by proteolytic bacteria. No specific bacteria have been implicated, the infection being of mixed type.

Food debris, saliva, and bacteria collect in the empty socket, the bone of which becomes infected and necrotic. The inflammatory reaction in the adjacent marrow localizes the infection to the walls of the socket, as otherwise osteomyelitis would ensue. The dead bone is gradually separated by osteoclasts and a number of tiny sequestra may be formed. Healing is extremely slow and follows the proliferation of granulation tissue from the surrounding vital bone.

A dry socket is associated with severe pain developing a few days after the extraction. The socket often contains foul tasting and smelling decomposing food debris which can be washed away to reveal the denuded bone lining the cavity.

Focal sclerosing (condensing) osteitis

As discussed in Chapter 5 osteosclerosis is one of the sequelae of periapical inflammation and may result from low-grade irritation and/or high tissue resistance. It is generally seen at the apex of a tooth, most commonly the first permanent molar, and may remain as a sclerotic area of bone following extraction. It is usually asymptomatic. Histologically, a localized increase in the number and thickness of the bone trabeculae is seen and there may be scattered lymphocytes and plasma cells in the surrounding scanty fibrosed marrow.

Osteomyelitis

Although osteomyelitis of the jaws was a common complication of dental sepsis before the advent of antibiotics, it is now a rare disease. Various clinical subtypes were recognized, leading to confusion in terminology and classification, but some are now obsolete. However, rather than representing distinct forms of the disease, the variation in the clinical and pathological features of osteomyelitis are best considered as comprising a spectrum of inflammatory and reactive changes in bone and periosteum. These reflect the balance between the nature and severity of the irritant, the host defences, and local and systemic predisposing factors. The latter are listed in Table 16.3 and relate mainly to local factors which compro-

Table 16.3   Factors predisposing to osteomyelitis of the jaws

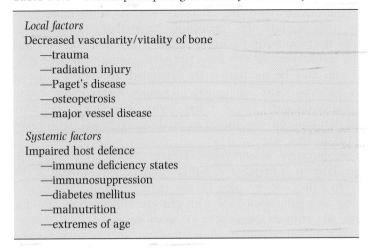

Local factors
Decreased vascularity/vitality of bone
 —trauma
 —radiation injury
 —Paget's disease
 —osteopetrosis
 —major vessel disease

Systemic factors
Impaired host defence
 —immune deficiency states
 —immunosuppression
 —diabetes mellitus
 —malnutrition
 —extremes of age

mise the vascularity and vitality of bone and to systemic conditions that compromise the defence systems of the host. Nevertheless, it is usual to distinguish between suppurative and sclerotic forms of osteomyelitis.

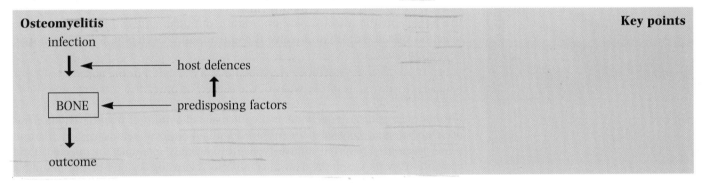

Osteomyelitis   **Key points**

 infection
     ↓ ←——— host defences
             ↑
  BONE ←——— predisposing factors
     ↓
 outcome

Suppurative osteomyelitis

Suppurative osteomyelitis is usually divided clinically into acute and chronic types depending on the severity of symptoms and on the course of the disease over time. Disease persisting for longer than a month is usually referred to as chronic suppurative osteomyelitis.

The source of the infection is usually an adjacent focus of infection associated with teeth (for example a dental abscess) or with local trauma (for example fractures, penetrating wounds, and extractions). A wide range of organisms may be involved and osteomyelitis of the jaws is usually a polymicrobial infection. Anaerobic organisms for example peptostreptococci and members of the 'black-pigmented bacteroides' group predominate. The mandible with its thick trabeculae and cortical plates and its main blood supply derived from the mandibular artery, an end artery, is much more frequently involved than the maxilla because the vascular supply is readily compromised. Thrombosis of the mandibular artery or of its branching loops can lead to extensive necrosis of bone. In contrast, there is a rich collateral circulation in the mid-face area and osteomyelitis of the maxilla is rare.

Following entry into the bone the organisms proliferate in the marrow spaces giving rising to an acute inflammatory reaction. Tissue necrosis and suppuration rapidly ensue and the necrosis may be widespread because of thrombosis of neighbouring vessels. Inflammation, suppuration, and necrosis continue and the marrow spaces become filled with pus. The suppurative inflammation tends to

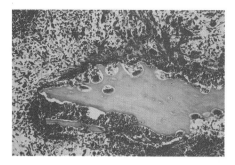

Fig. 16.22 Acute osteomyelitis showing osteoclastic resorption of necrotic bone and surrounding suppurative inflammation.

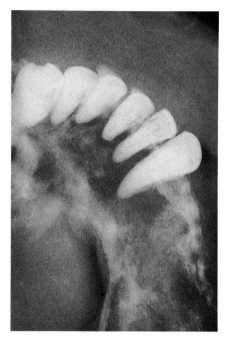

Fig. 16.23 Extensive destruction and moth-eaten appearance of bone in acute osteomyelitis of the mandible.

spread through the adjacent marrow spaces and may extend through the cortical bone to involve the periosteum. Stripping of the periosteum compromises the blood supply to the cortical plate and predisposes to further bone necrosis. Eventually a mass of necrotic bone (a sequestrum) which is bathed in pus becomes separated by osteoclastic activity from the surrounding vital bone (Fig. 16.22). The sequestrum may be spontaneously exfoliated through a sinus or have to be surgically removed before healing can take place. Radiographic examination may be normal in the early stages of the disease, but after 10–14 days sufficient bone resorption may have occurred to produce irregular, moth-eaten areas of radiolucency (Fig. 16.23).

Clinically, acute suppurative osteomyelitis presents with pain, swelling, pyrexia, and malaise. Trismus is frequent and there may be paraesthesia of the lip and mobility of teeth if they are involved. Disease of more chronic nature also presents with swelling and pain associated with chronic suppuration and discharge of pus through one or more intraoral or extraoral sinuses.

In contrast to adults, infantile osteomyelitis characteristically involves the maxilla, but this is now a rare disease. It is also referred to as neonatal maxillitis, but may present any time up to about nine months of age, and probably results from infection introduced during delivery or feeding. *Staphylococcus aureus* is the most common cause. Clinically, the disease is of sudden onset and presents with acute swelling, periorbital oedema, and severe constitutional symptoms. Pus in the nostril on the affected side and, later, multiple sinuses may be seen. The infection spreads rapidly to involve the antrum and developing teeth which may be sequestrated.

Sclerosing osteomyelitis

Chronic sclerosing osteomyelitis is a controversial condition whose existence has been questioned. Localized lesions are identical to focal sclerosing osteitis and some previously reported diffuse types are probably examples of infected florid cemento-osseous dysplasia. However, diffuse sclerosing lesions of the mandible have occasionally been reported as a complication of spread from a contiguous focus of low-grade infection/inflammation such as a periapical granuloma or pulse granuloma (see later).

So-called Garré's osteomyelitis is a distinct clinicopathological entity characterized by a proliferative subperiosteal reaction rather than inflammation of the interior of the bone. It is essentially a periostitis rather than osteomyelitis and is considered separately below.

Chronic osteomyelitis with proliferative periostitis (Garré's osteomyelitis, periostitis ossificans)

This type of sclerosing osteomyelitis is seen almost exclusively in the mandible in children and young adults. As discussed above, it is essentially a periosteal osteosclerosis presenting clinically as a bony hard swelling on the outer surface of the mandible. The periosteal reaction is thought to result from the spread of a low-grade, chronic apical inflammation through the cortical bone, stimulating a proliferative reaction of the periosteum. Occlusal radiographs show a focal subperiosteal overgrowth of bone with a smooth surface on the outer cortical plate. The subperiosteal mass consists of irregular trabeculae of actively forming woven bone with scattered chronic inflammatory cells in the fibrous marrow.

Occasionally, a proliferative periostitis may develop from overlying soft-tissue infection, or from the mechanical irritation of a denture. In these cases the endosteal bone is normal.

Chronic periostitis associated with hyaline bodies (pulse granuloma, vegetable granuloma)

An unusual form of chronic periostitis in the jaws is associated histologically with hyaline ring-shaped bodies accompanied by a foreign body, giant-cell reaction (Fig. 16.24). The nature and origin of these bodies is still debated, but there is now considerable evidence that they represent, at least in part, vegetable material, especially pulses, that has been implanted in the tissues. The type of inflammatory reaction is variable. In most cases it is associated with fibrous thickening of the periosteum, a proliferative periostitis, but in others there is chronic suppuration.

The vegetable material could gain access to the tissues via a tooth socket (when it may also cause delayed healing), a surgical flap, open root canal, or through some other breach in the mucosa, such as traumatic ulceration associated with ill-fitting dentures. Similar hyaline bodies are occasionally seen in association with apical granulomas and the capsules of odontogenic cysts following impaction of food debris down a root canal.

Radiation injury and osteoradionecrosis

Radiation, as part of the therapy of oral malignancy, affects the vascularity of the bone by causing a proliferation of the intima of the blood vessels (endarteritis obliterans). This can have serious consequences in the mandible with its end-artery supply, and the inferior dental artery or its branches may become thrombosed. The non-vital bone which results from the reduction in blood supply is sterile and asymptomatic (Fig. 16.25) but is very susceptible to infection and to trauma from a denture. Infection may spread rapidly through the irradiated bone, resulting in extensive osteomyelitis and painful necrosis of the bone, often associated with sloughing of the overlying oral and occasionally facial soft tissues. Modern methods of radiotherapy have greatly reduced the incidence of this condition.

METABOLIC AND ENDOCRINE DISORDERS OF BONE

The normal process of osteogenesis involving the formation of a collagenous matrix in which bone salts are deposited may be affected by a variety of metabolic diseases. For example, the formation of a collagenous matrix may be impaired by vitamin C deficiency (scurvy) or unknown factors as in idiopathic

Fig. 16.24 Chronic periostitis associated with hyaline bodies showing chronic inflammation and fibrosis. The hyaline ring or doughnut-shaped bodies are probably of vegetable origin.

Fig. 16.25 Partly resorbed osteoradionecrotic mandibular bone.

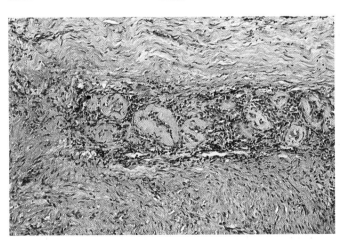

Fig. 16.24

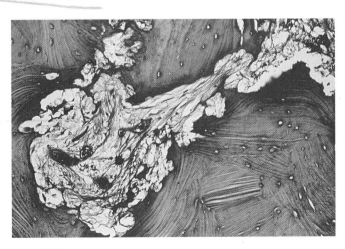

Fig. 16.25

osteoporosis, and an inadequate supply of bone salts such as in vitamin D deficiency (rickets) may affect the normal process of calcification. Homeostasis of calcium and phosphate metabolism is affected by the activity of the parathyroid glands, disturbances of which are associated with changes in bone.

Osteoporosis

Bone is in a state of constant turnover and in adult life bone loss gradually predominates over bone apposition. Osteoporosis results either when the bone loss is excessive or when the apposition of bone is reduced. A variety of risk factors have been identified, but the disease presents most commonly in postmenopausal women and in this group hormone replacement therapy significantly reduces the extent of bone loss. The rate of loss of bone mineral is variable but in most postmenopausal women is about 1–2 per cent per year. In about a quarter of cases more rapid loss, up to 5–8 per cent per year, may occur. The rate of loss is about twice as fast in women as in men. Osteoporosis is also accentuated in several other diseases, particularly Cushing syndrome, thyrotoxicosis, and primary hyperparathyroidism.

Osteoporotic bone is of normal composition but it is reduced in quantity. There is an increased radiolucency of bone, the cortex is thinned, and there are more marrow spaces in the cancellous bone associated with thin trabeculae.

The jaws may be involved, as may any other bone, but the condition is often asymptomatic. Bone pain, usually in the lumbar region following vertebral involvement, is a common complaint and fractures are much more frequent than in individuals with a normal bone structure. Osteoporosis occurring in edentulous patients may result in total disappearance of the alveolar ridges and loss of much of the basal bone. The mandible may be reduced to a thin fragile strip of bone, and in the maxilla there may be places where there is absence of bone separating the oral from the antral mucosa. It has been suggested that osteoporosis is a risk factor in chronic periodontal disease, but there is little supporting evidence.

Primary hyperparathyroidism

This relatively common disease is seen predominantly in middle-aged women and results from excessive parathormone secretion, usually from an adenoma but occasionally from carcinoma or idiopathic hyperplasia of a parathyroid gland. The effects of parathormone include stimulation of intestinal absorption of calcium, reabsorption of calcium by the renal tubules, and bone resorption by osteoclasts. Thus, excess secretion of the hormone results in hypercalcaemia and hypercalciuria. Pathological metastatic calcification may occur, commonly as urinary calculi but also in blood vessel walls and lungs.

Histologically, osteoclastic activity is increased throughout the skeleton and there is fibrosis of marrow (osteitis fibrosa). On occasions, focal areas of bone resorption result in the formation of lesions called brown tumours which consist of large numbers of multinucleate, osteoclast-like giant cells scattered in a highly cellular, vascular fibroblastic connective tissue stroma. There is much haemosiderin pigment present, hence the brown colour of these lesions seen macroscopically (Figs 16.26, 16.27). Histologically, it is impossible to distinguish a brown tumour of hyperparathyroidism from other giant-cell lesions of bone. Very rarely a focal collection of osteoclasts (brown tumour) may occur in relation to the periosteum and be indistinguishable from a peripheral giant-cell granuloma (giant-cell epulis, see Chapter 8). The possibility of hyperparathyroidism should be considered in patients with recurrent or multiple epulides.

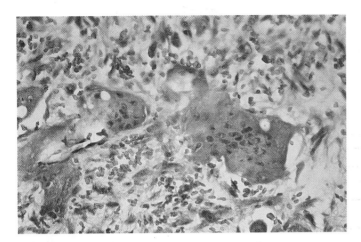

Fig. 16.26

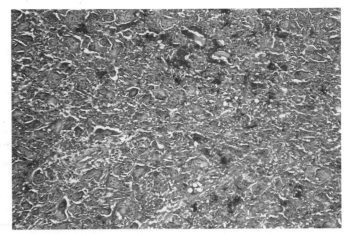

Fig. 16.27

Radiographic examination may show no detectable changes or a generalized osteoporosis. Partial loss of the lamina dura around the teeth may occur but it is not a constant feature. If focal lesions (brown tumours) develop, they present as sharply defined, round or oval radiolucent areas which may appear multilocular. Such lesions occur more frequently in the mandible than in the maxilla.

The biochemical changes of hyperparathyroidism have to be demonstrated for confirmation of the diagnosis. In addition to elevated levels of parathormone, they include a raised serum calcium level, a reduced serum phosphate level, and an increased urinary excretion of phosphate and calcium. Serum alkaline phosphatase levels may also be elevated.

Fig. 16.26 Brown tumour of hyperparathyroidism showing multinucleated, osteoclast-like giant cells.

Fig. 16.27 Brown tumour of hyperparathyroidism showing deposits of haemosiderin (brown).

Secondary hyperparathyroidism

Secondary hyperparathyroidism occurs in response to chronic hypocalcaemia, most frequently as a result of chronic renal failure but also in association with rickets and osteomalacia. The bone changes are complex and are a mixture of those associated with osteomalacia (see below) and hyperparathyroidism. Involvement of the jaws has been reported.

Key points

Metabolic bone disease
- osteoporosis is associated with enhanced atrophy of alveolar ridges
- hyperparathyroidism may present as a central giant-cell lesion of the jaws
- rickets is associated with dental abnormalities

Rickets and osteomalacia

Classically, rickets and its adult counterpart osteomalacia are due to deficiency of, or resistance to the action of, vitamin D. Deficiency may be due to lack of exposure to sunlight or dietary causes. In the UK dietary deficiency is seen mainly among the Asian immigrant population. In addition, the high cereal content of their diet and the use of wholemeal grains containing phytates impairs calcium absorption. Other causes of hypocalcaemia, such as renal failure or malabsorption, may also be associated with osteomalacia.

The radiographic changes are similar to those seen in osteoporosis, but in contrast to the latter, where the bone present is normally mineralized, in rickets and osteomalacia there is a failure of mineralization of osteoid and of cartilage.

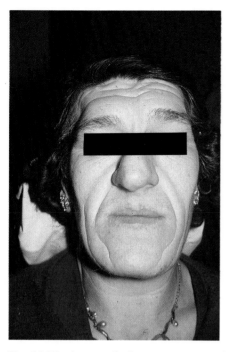

Fig. 16.28 Acromegaly showing coarsening of facial features.

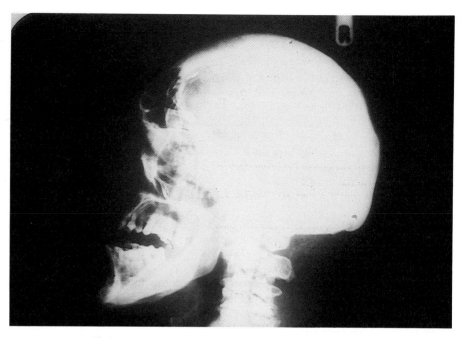

Fig. 16.29 Mandibular prognathism associated with acromegaly.

Histologically, the bony trabeculae in rickets and osteomalacia are characterized by wide seams of uncalcified osteoid.

Dental abnormalities in rickets include enamel hypoplasia, increased width of the predentine, and large amounts of interglobular dentine similar to the changes seen in vitamin D-resistant rickets—hypophosphataemia (see Chapter 1). In rickets and osteomalacia involvement of the jaws has been reported. In addition, in rickets, deficient growth of the condylar cartilage may lead to lack of growth of the vertical ramus of the mandible.

Acromegaly

This disease is caused by prolonged and excessive secretion of growth hormone, usually due to a secreting adenoma of the anterior lobe of the pituitary developing after the epiphyses have closed. There is renewed growth of the bones of the jaws, hands, and feet with overgrowth of some soft tissues. Activation of the condylar growth centre of the mandible causes the jaw to become enlarged and protrusive and if teeth are present they become spaced. The soft tissues of the face, particularly the lips and nose, become thickened and enlarged (Figs 16.28, 16.29).

FURTHER READING

Bjorvatn, K., Gilhuus-Moe, O., and Aarskog, D. (1979). Oral aspects of osteopetrosis. *Scandinavian Journal of Dental Research*, **87**, 245–52.

Devlin, H. and Ferguson, M. W. J. (1991). Alveolar ridge resorption and mandibular atrophy. A review of the role of local and systemic factors. *British Dental Journal*, **170**, 101–4.

Groot, R. H., van Merkesteyn, J. P. R., and Bras, J, (1996). Diffuse sclerosing osteomyelitis and florid osseous dysplasia. *Oral Surgery, Oral Medicine, Oral Pathology, Oral Radiology and Endodontics*, **81**, 333–42.

Harrison, J. D. and Martin, I. C. (1986). Oral vegetable granuloma: ultrastructural and histological study. *Journal of Oral Pathology*, **15**, 322–6.

Hudson, J. W. (1993). Osteomyelitis of the jaws: a 50-year perspective. *Journal of Oral and Maxillofacial Surgery*, **51**, 1294–301.

Koorbusch, G. F., Fotos, P., and Goll, K. T. (1992). Retrospective assessment of osteomyelitis. Etiology, demographics, risk factors, and management in 35 cases. *Oral Surgery, Oral Medicine, Oral Pathology*, **74**, 149–54.

Lockington, T. J. and Bennett, G. C. (1994). Osteoporosis and the jaws: questions remain to be answered. *Gerodontology*, **11**, 67–75.

Loza, J. C., Carpio, L. C., and Dziak, R. (1996). Osteoporosis and its relationship to oral bone loss. *Current Opinion in Periodontology*, **3**, 27–33.

Lukinman, P-J., Ranta, H., Ranta, K., and Kaitila, I. (1987). Dental findings in osteogenesis imperfecta (parts I and II). *Journal of Craniofacial Genetics and Development*, **7**, 115–25 and 127–35.

MacDonald, D. G. and Boyle, I. T. (1990). Skeletal diseases. In *Oral manifestations of systemic disease* (2nd edn) (ed. J. H. Jones and D. K. Mason), pp. 616–59. W. B. Saunders, London.

Nortje, C. J., Wood, R. E., and Grotepass, T. (1988). Periostitis ossificans versus Garré's osteomyelitis, Part II. Radiologic analysis of 93 cases in the jaws. *Oral Surgery, Oral Medicine, Oral Pathology*, **66**, 249–60.

Peters, W. J. N. (1979). Cherubism. A study of twenty cases from one family. *Oral Surgery, Oral Medicine, Oral Pathology*, **47**, 307–11.

Richardson, A. and Deussen, F. F. (1994). Facial and dental anomalies in cleidocranial dysplasia: a study of 17 cases. *International Journal of Paediatric Dentistry*, **4**, 225–31.

Waldron, C. A. (1993). Fibro-osseous lesions of the jaws. *Journal of Oral and Maxillofacial Surgery*, **51**, 828–35.

Waldron, C. A., Giansanti, J. S., and Browand, B. C. (1975). Sclerotic cemental masses of the jaws (so-called sclerosing osteomyelitis, sclerosing osteitis, multiple enostosis and gigantiform cementoma). *Oral Surgery, Oral Medicine, Oral Pathology*, **39**, 590–604.

Zachariades, N., Papanicolaou, S., Xypolyta, A., and Constantinidis, I. (1985). Cherubism. *International Journal of Oral Surgery*, **14**, 138–45.

17 Paget's disease, tumours, and tumour-like lesions of bone

17 Paget's disease, tumours, and tumour-like lesions of bone

PAGET'S DISEASE OF BONE

Paget's disease of bone was described by an English surgeon, Sir James Paget, in 1877 who proposed calling the condition 'osteitis deformans'. However, the disease is not inflammatory but is a form of osteodystrophy characterized by disorganized formation and remodelling of bone, unrelated to functional requirements. The aetiology of the disease still remains unclear, but it is thought to be due to a primary dysfunction of osteoclasts and there is evidence that the disease has a viral aetiology. Viral-like inclusions similar to those seen in paramyxovirus infections have been identified which resemble those of measles virus or respiratory syncytial virus. Measles virus DNA and RNA have also been identified in osteoclasts and other bone cells in Paget's disease using *in situ* hybridization techniques. The paramyxoviruses also include canine distemper and dog ownership has been linked with Paget's disease. It has been suggested that Paget's disease is a slow-virus disorder and that following childhood infection with a paramyxovirus viral DNA becomes integrated into the genome of osteoclast progenitor cells. A variety of other cofactors, including genetic factors, may then be involved before the disease becomes manifest in adult life.

The natural history of the disease can be divided into three progressive and overlapping phases:

(1) an initial predominantly osteolytic phase;

(2) an active stage of mixed osteolysis and osteogenesis; and

(3) a predominantly osteoblastic or sclerotic phase.

In the first two phases the bones become softened and distorted and their overall size may be markedly increased. In the sclerotic phase, the distorted bones become fixed in their deformed state (hence 'deformans').

Paget's disease of bone
Key points
- probably a slow-virus infection
- enlargement and deformity of bones
- rare under 40 years of age
- geographical variations in incidence

Clinical and radiographic features

Paget's disease occurs predominantly in patients over 40 years of age and there is a slight preponderance of males. Subclinical disease is not uncommon and radiological surveys and autopsy studies have demonstrated an incidence of about 3 per cent in all persons over 40 years of age. However, there are striking

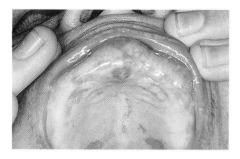

Fig. 17.1 Enlargement of the maxilla in Paget's disease of bone.

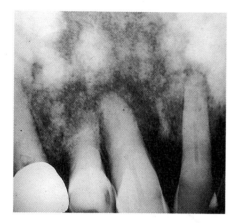

Fig. 17.2 Cotton-wool appearance of bone in Paget's disease.

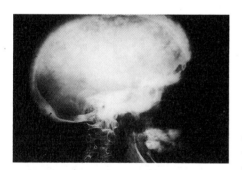

Fig. 17.3 Paget's disease of the skull showing thickening of the calvarium, with loss of distinction between the tables and the diploe, and maxillary lesions.

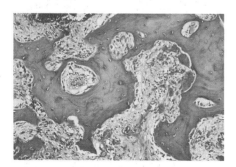

Fig. 17.4 Disorganized remodelling of bone in Paget's disease with simultaneous osteoclastic and osteoblastic activity.

differences in geographical incidence; it is rare in Russia, Asia, and parts of Europe but is common in the United Kingdom, Australasia, and North America. The lesions may involve a single or small number of bones or, less commonly, may be disseminated widely throughout the skeleton. They are commonest in the weight-bearing bones of the axial skeleton particularly the sacrum, followed by lumbar, thoracic, and cervical vertebrae. The skull and femur are the next most frequent sites. Jaw lesions are more common in the maxilla than mandible and although monostotic lesions have been reported, when the jaws are involved the skull is almost invariably affected.

Clinically, patients with Paget's disease show varying degrees of bony deformity and distortion of the weight-bearing portions of the skeleton with curvature of the spine and bowing of the legs being common. The latter results in a characteristic waddling gait. Despite the gross thickening of bones that occurs, they are mechanically weaker than normal and pathological fractures are not infrequent. The progressive enlargement of the skull and facial bones can produce marked deformity, and in the past the need to buy hats of progressively increasing size was one of the classical presenting symptoms. Other common complaints are bone pain, and sensory and motor disturbances related to cranial nerves. These include blindness, deafness, and facial paralysis and are due to compression of nerves as they exit through foramina in the base of the skull. With progressive enlargement of the maxilla, the alveolar ridge becomes thickened and widened, the palate flattened (Fig. 17.1), and there is increasing facial deformity. The bony enlargement may lead to incompetence of the lips. In dentate patients, derangement of the occlusion, spacing of the teeth, and retroclination of incisors and palatoversion of posterior teeth may be striking. In edentulous patients, difficulties in wearing dentures and the need to have these remade periodically as the jaws increase in size, are common complaints. Other important oral manifestation are related to involvement of the teeth which often show hypercementosis and may become ankylosed, leading to difficulty in extraction. Root resorption may also occur in the osteolytic phase. In the active stages of the disease, postextraction haemorrhage may be a problem because of the highly vascular marrow which contains extensive arteriovenous communications. In contrast, in the later sclerotic phase the bone is relatively dense and avascular and extraction sockets are prone to infection.

The radiographic features are variable but reflect the different stages of the disease. Osteoporosis is the earliest change, followed by patchy osteosclerosis and the appearance of ill-defined and irregular radiopaque areas producing a characteristic cotton-wool appearance (Fig. 17.2). In the skull, thickening of the outer table of the vault and loss of distinction between the tables and diploe are also typical features (Fig. 17.3). In the jaws, loss of the lamina dura, hypercementosis, and ankylosis may be noted.

Pathology

The microscopic features of Paget's disease reflect the disorganized bone remodelling which is a feature of the disease, and the lesions show combinations of osteoclastic and osteoblastic activity unrelated to normal function. During the early osteoporotic phase, osteoclastic resorption predominates. The resorbed areas are filled by cellular and vascular fibrous marrow within which new bone forms and this in turn is remodelled and replaced by further new bone. This disorganized remodelling activity is repeated and in fully developed active lesions there is simultaneous osteoclastic and osteoblastic activity involving most of the trabeculae (Fig. 17.4). The osteoclasts are often much larger than normal and contain a great many nuclei. As a result of the remodelling activity the bone trabeculae show numerous criss-crossing, resting, and scalloped reversal lines which stain deeply with haematoxylin. These criss-crossing lines give the bone a characteristic mosaic appearance (Fig. 17.5). Reversal lines indicate junctions where there has been reversal of osteoclastic to osteoblastic activity and their scalloped outlines represent the margins of the previously existing Howship's lacunae. As more and more bone is formed within the lesion, the disjointed trabeculae fuse to form dense sclerotic masses of mosaic bone. As the disease becomes less active so the marrow becomes less vascular, and osteoclastic and osteoblastic activity is decreased. In the jaws, the new bone is often in the form of acellular globular deposits which enlarge and fuse to form dense sclerotic masses (Fig. 17.6). These, in turn, may fuse with the hyperplastic cementum covering the roots of the teeth, resulting in ankylosis (Fig. 17.7).

The cementum may also undergo disorganized remodelling and consequently may show the characteristic mosaic appearance.

Investigation of the blood chemistry is important in the diagnosis of Paget's disease. The serum calcium and serum phosphorus levels are usually within normal limits but the serum alkaline phosphatase level is often raised, sometimes markedly so in patients with widespread active disease.

Complications

In addition to complications which may arise because of the bone alterations, patients with Paget's disease may develop high output cardiac failure as a result of shunting of blood through arteriovenous anastomoses in the marrow of affected bones. Sarcomatous change is a rare complication occurring in about 0.1–0.2 per cent of patients overall. The risk is higher in those with widespread disease as opposed to those where only one or a small number of bones are affected. Osteosarcoma is the commonest type of malignancy.

Paget's disease of bone   **Key points**

- jaw lesions more common in maxilla
- cotton-wool appearance on radiographs
- reversal lines; mosaic bone
- complications with dental extractions
- cranial nerve compressions

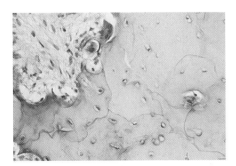

Fig. 17.5 Mosaic appearance of bone in Paget's disease.

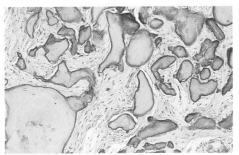

Fig. 17.6 Acellular globular masses of cementum-like tissue in Paget's disease of the jaws.

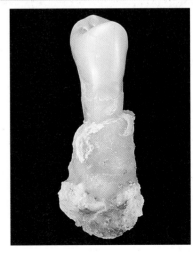

Fig. 17.7 Hypercementosis with ankylosis to aveolar bone in Paget's disease of the jaws.

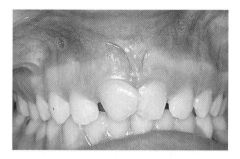

Fig. 17.8

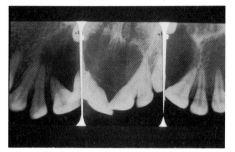

Fig. 17.9

Figs 17.8, 17.9 Central giant-cell granuloma presenting with displacement of the central incisors associated with well-defined radiolucent lesion.

CENTRAL GIANT-CELL GRANULOMA

This condition may occur at any age but presents most frequently in the second and third decades. There is a female predominance. It involves the mandible more frequently than the maxilla and most arise in the anterior part of the jaws. The lesion usually presents clinically as a swelling of the bone, and growth may sometimes be rapid. When the cortical plate is perforated the lesion may present as a peripheral giant-cell granuloma (see Chapter 8). Some cases are symptomless and are first detected on routine radiological examination. Radiographically, the lesion appears as a well-defined radiolucent area with thinning and often expansion of the cortex. Some are characteristically multilocular but the appearances are not specific and cannot be distinguished from other causes of multilocular radiolucent areas. Involved teeth may be displaced and their roots may show resorption (Figs 17.8, 17.9).

Histological examination shows large numbers of multinucleate, osteoclast-like giant cells lying in a vascular stroma which is rich in small, spindle-shaped cells having oval or fusiform nuclei (Fig. 17.10). The giant cells may be arranged in focal aggregates or be scattered throughout the lesion, although they are often related to vascular channels. The spindle cell component probably consists predominantly of mononuclear precursors of the giant cells, but includes fibroblasts and endothelial cells. Foci of extravasated erythrocytes and granules of haemosiderin pigment are common in the stroma. Sparse strands of collagen fibres partly subdivide the lesion which may also contain a few trabeculae of osteoid or bone (Fig. 17.11).

Key points	Central giant-cell granuloma
	• most patients less than 30 years of age
	• more common in mandible than maxilla
	• histologically indistinguishable from other giant-cell lesions of bone: —cherubism —brown tumour of hyperparathyroidism —giant-cell tumour —aneurysmal bone cyst

Central giant-cell granuloma is a condition of unknown aetiology. It has been suggested that it could be a reaction to some form of haemodynamic disturbance in bone marrow perhaps associated with trauma and haemorrhage. The majority respond well to simple enucleation and curettage, but some pursue a more aggressive course and have a tendency to recur. The central giant-cell

Fig. 17.10 Central giant-cell granuloma showing collections of multinucleated osteoclast-like giant cells in a vascular spindle cell stroma.

Fig. 17.11 Trabeculae of newly forming bone in a central giant-cell granuloma.

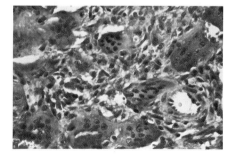

Fig. 17.10

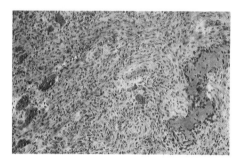

Fig. 17.11

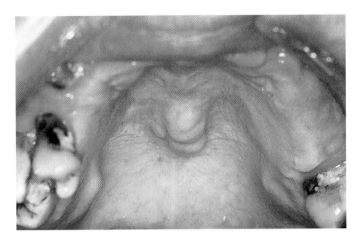

Fig. 17.12 Torus palatinus.

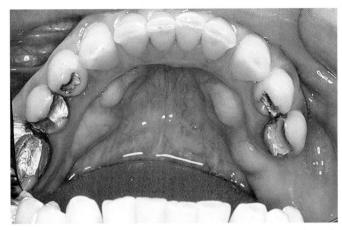

Fig. 17.13 Torus mandibularis.

granuloma is impossible to distinguish histologically from a focal lesion of hyper-parathyroidism (brown tumour—see Chapter 16) which must be excluded by biochemical investigations.

TORUS PALATINUS, TORUS MANDIBULARIS, AND OTHER EXOSTOSES

The term exostosis is used clinically to describe a variety of bony outgrowths. It implies a non-neoplastic lesion that may be of developmental origin or that may have arisen in response to a stimulus such as a chronic trauma (a reactive exostosis).

A torus is an exostosis which occurs at a characteristic site, either in the midline of the palate (torus palatinus) (Fig. 17.12) or on the lingual surface of the mandible, usually in the premolar region above the mylohyoid line (torus mandibularis) (Fig. 17.13). Mandibular tori are frequently bilateral. Palatal tori are more common than mandibular tori. Their aetiology is unknown and the two conditions do not appear to be related except for evidence suggesting heredi-tary factors, an autosomal dominant pattern of inheritance being reported in some patients.

Tori are rarely seen in childhood and have a slow growth. They may vary considerably in size and shape, ranging from flat and small elevations to large, nodular growths. They may be composed entirely of dense, cortical bone or consist of cancellous bone with a shell of cortical bone. The lesions are entirely benign and need to be removed only for cosmetic reasons or before the construc-tion of a denture.

Exostoses are seen occasionally in other parts of the jaw and may be multiple, particularly on the buccal alveolus in the molar region of the maxilla (Fig. 17.14). Irregularities of the alveolus following tooth extraction are also often described clinically as exostoses, as is enlargement of the genial tubercle in eden-tulous patients. The distinction between an exostosis and an osteoma is often difficult to determine.

TUMOURS OF BONE

Primary tumours of bone are uncommon lesions in the jaws. They may arise from any of the number of different cells and tissues present in bone, including

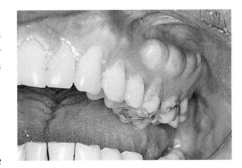

Fig. 17.14 Multiple exostoses of the maxilla.

Table 17.1   Classification of tumours of bone

Bone-forming tumours
  (a) Benign: osteoma
                   osteoblastoma
  (b) Malignant: osteosarcoma

Cartilage-forming tumours
  (a) Benign: chondroma
                   osteochondroma
  (b) Malignant: chondrosarcoma

Giant-cell tumour

Marrow tumours
  (a) Myeloma
  (b) Other types

Fibrous tumours
  (a) Benign: cemento-ossifying
                   fibroma
  (b) Malignant: fibrosarcoma of
                   bone

Tumour-like lesions in bone
  (a) Langerhans cell histiocytosis
  (b) Haemangioma of bone

Metastatic tumours

cartilage, marrow, vascular, and fibrous tissues. Their classification is complex, and while many lesions are recognized not all have been recorded in the jaws. The abridged classification used in this chapter is given in Table 17.1. It is based on that recommended by the World Health Organization, which seeks to define the tumours in terms of the type of differentiation of the tumour cells and especially the differentiation of the intercellular material (if any) formed by them. For convenience, the Langerhans cell histiocytosis group has been included in the classification since destructive lesions in the jaws are a feature of these disorders.

Osteoma

An osteoma is a benign, slow-growing tumour consisting of well-differentiated mature bone. It may arise as a central or subperiosteal lesion and is more frequent in the mandible than maxilla. The majority of tumours are diagnosed in adult life. Differentiation of a subperiosteal osteoma from a reactive exostosis and of a central lesion from enostosis (sclerosis) is difficult, but persistent slow growth and radiographic evidence of a clearly circumscribed lesion suggest a benign neoplasm (Figs 17.15, 17.16). Histologically, osteomas can be divided into compact (or ivory) and cancellous types. The compact osteoma (Fig. 17.17) consists of a mass of dense lamellar bone with few marrow spaces, the cancellous (Fig. 17.18) type is made up of interconnecting trabeculae enclosing fatty or fibrous marrow.

Although usually solitary, multiple osteomas of the jaws occur as a feature of Gardner syndrome. The latter is a rare familial disorder transmitted as an autosomal dominant trait. Other components of the syndrome include polyposis coli, which shows a marked tendency to undergo malignant change, and multiple fibrous tumours and epidermal/sebacaeous cysts of the skin. Multiple impacted supernumerary and permanent teeth may be found. Although rare, the initial signs are often in the facial region and it is important that they are recognized since a favourable prognosis depends on early diagnosis.

Osteoblastoma

Osteoblastoma is a rare tumour in the jaws (cementoblastoma is its odontogenic equivalent—see Chapter 15) and may present with dull, low-grade pain. Radiographically, it is well circumscribed and may be surrounded by a reactive sclerosis. The central area may appear radiolucent or speckled depending on the amount of calcified bone formed within the lesion.

Histologically, the tumour is richly cellular consisting of proliferating osteoblasts, multinucleated giant cells, and varying amounts of osteoid in a richly vascular fibrous stroma.

Osteosarcoma

Osteosarcoma is the commonest primary malignant tumour of bone but is relatively rare in the jaws. Most patients with jaw tumours are around 30 years of age at diagnosis and this is about a decade later than for osterosarcoma elsewhere in the skeleton. Occasionally, the tumour presents in older patients, for example in association with Paget's disease of bone, and rarely as a complication of radiotherapy given for the treatment of some other bone disease.

In the jaws, osteosarcoma is slightly more common in the mandible than maxilla. The tumour presents as a fairly rapidly enlarging swelling that may be accompanied by pain, numbness of the lip, trismus, and displacement and loosen-

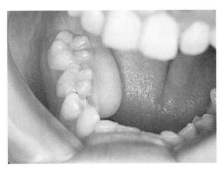

Fig. 17.15

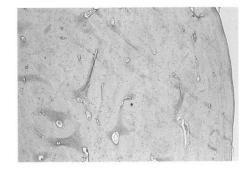

Fig. 17.17

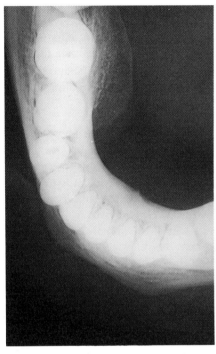

Fig. 17.16

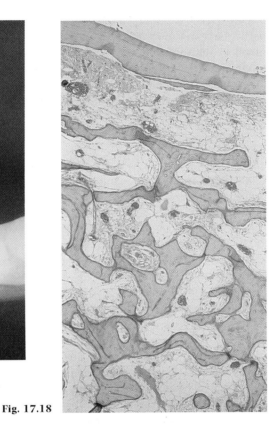

Fig. 17.18

Figs 17.15, 17.16 Clinical and radiographic appearance of a subperiosteal osteoma of the mandible.

Fig. 17.17 Compact (ivory) osteoma.

Fig. 17.18 Cancellous osteoma.

ing of teeth. Nasal obstruction and symptoms referable to the eye may also be features of maxillary tumours. Ulceration of overlying skin or mucosa is a late feature.

The radiographic appearances are variable and depend on the amount of normal bone destroyed by the tumour and the amount of neoplastic bone formed within the lesion. Predominantly osteolytic tumours produce irregular areas of radiolucency whereas sclerosing types, in which much tumour bone is formed, produce irregular areas of radiopacity (Fig. 17.19). The two patterns may coexist in different parts of the same tumour. When the cortical plates are perforated, the periosteum is raised and the tumour may extend into the surrounding soft tissues. This may be associated with a characteristic radiographic appearance in which trabeculae of bone radiate perpendicularly around the lesion producing the classical sun-ray appearance. A symmetrically widened periodontal ligament space has been reported as a feature of very early lesions.

Microscopically, osteosarcomas show considerable variation in pattern, but by definition are malignant tumours characterized by the direct formation of bone or

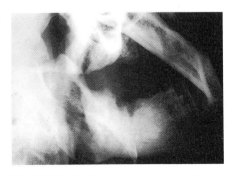

Fig. 17.19 Radiographic appearances of osteosarcoma of the mandible.

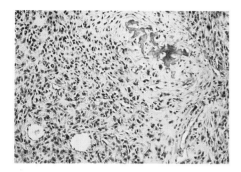

Fig. 17.20 Cytologically malignant cells associated with direct formation of malignant bone (top right) in osteosarcoma.

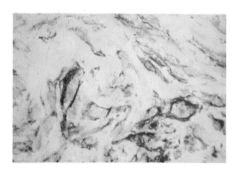

Fig. 17.21 Alkaline phosphatase activity (red reaction product) in malignant osteoblasts.

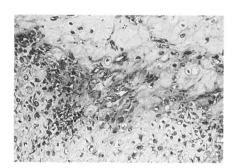

Fig. 17.22 Chondrosarcoma.

osteoid by the tumour cells (Fig. 17.20). In addition to bone and osteoid (osteoblastic type) the malignant cells may produce abundant fibrous tissue (fibroblastic type) and/or cartilage (chondroblastic type) and the appearances may simulate fibrosarcoma or chondrosarcoma. The histochemical demonstration of alkaline phosphatase activity helps to identify the malignant osteoblasts, which are strongly positive (Fig. 17.21).

The various histological patterns seen in osteosarcoma do not appear to affect the prognosis to any great extent, but chondroblastic and fibroblastic types have slightly better survival rates. The overall 5-year survival rate for osteosarcoma of the jaws is about 40 per cent. In contrast to osteosarcomas at other sites, jaw lesions metastasize infrequently but local recurrence rates are high, leading eventually to death from uncontrolled local disease.

The juxtacortical, or parosteal, osteosarcoma is a rare form of osteosarcoma, particularly in the jaws, but is considered as a distinct type since the prognosis is much better than for other osteosarcomas. As the term indicates, the tumour grows from the external surface of a bone. Histologically, it is a well-differentiated, highly ossified lesion and the neoplastic cells show little pleomorphism, which reflects the low-grade malignancy of the tumour. The 5-year survival rate is 85 per cent or better.

Chondroma and chondrosarcoma

Chondroma and chondrosarcoma are rare tumours in the jaws but they present problems to the diagnostic histopathologist, since it may be difficult to distinguish in some cases between benign and malignant growths. Any intraosseous cartilagenous tumour in the jaws should be regarded with suspicion.

The anterior part of the maxilla and posterior part of the mandible are the most common sites of occurrence, but mandibular tumours may also originate at the symphysis and in the condylar and coronoid processes. In the condylar processes, diagnosis is further complicated because of the difficulty in distinguishing cartilagenous hyperplasia from true benign neoplasia. However, these are rare sites for primary chondrosarcoma. In the anterior maxilla, cartilage-forming tumours must be distinguished from cartilagenous rests which may be found in the incisive fossa.

Histologically, a chondroma is a benign tumour characterized by the formation of mature cartilage. However, the presence of a high degree of cellularity and of plump, often binucleate cells should alert suspicion that the tumour is a well-differentiated chondrosarcoma. Less well-differentiated chondrosarcomas may show obvious cytological features of malignancy (Fig. 17.22). Calcification and endochondral ossification may occur in both benign and malignant tumours and this is reflected in their variable radiographic appearances. It is important to differentiate ossification in a chondrosarcoma from a chondroblastic osteosarcoma; direct bone formation by malignant cells is seen only in osteosarcoma.

The prognosis for chondrosarcoma of the jaws is better for mandibular compared to maxillary lesions (reflecting the problems of achieving clearance by radical surgery) and for well-differentiated compared to poorly differentiated neoplasms. Five-year survival rates vary from about 30 per cent to 80 per cent in different reported series. Metastases are rare, but local recurrences are common and may show a higher grade of malignancy than the original tumour. Most patients die as a result of uncontrolled local disease.

Osteochondroma

Osteochondroma usually presents in childhood or adolescence and may be hamartomatous rather than truly neoplastic. The tumour is usually pedunculated and consists of a core of mature bone capped by hyaline cartilage with active endochondral ossification at its junction. It tends to stop enlarging with cessation of skeletal growth. Osteochondroma is rare in the jaws but has been reported in association with the coronoid process and mandibular condyle.

Giant-cell tumour (osteoclastoma)

There is considerable controversy as to whether or not true giant-cell tumour occurs in the jaws. In contrast, central giant-cell granuloma is relatively common. There are no reliable histological differences between the two (or from other giant-cell lesions of bone). However, in the giant-cell tumour and in those central giant-cell granulomas that pursue a more aggressive course, the giant cells tend to be uniformly dispersed throughout, rather than being focally grouped, and it is unusual to find foci of bone or osteoid formation within the lesion. Despite these similarities the vast majority of giant-cell lesions in the jaws do not behave like giant-cell tumours. The latter typically involve the ends of long bones and are aggressive, locally invasive tumours with a high recurrence rate following curettage. In a small percentage of cases they pursue a frankly sarcomatous course with metastases. On the other hand, giant-cell granulomas never metastasize and are seldom as locally aggressive as giant-cell tumours. They can be treated satisfactorily by curettage and do not require the radical treatment that may be necessary to effect cure with a giant-cell tumour. Moreover, the granuloma tends to present in a younger age group than the giant-cell tumour.

In summary, although there are similarities between a central giant-cell granuloma and giant-cell tumour the differences in clinical features and behaviour, and to some extent the histological patterns, indicate that they are best considered as separate entities.

Myeloma

Myeloma is a neoplasm composed of plasma cells and generally occurs as a disseminated disease involving many bones (multiple myeloma or myelomatosis). Less commonly the condition occurs as a solitary lesion within bone or, more rarely, soft tissue (solitary myeloma or plasmacytoma). Some, but not all, patients with solitary lesions eventually develop multiple myeloma.

Jaw lesions may occur as part of multiple myeloma or as a solitary lesion, and extramedullary plasmacytoma may also occur in the oral soft tissues.

Multiple myeloma is a chronic, progressive, and invariably fatal disorder. It is the result of neoplastic proliferation of a single clone of immunoglobulin-producing cells and is characterized, therefore, by the production of large amounts of a single homogeneous type of immunoglobulin, most commonly IgG; that is, it is a monoclonal gammopathy. Abnormally high levels of the homogeneous immunoglobulin and/or its constituent polypeptide chains appear in serum, and are termed paraproteins or 'M' components (in reference to myeloma). As well as complete immunoglobulin molecules, excess light and/or heavy polypeptide chains are synthesized. The light chains are sufficiently small in size to be excreted in the urine and are known as Bence-Jones protein which has characteristic thermolabile properties.

Clinically, multiple myeloma occurs most frequently in patients between 50 and 70 years of age. Although any bone may be involved the skull, vertebrae, sternum, ribs, and pelvic bones are most commonly affected. These are sites where red marrow is normally present. Jaw lesions are not uncommon and although they may be the initial manifestation of disease, more commonly they

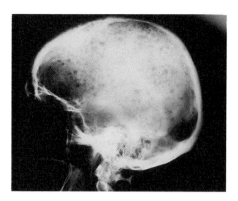

Fig. 17.23   Radiograph of the skull in multiple myeloma showing punched-out radiolucencies.

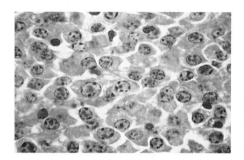

Fig. 17.24   A well-differentiated myeloma showing resemblance of neoplastic cells to mature plasma cells.

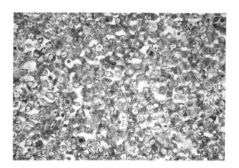

Fig. 17.25   Immunohistochemical demonstration of kappa light-chain production (brown reaction product) by neoplastic cells. All cells are positive confirming a monoclonal proliferation.

are purely incidental to the overall picture. The mandible is much more commonly affected than the maxilla and the lesions usually occur in the posterior region. The general features are diverse but include bone pain, anaemia, infections, hypercalcaemia, and renal failure, and can be related to focal osteolytic lesions, diffuse marrow replacement with pancytopenia, paraproteinaemia, and proteinuria. Amyloidosis may occur (see Chapter 13) and a resulting macroglossia may be an early feature. Jaw lesions may also be associated with pain, and other features may include numbness or paraesthesia over the distribution of the mental nerve, loosening of teeth, pathological fracture, and postextraction hemorrhage. As the lesions enlarge the cortical plates may be perforated and the tumour may present as a fleshy extraosseous mass. The classical radiographic feature is of sharply demarcated, round or oval osteolytic lesions with a characteristic punched-out appearance (Fig. 17.23).

Microscopically, the lesions are densely cellular with little or no supporting stroma and consist of sheets of myeloma cells which bear a striking resemblance to mature plasma cells or their immediate precursors (Fig. 17.24). Binucleate, and occasionally multinucleated, forms are present. Immunohistochemistry using monoclonal antibodies to different heavy and light chains is used to characterize the immunoglobulin production by the neoplastic cells (Fig. 17.25).

Solitary myeloma of the jaws and extramedullary plasmacytoma are uncommon, although the great majority of the latter arise in the head and neck region. They too are usually solitary and present as soft tissue, often polypoid swellings which can occur anywhere in the oral cavity, not just in mucosa overlying bone. Immunohistochemistry for heavy and light chains demonstrates the monoclonal nature of the proliferation which distinguishes such lesions from inflammatory infiltration. The behaviour of solitary osseous and of extramedullary lesions is unpredictable. Some regress after local radiotherapy but others progress eventually to multiple myeloma, perhaps after a latent period of many years.

Other primary marrow tumours are uncommon, particularly in the jaws. Ewing's sarcoma occurs in patients between the ages of 5 and 15 years and is more common in males. When the jaws are involved the lesions are seen most frequently in the mandible. The prognosis is very poor and most patients die within 2 years.

Cemento-ossifying fibroma

The cemento-ossifying fibroma now encompasses lesions previously designated as ossifying or as cementifying fibromas. A cemento-ossifying fibroma can be defined as a well-demarcated or rarely encapsulated benign neoplasm consisting of fibrous tissue containing varying amounts of metaplastic bone and mineralized masses resembling cementum. Its demarcated nature is an important feature distinguishing it from fibrous dysplasia.

Clinically, it presents as a slowly enlarging and progressive swelling (Fig. 17.26) most often in the premolar-molar region of the mandible, and can occur over a wide age-range. Some authors have reported a definite female predilection. Radiologically the appearances vary with the stage of development of the lesion. Initially there is a well-demarcated radiolucent area within which, as the lesion matures, varying amounts of calcified tissue are deposited (Fig. 17.27).

Histologically, the lesion is well circumscribed (Fig. 17.28). It consists of cellular fibrous tissue containing trabeculae of bone and, rather characteristically, numerous spherical deposits or rounded masses of homogeneous acellular calcified material resembling cementum. In these respects it is indistinguishable from fibrous dysplasia (Fig. 17.29). Clinical and radiographic features are important in establishing the diagnosis.

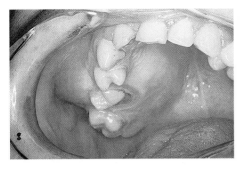

Fig. 17.26

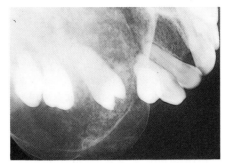

Fig. 17.27

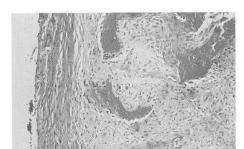

Fig. 17.28

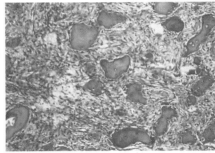

Fig. 17.29

Figs 17.26, 17.27 Clinical and radiographic appearances of cemento-ossifying fibroma. The tumour is well demarcated and contains varying amounts of mineralized tissue.

Fig. 17.28 Cemento-ossifying fibroma showing encapsulation.

Fig. 17.29 Metaplastic bone and cementum-like tissue forming in fibrous tissue in cemento-ossifying fibroma.

The majority of ossifying fibromas are slow growing but some, mainly in children and adolescents, show rapid growth. Histologically, they are characterized by richly cellular, mitotically active fibrous tissue with trabeculae of immature-looking woven bone and must be distinguished from osteosarcomas. The term juvenile ossifying fibroma has been applied to such lesions. In contrast to the more usual type of cemento-ossifying fibroma above, which has a negligible recurrence rate, juvenile ossifying fibroma has a recurrence rate of about 30–60 per cent.

Fibrosarcoma of bone

Medullary fibrosarcoma of bone is generally accepted as a distinct entity and should be differentiated from fibroblastic osteosarcoma. It is an uncommon lesion in the jaws but most have occurred in the mandible. Like fibrosarcoma of the oral soft tissues, it tends to occur in adult life and histologically resembles its soft-tissue counterpart. The important difference between the two lesions is in their clinical behaviour. Fibrosarcoma of bone has a propensity for local recurrence and eventual metastatic spread. A 5-year survival rate for intraosseous jaw tumours of about 30 per cent has been reported compared to around 70 per cent for soft-tissue sarcomas.

Tumours of bone   **Key points**

- osteomas difficult to distinguish from exostoses
- osteosarcoma and chondrosarcoma rare
- direct formation of bone by malignant cells in osteosarcoma
- endochondral ossification occurs in chondrosarcoma
- myeloma may be multiple or solitary
- cemento-ossifying fibroma must be distinguished from fibrous dysplasia

LANGERHANS CELL HISTIOCYTOSIS

This group of diseases with similar histological appearances but diverse clinical manifestations, was previously known as histocytosis-X or the idiopathic histiocytoses. The diseases range in severity from a fatal, leukaemia-like disorder to an isolated, lytic lesion of bone, with intermediate forms characterized by multiorgan involvement. The histological feature common to the group is the infiltration of various tissues and organs by tumour-like masses of proliferating histiocytes admixed with a variable number of eosinophils. The prevailing opinion is that the cell of origin is the Langerhans cell, a dendritic antigen-presenting cell that shares many features with cells of the mononuclear phagocytic system. The disease presents clinically in one of three main ways:

(1) unifocal (solitary) eosinophilic granuloma;
(2) multifocal eosinophilic granuloma;
(3) progressive (acute) disseminated histiocytosis.

Unifocal (solitary) eosinophilic granuloma

Unifocal eosinophilic granuloma predominantly affects patients under 20 years of age and is more common in males. Any bone may be involved but the cranium, jaws, ribs, and long bones are the most common sites. Jaw lesions are most frequent in the mandible. Radiographs show a focal osteolytic lesion that may be well or poorly demarcated. In some patients the lesions undergo spontaneous fibrosis and regression but in others, curettage, excision, or local radiotherapy are required to effect a cure. However, patients must be followed for long periods since some with an apparently unifocal lesion have presented eventually with multifocal disease.

Multifocal eosinophilic granuloma

The lesions of multifocal esoinophilic granuloma involve several bones and often other organs. The skull, especially the temporal bone, is a favoured site and recurrent otitis media is a common feature. Jaw lesions are more common in the mandible and extensive destruction results in loss and/or loosening of teeth which on radiographs may appear to be floating in air (Fig. 17.30). Visceral lesions are variable in extent but hepatosplenomegaly and lymphadenopathy may be present. When the orbit and posterior pituitary are also involved the patient presents with the classical triad of Hand–Schuller–Christian syndrome—skull defects, exophthalmos, and diabetes insipidus. The prognosis is generally good, particularly with the advent of modern chemotherapeutic regimes.

Progressive (acute) disseminated histiocytosis

Progressive disseminated histiocytosis (Letterer-Siwe disease) presents with fever, skin rashes, hepatosplenomegaly, lymphadenopathy, and pancytopenia. Radiographically, there are localized or diffuse osteolytic lesions in many bones, especially the skull, pelvis, and long bones. In the jaws, diffuse bone destruction may cause loosening and exfoliation of teeth and the teeth may appear to be floating in air. Death is related to intercurrent infections and progressive anaemia and debility.

Histopathology

Histologically, the lesions of this group of diseases consist of poorly defined collections of histiocytes mixed with variable numbers of granulocytes (both

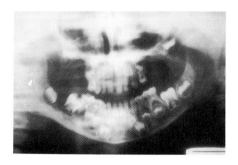

Fig. 17.30 Osteolytic lesion associated with developing first permanent molar in the right mandible of a five-year-old child with multifocal eosinophilic granuloma. Similar lesions resulted in exfoliation of both maxillary first permanent molars at age three years.

eosinophils and neutrophils) and lymphocytes (Fig. 17.31). Areas of haemorrhage, necrosis, and fibrosis may be seen and multinucleated giant cells are prominent in some lesions.

Ultrastructural examination shows that some of the histiocytes contain cytoplasmic granules similar to the Birbeck granules of Langerhans cells (Fig. 17.32). These granules are rod-shaped structures with a central striated line. Vesicular expansion of the membrane at the ends of the rods often gives the granules a racquet shape. The cells also express surface antigens shared by normal Langerhans cells.

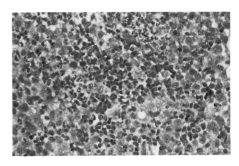

Fig. 17.31 Eosinophilic granuloma showing sheets of histiocytes with scattered eosinophils and neutrophils.

HAEMANGIOMA OF BONE

Although haemangioma of bone is a rare lesion, it is important that the lesion is considered in the differential diagnosis of a radiolucent area in the jaws before operative intervention, including extraction of associated teeth. Haemangioma of the jaws is more common in the mandible than in the maxilla and may present as a slowly enlarging painless swelling, but other features, such as haemorrhage around the necks of the teeth in the involved area or severe postextraction haemorrhage, may give clues as to the nature of the lesion. Other haemangiomas are discovered as incidental findings on routine radiographic examination and appear as osteolytic defects that may have a multilocular honeycomb appearance. Aspiration will reveal fresh blood. Microscopically, most haemangiomas of bone are of the cavernous type and they may arise either from the periosteum and resorb the underlying bone, or from medullary vessels. Extraction of teeth from the area may be followed by severe and possibly uncontrollable haemorrhage. Death from exsanguination may occur.

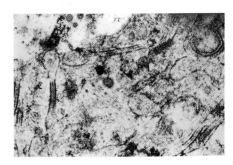

Fig. 17.32 Electronmicrograph of histiocytic cells in eosinophilic granuloma showing rod and racquet-shaped Birbeck granules.

METASTATIC TUMOURS

It has been estimated that metastatic tumours in the oral soft tissues and jaws account for about 1 per cent of malignant tumours occurring in the oral cavity. Metastasis to bone is more common than to the soft tissues, the mandible being much more frequently affected than the maxilla. The most common primary tumours reported as metastasizing to the jaws are carcinomas of the breast, bronchus, and kidney. Presenting features of metastatic tumours may be pain, loose teeth, swelling, and paraethesia or anaesthesia of the lip due to involvement of the inferior dental nerve, but many lesions are asymptomatic.

Most metastatic tumours are osteolytic but some, such as carcinomas of breast and prostate, may be osteoblastic and appear radiographically as an area of radiopacity rather than radiolucency.

The most common sites for metastases to the oral mucosa are the gingiva or alveolar mucosa, followed by the tongue.

FURTHER READING

Chu, T. and Jaffe. R. (1994). The normal Langerhans cell and the LCH cell. *British Journal of Cancer—Supplement*, **23**, S4–10.

Clark, J. L., Umni, K. K., Dahlin, D. C., and Devine, K. D. (1983). Osteosarcoma of the jaw. *Cancer*, **51**, 2311–16.

Cleveland, D. B., Goldberg, K. M., Greenspan, J. S., Seitz, T. E., and Miller, A. S. (1996). Langerhans' cell histiocytosis. *Oral Surgery, Oral Medicine, Oral Pathology, Oral Radiology and Endodontics*, **82**, 541–8.

Furutani, M., Ohnishi, M., and Tanaka, Y. (1994). Mandibular involvement in patients with multiple myeloma. *Journal of Oral and Maxillofacial Surgery*, **52**, 23–5.

Garrington, G. E. and Collett, W. K. (1988). Chondrosarcoma I. A selected literature review. *Journal of Oral Pathology*, **17**, 1–11.

Garrington, G. E. and Collett, W. K. (1988). Chondrosarcoma II. Chondrosarcoma of the jaws: analysis of 37 cases. *Journal of Oral Pathology*, **17**, 12–20.

Hartman, K. S. (1980). Histiocytosis X: A review of 114 cases with oral involvement. *Oral Surgery, Oral Medicine, Oral Pathology*, **49**, 38–54.

Hirshberg, A., and Buchner, A. (1995). Metastatic tumours to the oral region. An overview. *Oral Oncology, European Journal of Cancer*, **31B**, 355–60.

Hirshberg, A., Leibovich, P., and Buchner, A. (1993). Metastases to the oral mucosa: analysis of 157 cases. *Journal of Oral Pathology and Medicine*, **22**, 385–90.

Kramer, I. R. H., Pindborg, J. J., and Shear, M. (1992). *Histological typing of odontogenic tumours* (2nd edn). World Health Organization International Classification of Tumours. Springer-Verlag, Berlin.

O'Malley, M., Pogrel, M. A., Stewart, J. C. B., Silva, R. G., and Regezi, J. A. (1997). Central giant cell granulomas of the jaws: phenotype and proliferation-associated markers. *Journal of Pathology and Medicine*, **26**, 159–63.

Raubenheimer, E. J., Dauth, J., and van Wilpe, E. (1987). Multiple myeloma: study of 10 cases. *Journal of Oral Pathology*, **16**, 383–8.

Saito, K., Unni, K. K., Wollan, P. C., and Lund, B. A. (1995). Chondrosarcoma of the jaw and facial bones. *Cancer*, **76**, 1550–8.

Smith, B. J. and Eveson, J. W. (1981). Paget's disease of bone with particular reference to dentistry. *Journal of Oral Pathology*, **10**, 233–47.

Thomas, D. W. and Shepherd, J. P. (1994). Paget's disease of bone: current concepts in pathogenesis and treatment. *Journal of Oral Pathology and Medicine*, **23**, 12–16.

Whitaker, S. B. and Waldron, A. (1993). Central giant cell lesions of the jaws. *Oral Surgery, Oral Medicine, Oral Pathology*, **75**, 199–208.

18 Diseases of the temporomandibular joint

18   Diseases of the temporomandibular joint

Many of the diseases affecting other joints in the body can involve the temporo-mandibular joint (TMJ) but they may be modified by particular structural and functional features of this joint. Some aspects of the structure of the joint are discussed below.

Three distinct cell zones can be distinguished in the articular surface of the mandibular condyle during growth:

(1) the articular zone of dense fibrous tissue covering the surface;
(2) the proliferative or cellular zone which is the main centre for growth and chondrogenesis;
(3) the hypertrophic zone, where the differentiated chrondrocytes and cartilage matrix undergo endochondral ossification.

In adults the proliferative zone is reduced to a narrow band of cells and the hypertrophic zone is replaced by fibrocartilage with few hypertrophied cells. With advancing age the articular surface becomes increasingly fibrous. Remodelling of the articular surface takes place throughout life to compensate for occlusal wear or the loss of teeth.

The articular fossa is covered by a thin layer of fibrous tissue which thickens over the articular eminence, but pathological changes involve the surface of the fossa much less frequently than the condyle.

Components of the temporomandibular joint   **Key points**

- mandibular condyle
  —articular zone
  —proliferative or cellular zone
  —hypertrophic zone
- articular fossa
- articular disc
  —anterior band
  —intermediate zone
  —posterior band
  —retrodiscal tissues

The articular disc is composed of fibrocartilage, comprising compact collagen fibres, small elastic fibres, and glycosaminoglycans, arranged in anterior and posterior bands connected by a narrower intermediate zone. The lateral pterygoid muscle is attached to the medial part of the anterior band, the lateral part being related to masseter and temporalis muscles. The posterior attachment of the disc is formed by the retrodiscal tissue which comprises a loosely organized meshwork of collagen fibres and large branching elastic fibres with fat, numerous

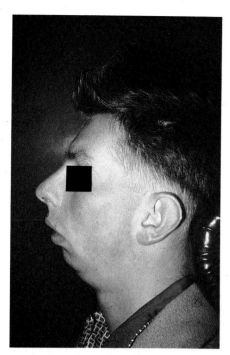

Fig. 18.1 Facial deformity associated with bilateral condylar hypoplasia.

blood vessels, and nerves. This connects the posterior band to the temporal bone, auditory meatus, and condyle. The stiff articular disc contrasts with the easily deformable posterior attachment. In normal joints the posterior band of the disc covers the summit of the condyle when the mouth is in a closed position. As the mouth is opened the posterior attachment expands to fill the joint space.

DEVELOPMENTAL DISORDERS

Aplasia of the condyle is extremely rare and may be unilateral or bilateral. Most of the reported cases have occurred in association with other facial anomalies.

Hypoplasia or underdevelopment of the condyle may be congenital or acquired. The cause of congenital hypoplasia is not known, but either one or both condyles may be involved. Acquired hypoplasia is due to an agent which interferes with the normal development of the condyle, such as trauma (from birth injury or fracture), radiation, or infection, usually resulting from extension of infection in the middle ear. The earlier the damage, the more severe is the resulting facial deformity (Fig. 18.1).

Hyperplasia of the mandibular condyle is a rare and self-limiting condition, the cause of which is not known. It is generally unilateral and results in facial asymmetry, deviation of the mandible to the opposite side, and malocclusion. It usually becomes apparent during the second decade of life, when one condyle continues to grow while the other is no longer active.

INFLAMMATORY DISORDERS

Traumatic arthritis

Damage to the joint following acute trauma to the mandible may lead to a traumatic arthritis or haemarthrosis. The condition usually revolves if the tissue damage is not severe, otherwise scar tissue formation may lead to ankylosis.

Infective arthritis

Infective arthritis of the temporomandibular joint is rare. Micro-organisms may reach the joint by various routes:

(1) direct spread from an adjacent focus of infection, for example from the middle ear or from a surrounding cellulitis;
(2) haematogenous spread from a distant focus of infection;
(3) facial trauma.

A variety of organisms has been implicated but *Staphylococcus aureus* is the most common isolate. The joint may also be involved in patients who develop a widespread infective polyarthritis such as in gonococcal arthritis or viral arthritis.

Patients usually present with pain, trismus, deviation on opening, and signs of acute infection. Complications include fibrous and occasionally bony ankylosis.

Rheumatoid arthritis

This is a disease of unknown aetiology, but autoimmune mechanisms and immune-complex formation have been implicated. The disease commonly begins in early adult life and affects women more frequently than men. It has a systemic distribution in which the involvement of joints is the major feature, but anaemia, weight loss, and subcutaneous nodules over bony prominences or in the vicinity of joints also occur. About 10 per cent of patients may show features of Sjögren syndrome. The smaller joints are mainly affected, particularly those of the hand, and the distribution tends to be symmetrical.

Although few patients with rheumatoid arthritis spontaneously complain of pain from their temporomandibular joints, clinical examination has shown involvement of these joints in 50–70 per cent of cases. Limitation of opening, stiffness, crepitus, referred pain, and tenderness on biting are the usual symptoms, but severe disability is unusual.

Joint involvement starts as a synovitis with an intense infiltration of lymphocytes and plasma cells in the hyperaemic synovial tissues. The synovial tissues proliferate and the hyperplastic and inflamed synovial membrane is thrown into folds which extend over the articular surfaces, clothing them in a vascular pannus. The articular surfaces become eroded by the pannus which may also extend into and cause resorption of the adjacent bone. Erosion of the condyle may be seen on radiographs. The articular surfaces become very irregular and fibrous ankylosis may result, either involving the lower joint compartment only or with total destruction of the articular disc and complete ankylosis.

Rheumatoid factor is mainly an IgM-class autoantibody against chemical groups on IgG molecules. It can be demonstrated in 85 per cent of patients with rheumatoid arthritis. Although its significance in the pathogenesis of the disease is not known, many of the features of rheumatoid arthritis are thought to be attributable to immune-complex deposition. The erythrocyte sedimentation rate is raised in rheumatoid arthritis because of the hypergammaglobulinaemia.

OSTEOARTHROSIS

This is primarily a degenerative disease which mainly affects weight-bearing joints. The disease in the temporomandibular joint differs in some respects from that elsewhere, probably because the joint is not weight-bearing and the articular surface is covered with a layer of mature fibrous tissue and not hyaline cartilage. Histologically, the disease is rare in the temporomandibular joint before the beginning of the fifth decade of life, but then increases proportionately with age. It may present clinically with pain, crepitus, limitation of jaw movement, and deviation on opening, but as in other joints many cases are clinically silent. Clinical studies have suggested a relationship in some cases between untreated myofascial pain–dysfunction syndrome or disc displacement and the later development of osteoarthrosis. Spontaneous resolution of symptoms is common.

The earliest histological changes in the temporomandibular joint are uneven distribution of the cells in the articular covering of the condyle which may be associated with some osteoclastic resorption of the subarticular bony end-plate. Vertical splits (fibrillation) develop in the articular layer (Fig. 18.2), followed by fragmentation and loss of the articular surface with eventual exposure (denudation) of the underlying bone (Fig. 18.3). Reactive changes in the exposed subarticular bone lead to thickening of trabeculae and the formation of a dense surface layer, referred to as eburnation. Osteophytic lipping on the anterior surface also occurs, but this is seldom prominent (Fig. 18.4). The rough exposed bone on the condylar surface may lead to disruption and eventual perforation of the articular disc.

The radiographic changes are variable and not pathognomonic. They include focal or diffuse areas of bone loss on the articular surface of the condyle, flattening and reduction in the total bony size of the condyle, and reduction in the joint space. Osteophytes may be seen at the anterior edge of the condyle. If large, they may fracture off and present on radiographs as loose bodies (see later).

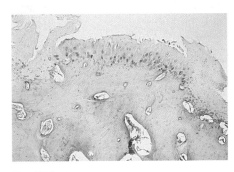

Fig. 18.2

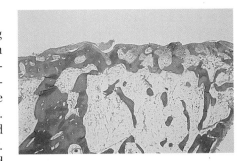

Fig. 18.3

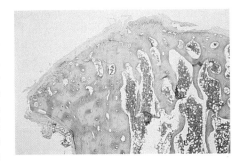

Fig. 18.4

Figs 18.2–18.4 Osteoarthritic changes in the temporomandibular joint showing fibrillation and fragmentation of articular cartilage (Fig. 18.2), denudation and exposure of underlying bony end-plate (Fig. 18.3), and osteophytic lipping of the condyle (Fig. 18.4).

Key points	**Arthritic conditions of TMJ**
	• infective
	—rare
	—acute symptoms
	—bacterial access: direct spread/ blood spread/trauma
	• rheumatoid arthritis
	—common in patients with generalized rheumatoid arthritis
	—stiffness, limitation of movement
	—erosion of condyle by vascular pannus
	• osteoarthrosis
	—increasing incidence after 50 years
	—pain, crepitus, limitation of movement, or symptomless
	—may be preceded by pain–dysfunction syndrome/disc displacement
	—degenerative changes, denudation, and eburnation of condyle

FUNCTIONAL DISORDERS

Myofascial pain-dysfunction syndrome

This is the commonest cause of complaint involving the temporomandibular joint and it has three cardinal symptoms: pain associated with the joint or its musculature, clicking of the joint, and limitation of jaw movement. Symptoms vary in intensity during the day and are most common in the morning. Tenderness to palpation of the origins and insertions of the masticatory muscles is usual. The condition is seen more frequently in women than in men, and the mean age of presentation is about 30 years. Unilateral tooth loss or other dental irregularities are very common, but there is no consistent relationship between the side of such occlusal disharmony and the side of joint symptoms. The incidence of the condition is said to decrease if more than six teeth are missing. There is a strong clinical impression that the syndrome has a relationship with various types of emotional stress. Bruxism is common and many sufferers have nocturnal tooth-grinding habits. No consistent radiological changes have been described, and examination of the condylar surface by light microscopy shows no abnormal features. Many patients respond well to reassurance and training in relaxed jaw movements, but some require bite plates or adjustments of the natural occlusion. It is now thought that the principal factor responsible for the symptoms in this condition is masticatory muscle spasm, which may be precipitated by muscular overextension, contraction, or fatigue. Little is known about the subsequent histories of patients with this syndrome.

Disc displacement

Disc displacement, defined as an abnormal positional relationship between the articular disc, the head of the condyle, and the articular fossa of the temporal bone has been reported in from about 25 to 65 per cent of elderly patients. It is also prevalent in patients with pain-dysfunction syndrome and/or osteoarthritic changes in the joint, but whether the displacement precedes or follows such changes is unclear. However, not all patients with displacements have or develop signs or symptoms of disease.

The displacement may initially be an adaptive change and reflect remodelling of the disc to prevent tissue injury. Remodelling is associated with changes in the external shape and proportions of the disc and its posterior attachment, and with reactive changes in the tissues, such as increasing fibrosis and hyalinization in the retrodiscal tissues (see also the discussion on age changes below). In patients where remodelling has been unable to prevent tissue injury various pathological changes may also be seen. These include haemorrhage, myxomatous change, thickening of blood vessel walls, cartilage formation, and perforation of the posterior attachment, usually at its junction with the remodelled posterior band. Disc displacement generally appears necessary for the development of perforations.

LOOSE BODIES

Radiopaque bodies apparently lying free within the joint space are relatively common in major joints but are rare in the temporomandibular joint. They may give rise to discomfort, crepitus, and limitation of opening. Although a variety of diseases may be associated with intra-articular loose bodies in other joints the main causes within the temporomandibular joint are intracapsular fractures, fractured osteophytes in osteoarthrosis (Fig. 18.5), and synovial chrondromatosis. The latter is a disease of unknown aetiology characterized by the formation of multiple nodules of metaplastic cartilage, which may calcify and ossify, scattered throughout the synovium. As the disease progresses they are released into the joint space as multiple loose bodies.

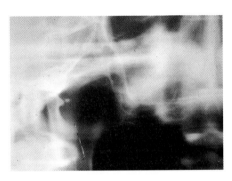

Fig. 18.5 Loose body, probably a fractured osteophyte, within the right temporomandibular joint

NEOPLASMS

Primary neoplasms arising from the structures of the temporomandibular joint are extremely rare. Benign tumours such as chondromas and osteomas are more frequent than sarcomas arising from bone or synovial tissues.

AGE CHANGES IN THE JAWS AND TEMPOROMANDIBULAR JOINT

As discussed in Chapter 16 increasing age is associated with progressive reduction in bone mass resulting in osteoporosis. Age-related osteoporosis is common, and in edentulous patients could play a role in atrophy of alveolar and possibly basal bone, although no clear relationship has been established. Atrophy of alveolar bone is related mainly to the loss of teeth, and its extent increases with age resulting, in the absence of dentures, in loss of facial height and upwards and forwards posturing of the mandible. Loss of alveolar bone is more extensive and occurs more rapidly in the mandible than in the maxilla.

With regard to the temporomandibular joint, it is difficult to distinguish changes due to ageing from those related to osteoarthrosis. If the latter are excluded the main age changes in the joint are related to remodelling of the articular surfaces and disc in response to functional changes following tooth loss. As discussed above, remodelling may result in disc displacement, particularly anterior displacement. The posterior band of the disc may then lie anterior to the condyle when the mouth is closed, the posterior attachment being drawn in between the bearing surfaces of the condyle and articular eminence. The retrodiscal tissues may show adaptive changes associated with decreased cellularity and vascularity, and increased density of collagen, and may eventually function as an articular disc. However, in some cases the displacement may lead to perforation of the disc, particularly of its posterior attachment, resulting in progressive joint damage and osteoarthrosis.

TRISMUS

Trismus means limitation of movement, which in the temporomandibular joint may be due either to factors within the joint (intra-articular) or outside the joint (extra-articular). Temporary trismus is much more common than permanent trismus. The main causes of trismus are listed in Table 18.1.

Table 18.1   Causes of trismus

Intra-articular	—Traumatic arthritis
	—Infective arthritis
	—Rheumatoid arthritis
	—Dislocation
	—Intracapsular fracture
	—Fibrous or bony ankylosis following trauma or infection
Extra-articular	—Adjacent infection, inflammation, and abscesses (e.g. mumps, pericoronitis, submasseteric abscess)
	—Extracapsular fractures (mandible, zygoma, middle third)
	—Overgrowth (neoplasia) of the coronoid process
	—Fibrosis from burns or irradiation
	—Haematoma/fibrosis of medial pterygoid (e.g. following inferior dental block)
	—Myofascial pain-dysfunction syndrome
	—Drug-associated dyskinesia and psychotic disturbances
	—Tetanus
	—Tetany

FURTHER READING

Bjornland, T. and Refsum, S. B. (1994). Histopathologic changes in the temporomandibular joint disk in patients with chronic arthritic disease. A comparison with internal derangement. *Oral Surgery, Oral Medicine, Oral Pathology*, **77**, 572–8.

Delfino, J. J. and Eppley, B. L. (1986). Radiographic and surgical evaluation of internal derangements of the temporomandibular joint. *Journal of Oral and Maxillofacial Surgery*, **44**, 260–7.

Dolwick, M. F. (1995). Intra-articular disc displacement part 1: its questionable role in temporomandibular joint pathology; part II: its significant role in temporomandibular joint pathology. *Journal of Oral and Maxillofacial Surgery*, **53**, 1069–72; 1073–9.

Fanibunda, K. B., Moore, U. J., and Soames, J. V. (1994). Bilateral osteochondral loose bodies of the temporomandibular joints with unilateral enlargement of the condyle. *British Journal of Oral and Maxillofacial Surgery*, **32**, 248–50.

Holmlund, A. B., Gynther, G., and Reinholt, F. P. (1992). Rheumatoid arthritis and disk derangement of the temporomandibular joint. A comparative arthroscopic study. *Oral Surgery, Oral Medicine, Oral Pathology*, **73**, 273–7.

Leighty, S. M., Spach, D. H., Myall, R. W., and Burns, J. L. (1993). Septic arthritis of the temporomandibular joint: review of the literature and report of two cases in children. *International Journal of Oral and Maxillofacial Surgery*, **22**, 292–7.

Marchetti, C., Piacentini, C., Farina, A., Bernasconi, G., and Calligaro, A. (1995). A microscopic and immunocytochemical study of structural changes in dysfunctional human temporomandibular joint discs. *Archives of Oral Biology*, **40**, 549–57.

Ogus, H. (1980). Degenerative disease of the temporomandibular joint in young persons. *British Journal of Oral Surgery*, **17**, 17–26.

Pereira, F. J. Jr, Lundh, H., Eriksson, L., and Westesson, P.-L. (1996). Microscopic changes in retrodiscal tissues of painful temporomandibular joints. *Journal of Oral and Maxillofacial Surgery*, **54**, 461–8.

Pereira, F. J. Jr, Lundh, H., and Westesson, P.-L. (1994). Morphologic changes in the temporomandibular joint in different age groups. An autopsy investigation. *Oral Surgery, Oral Medicine, Oral Pathology*, **78**, 279–87.

Pereira, F. J. Jr, Lundh, H., and Westesson, P.-L. (1996). Age-related changes in retrodiscal tissues in the temporomandibular joint. *Journal of Oral and Maxillofacial Surgery*, **54**, 55–61.

Widmalm, S. E., Westesson, P.-L., Kim, I. K., Pereira, F. J. Jr, Lundh, H., and Tsaki, M. M. (1994). Temporomandibular joint pathosis related to sex, age, and dentition in autopsy material. *Oral Surgery, Oral Medicine, Oral Pathology*, **78**, 416–25.

Index